Modern Management of Benign and Malignant Pancreatic Disease

Guest Editor

JACQUES VAN DAM, MD, PhD

GASTROENTEROLOGY CLINICS OF NORTH AMERICA

www.gastro.theclinics.com

March 2012 • Volume 41 • Number 1

SAUNDERS an imprint of ELSEVIER, Inc.

W.B. SAUNDERS COMPANY
A Division of Elsevier Inc.

Elsevier Inc. • 1600 John F. Kennedy Blvd., Suite 1800 • Philadelphia, Pennsylvania 19103-2899

http://www.theclinics.com

GASTROENTEROLOGY CLINICS OF NORTH AMERICA Volume 41, Number 1
March 2012 ISSN 0889-8553, ISBN-13: 978-1-4557-3863-2

Editor: Kerry Holland
Developmental Editor: Donald Mumford

Gastroenterology Clinics of North America (ISSN 0889-8553) is published quarterly by Elsevier Inc., 360 Park Avenue South, New York, NY 10010-1710. Months of issue are March, June, September, and December. Business and Editorial Offices: 1600 John F. Kennedy Blvd., Suite 1800, Philadelphia, PA 19103-2899. Customer Service Office: 6277 Sea Harbor Drive, Orlando, FL 32887-4800. Periodicals postage paid at New York, NY and additional mailing offices. Subscription prices are $305.00 per year (US individuals), $153.00 per year (US students), $488.00 per year (US institutions), $335.00 per year (Canadian individuals), $594.00 per year (Canadian institutions), $423.00 per year (international individuals), $211.00 per year (international students), and $594.00 per year (international institutions). Foreign air speed delivery is included in all *Clinics* subscription prices. All prices are subject to change without notice. **POSTMASTER:** Send address changes to *Gastroenterology Clinics of North America*, Elsevier Health Sciences Division, Subscription Customer Service, 3251 Riverport Lane, Maryland Heights, MO 63043. Telephone: 1-800-654-2452 (U.S. and Canada); 314-447-8871 (outside U.S. and Canada). Fax: 314-447-8029. E-mail: journalscustomerservice-usa@elsevier.com (for print support); journalsonlinesupport-usa@elsevier.com (for online support).

Reprints. For copies of 100 or more, of articles in this publication, please contact the Commercial Reprints Department, Elsevier Inc., 360 Part Avenue South, New York, New York 10010-1710. Tel. (212) 633-3813, Fax: (212) 462-1935, E-mail: reprints@elsevier.com.

Gastroenterology Clinics of North America is also published in Italian by Il Pensiero Scientifico Editore, Rome, Italy; and in Portuguese by Interlivros Edicoes Ltda., Rua Commandante Coelho 1085, 21250 Cordovil, Rio de Janeiro, Brazil.

Gastroenterology Clinics of North America is covered in *MEDLINE/PubMed (Index Medicus), Excerpta Medica, Current Contents/Clinical Medicine, Science Citation Index, ISI/BIOMED,* and *BIOSIS.*

Printed and bound by CPI Group (UK) Ltd, Croydon, CR0 4YY
Transferred to Digital Print 2012

Contributors

GUEST EDITOR

JACQUES VAN DAM, MD, PhD
Professor of Medicine, Keck School of Medicine, University of Southern California, Los Angeles, California

AUTHORS

NEERAJ ANAND, MD
Department of Gastroeneterology, Kaiser Permanente Los Angeles Medical Center, Los Angeles, California

WILLIAM R. BRUGGE, MD
Professor of Medicine, Harvard Medical School; Gastrointestinal Unit, Massachusetts General Hospital, Boston, Massachusetts

JAMES BUXBAUM, MD
Chief of Endoscopy, Los Angeles County Hospital, Division of Gastroenterology and Liver Diseases, The University of Southern California, Keck School of Medicine, Los Angeles, California

MARCIA IRENE CANTO, MD, MHS
Professor of Medicine and Oncology, Division of Gastroenterology and Hepatology, Johns Hopkins University School of Medicine, Baltimore, Maryland

DANIEL T. CHANG, MD
Department of Radiation Oncology, Stanford University School of Medicine and Cancer Center, Stanford, California

KIRAN K. DHANIREDDY, MD
Assistant Professor of Clinical Surgery, Director, Pancreas Transplantation, Chief of Service, Hepatobiliary Surgery, Los Angeles County and University of Southern California, Keck School of Medicine, University of Southern California, Los Angeles, California

YURI GENYK, MD
Assistant Professor of Clinical Surgery, Hepatobiliary/Pancreatic Surgery and Abdominal Transplantation Division, Department of Surgery, University of Southern California, Los Angeles, California

DANIEL M. HALPERIN, MD
Department of Medicine, Brigham and Women's Hospital, Boston, Massachusetts

R. BROOKE JEFFREY, MD
Professor and Vice Chairman, Chief of Abdominal Imaging, Department of Radiology, Stanford University Medical Center, Stanford, California

ALBERT C. KOONG, MD, PhD
Department of Radiation Oncology, Stanford University School of Medicine and Cancer Center, Stanford, California

MATTHEW H. KULKE, MD
Director, Carcinoid and Pancreatic Neuroendocrine Tumor Program, Dana-Farber Cancer Institute; Associate Professor of Medicine, Harvard Medical School, Boston, Massachusetts

MELISSA J. LABONTE, PhD
Division of Medical Oncology, University of Southern California/Norris Comprehensive Cancer Center, Keck School of Medicine, Los Angeles, California

HEINZ-JOSEF LENZ, MD, FACP
Division of Medical Oncology, University of Southern California/Norris Comprehensive Cancer Center, Keck School of Medicine, Los Angeles, California

SIMON K. LO, MD
Director of Endoscopy, Cedars-Sinai Medical Center; Clinical Professor of Medicine, David Geffen School of Medicine at University of California, Los Angeles, Los Angeles, California

LEA MATSUOKA, MD
Assistant Professor of Surgery, Hepatobiliary/Pancreatic Surgery and Abdominal Transplantation Division, Department of Surgery, University of Southern California, Los Angeles, California

PETER G. MAXIM, PhD
Department of Radiation Oncology, Stanford University School of Medicine and Cancer Center, Stanford, California

UDAYAKUMAR NAVANEETHAN, MD
Digestive Disease Institute, The Cleveland Clinic, Cleveland, Ohio

MOHAMED O. OTHMAN, MD
Assistant Professor, Division of Gastroenterology, Department of Internal Medicine, Texas Tech Health Science Center at El Paso, El Paso, Texas

DAVID PÁEZ, MD
Division of Medical Oncology, University of Southern California/Norris Comprehensive Cancer Center, Keck School of Medicine, Los Angeles, California; Medical Oncology Department, Hospital de la Santa Creu i Sant Pau, Barcelona, Spain

DILIP PAREKH, MD
Professor, Department of Surgery, University of Southern California, Los Angeles, California

JUNG H. PARK, MD
Department of Gastroeneterology, Kaiser Permanente Los Angeles Medical Center, Los Angeles, California

ANDREW L. SAMUELSON, MD
Gastroenterology Fellow, University of Colorado Anschutz Medical Campus, Aurora, Colorado

RICK SELBY, MD
Professor of Clinical Surgery, Hepatobiliary/Pancreatic Surgery and Abdominal Transplantation Division, Department of Surgery, University of Southern California, Los Angeles, California

RAJ J. SHAH, MD, FASGE
Associate Professor of Medicine, University of Colorado School of Medicine, Aurora, Colorado

EUN JI SHIN, MD
Assistant Professor of Medicine, Department of Internal Medicine, Division of Gastroenterology and Hepatology, Johns Hopkins University School of Medicine, Baltimore, Maryland

ARAVIND SUGUMAR, MD
Assistant Professor of Medicine, Division of Gastroenterology and Hepatology, University of Kansas Medical Center, Kansas City, Kansas

NICHOLAS TRAKUL, MD, PhD
Department of Radiation Oncology, Stanford University School of Medicine and Cancer Center, Stanford, California

GURU TRIKUDANATHAN, MD
Department of Internal Medicine, University of Connecticut Medical Center, Farmington, Connecticut

SANTHI SWAROOP VEGE, MD
Director, Pancreas Group, Professor of Medicine, Division of Gastroenterology, Mayo Clinic, Rochester, Minnesota

MICHAEL B. WALLACE, MD, MPH
Professor and Chief, Division of Gastroenterology, Department of Internal Medicine, Mayo Clinic, Jacksonville, Florida

BECHIEN U. WU, MD, MPH
Center for Pancreatic Disorders, Department of Gastroeneterology, Kaiser Permanente Los Angeles Medical Center, Los Angeles, California

WON JAE YOON, MD
Research Fellow, Gastrointestinal Unit, Massachusetts General Hospital, Boston, Massachusetts

Contents

> This article focuses on recent developments in the management of acute pancreatitis. Several prognostic scoring systems have been developed to aid in the evaluation of patients with acute pancreatitis. Recent data have shown that early fluid resuscitation and enteral nutrition are cornerstones to therapy during early management. Current practice guidelines do not recommend routine computed tomography or antibiotics in the early phase of management. The management of infected pancreatic necrosis now favors more conservative therapy, including a "step-up" approach using percutaneous drainage followed by minimally invasive retroperitoneal débridement if the patient fails to improve. This article focuses on recent developments in the management of acute pancreatitis.

> Autoimmune pancreatitis is a rare, newly recognized type of chronic pancreatitis. Its histopathology, clinical presentation, and diagnostic profile differ from those of other types of pancreatitis. Although its clinical presentation can vary, it most closely resembles pancreatic cancer. Numerous publications from Japan, United States, and Europe have helped define this hitherto ill-defined disease and described two histologically distinct subtypes. Both are exquisitely sensitive to steroid therapy. Type 1 has been well described in the literature and multiple diagnostic criteria exist. Less is known about type 2, and although it can be suspected clinically, histologic confirmation is needed for definitive diagnosis.

> Endoscopic retrograde cholangiopancreatography (ERCP) is now reserved as a therapeutic procedure for those with pancreatic disease. Among those with idiopathic pancreatitis, ERCP may be used to confirm and treat sphincter of Oddi dysfunction, microlithiasis, and structural anomalies, including pancreas divisum. Pancreatic endotherapy is a consideration to decrease pain in those with pancreatic

duct obstruction, although surgical decompression may be more durable. Pancreatic duct leaks may respond to endoscopic drainage, but optimal therapy is achieved if a bridging stent can be placed. Finally, using a wire-guided technique and pancreatic duct stents in high-risk patients, may minimize the risk of post-ERCP pancreatitis.

This review focuses on the endoscopic management of pancreatic pseudocysts utilizing endoscopic ultrasound guidance for transenteric and transpapillary drainage. Techniques and efficacy along with complications are addressed. Further, efficacy and comparative data with alternative techniques such as percutaneous and surgical drainage are discussed.

Chronic pancreatitis is a progressive fibroinflammatory process that can culminate in permanent impairment of exocrine and endocrine function. Pain is a cardinal feature. Pain management involves use of potent analgesics, pancreatic duct decompression by endoscopic or surgical techniques, and partial or total pancreatectomy. Micronutrients including methionine, vitamin C, selenium, and antioxidants are better at controlling pain and improving quality of life. Pancreatic exocrine and endocrine insufficiency and labile glycemic control associated with chronic pancreatitis require specific treatment modalities and present significant challenges. Future studies are needed to transcend symptomatic pain control, enzyme supplementation, and hyperglycemia control.

Laparoscopic pancreas surgery has developed rapidly. Although acceptance among traditional surgeons has been low, emerging specialty centers report excellent outcomes. As these procedures gain wider practice, outcomes need to be watched. Although many have suggested that studies comparing laparoscopic with open resections are necessary, cumulative data on the safety and efficacy of laparoscopic procedures argue against this approach. A reasonable approach is the establishment of a national registry to measure progress and record outcomes. Hepatobiliary training programs should also establish minimal standards of training so that the benefits of laparoscopic surgery can be made available widely.

Pancreatic cystic neoplasms are detected with increasing frequency. The management of such lesions is frequently hampered by limitations of current imaging techniques, difficulty in tissue acquisition, and the morbidity and mortality associated with pancreatic resection. Despite recent development in our understanding of the premalignant nature of mucinous lesions, the indications and timing of surgery remain controversial. More effort is needed to improve our diagnostic and treatment ability of pancreatic cystic neoplasms.

Pancreatic neuroendocrine tumors secrete hormones that can result in characteristic clinical syndromes; however, most remain clinically silent and are diagnosed at a late stage. Tumor stage and histologic grade are associated with prognosis and help guide therapeutic decisions. Surgical resection is generally attempted in patients with localized disease. In patients with surgically unresectable disease, treatment with somatostatin analogs, hepatic embolization, or cytotoxic chemotherapy may be recommended. Newer targeted therapies have been shown to improve progression-free survival durations and were recently approved for use in patients with advanced pancreatic neuroendocrine tumors, further expanding treatment options for patients with this disease.

Pancreas transplantation is the definitive treatment for type 1 diabetes and end-stage renal disease. Surgical techniques include systemic or portal venous drainage and enteric or bladder exocrine drainage. Major surgical complications such as graft thrombosis or enteric leak can lead to significant morbidity and mortality. Long-term pancreas graft survival is necessary to gain the maximal reduction in diabetes-related complications and improvement in overall survival.

Accumulating data indicate that clinically available abdominal imaging tests such as endoscopic ultrasound and magnetic resonance imaging/magnetic resonance cholangiopancreatography can detect asymptomatic precursor benign and invasive malignant pancreatic neoplasms, such as ductal adenocarcinoma, in individuals with an inherited predisposition. These asymptomatic familial pancreatic cancers detected have been more likely to be resectable, compared to symptomatic tumors. The most challenging part of screening high-risk individuals is the selection of individuals with high-grade precursor neoplasms for preventive treatment (ie, surgical resection before development of invasive cancer).

Although a variety of imaging techniques, such as multidetector computed tomography (MDCT), magnetic resonance imaging (MRI), endoscopic ultrasound, and fluorodeoxyglucose positron emission tomography have all been used in the initial diagnostic assessment of pancreatic lesions, in general, MDCT is the mainstay of diagnosis. This is due in large part to the high spatial resolution of its three-dimensional data sets that are indispensable in determining the local extent of tumor infiltration. This article describes MRI and MDCT techniques and accuracy and new horizons in MDCT in imaging of pancreatic cancer.

Endoscopic ultrasonography (EUS) has 85% to 99% sensitivity in detecting pancreatic cancer. In addition, EUS provides the opportunity of fine needle aspiration of suspected pancreatic lesions. EUS accuracy is decreased in chronic pancreatitis. Newer techniques, such as EUS elastography and contrast enhanced EUS, improved the accuracy of EUS in differentiating chronic pancreatitis from pancreatic cancer. Therapeutic applications of EUS in pancreatic cancer included EUS guided fiducial insertions for stereotactic body radiotherapy and EUS-guided delivery of antitumor agents locally.

The 5-year survival probability for pancreatic cancer is less than 5% for all stages. The only chance for cure or longer survival is surgical resection; however, only 10% to 20% of patients have resectable disease. Adjuvant systemic therapy reduces the recurrence rate and improves outcomes. There is a potential role for radiation therapy as part of treatment for locally advanced disease, although its use in both the adjuvant and neoadjuvant settings remains controversial. Palliative systemic treatment is the only option for patients with metastatic disease.

FORTHCOMING ISSUES

June 2012

Evaluation of Inflammatory Bowel Disease
Samir Shah, MD, and Edward Feller, MD,
Guest Editors

September 2012

Chronic Diarrhea
Heinz Hammer, MD,
Guest Editor

December 2012

**Clinical Applications of Probiotics in
Gastroenterology: Questions and Answers**
Gerald Friedman, MD, *Guest Editor*

RECENT ISSUES

December 2011

**Motility Consultation: Challenges in
Gastrointestinal Motility in Everyday
Clinical Practice**
Eammon M.M. Quigley, MD,
Guest Editor

September 2011

**Hepatology Update: Current Management
and New Therapies**
David A. Sass, MD, *Guest Editor*

June 2011

Women's Issues in Gastroenterology
Asyia Ahmad, MD, MPH,
and Barbara B. Frank, MD,
Guest Editors

THE CLINICS ARE NOW AVAILABLE ONLINE!
Access your subscription at:
www.theclinics.com

Preface

Modern Management of Pancreatic Disease

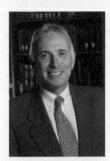

Jacques Van Dam, MD, PhD
Guest Editor

An issue devoted to the modern management of pancreatic disease? *Really*? Is there a cure for pancreatic cancer? *Well. . . no.* Have we found a cure for acute pancreatitis? *Well. . ..* Can we now prevent post endoscopic retrograde cholangiopancreatography (ERCP) pancreatitis? Can we definitively diagnose one particular type of cystic neoplasm of the pancreas from among the wide variety of potential etiologies? *Well. . . no.* So what could possibly be so new that a monograph on managing pancreatic disease could deign to use the term "modern" in its title? *Read on. . ..*

Researchers who study benign and malignant pancreatic disease have not hit the homeruns noted above (international readers will please forgive my American baseball analogy in this paragraph). Nonetheless, there are other ways to score major advances against diseases of this particularly enigmatic organ. The following monograph details the base hits and even the doubles and triples that have led to major advances in recent years.

The pancreas is unique. It serves both exocrine and endocrine functions. Its anatomy and location deep within the body allow benign and malignant changes to go unrecognized by its host, often until late in the course of a disease. And yet, the pancreas is so fragile that endoscopists can sometimes create havoc by simply working in its vicinity.

After reading this monograph, clinicians will learn the most prognostic scoring systems for acute pancreatitis, review the basics for early management of the disease, and see how current practice guidelines have evolved. Advances in radiological imaging when applied to the pancreas have resulted in enhanced staging and improved selection for surgical intervention. Endoscopy of the pancreas via both ERCP and endoscopic ultrasound has led to unprecedented access and potential for nonoperative intervention. Surgical advances have provided the most significant breakthroughs. Pancreatic surgery now takes advantage of both minimally invasive (laparoscopic)

Gastroenterol Clin N Am 41 (2012) xiii–xiv
doi:10.1016/j.gtc.2012.01.017
0889-8553/12/$ – see front matter © 2012 Elsevier Inc. All rights reserved.

approaches and techniques learned from organ transplantation. And noteworthy advances in medical and radiation oncology are extending life expectancy for patients with the most advanced malignant disease while limiting treatment toxicity.

I am indebted to the multidisciplinary team of authors, luminaries in their respective fields, who have graciously given their time and considerable expertise to this monograph. They represent gastroenterologists, endoscopists, radiologists, surgeons, oncologists, and radiation oncologists who have advanced the field and together have created a well-written, well-documented, and well-referenced manual for treating patients with benign and malignant diseases of the pancreas. I also wish to thank Kerry Holland for the opportunity to organize and edit this monograph and Lesley Simon for her outstanding editorial skills. Their support and guidance were essential to its success.

Jacques Van Dam, MD, PhD
Keck School of Medicine
University of Southern California
1510 San Pablo Street
HealthCare Consultation I; Suite 322R
Los Angeles, CA 90033, USA

Modern Management of Acute Pancreatitis

Neeraj Anand, MD, Jung H. Park, MD, Bechien U. Wu, MD, MPH*

KEYWORDS

- Acute pancreatitis • BISAP • Mortality • Management
- Complications • Fluid Resuscitation • Necrosis

BURDEN OF ACUTE PANCREATITIS IN THE MODERN ERA

Recent national survey data indicate a rising incidence of acute pancreatitis in the United States, attributed primarily to a rise in biliary pancreatitis. At present, there are more than 300,000 admissions for acute pancreatitis on an annual basis[1] at a direct cost exceeding $2 billion.[2] Although acute pancreatitis is typically a self-limited illness, up to 15% of patients experience a severe life-threatening form of disease.[3] Length of stay and direct costs vary considerably by severity of disease. In this age of cost containment, modern management of acute pancreatitis has evolved to emphasize effective interventions for prevention and management of complications, as well as appropriate resource utilization. This article addresses recent developments in the management of acute pancreatitis starting from initial hospital presentation extending through discharge and includes discussion of approaches secondary prevention.

INITIAL ASSESSMENT OF SEVERITY

Since the Ranson criteria were originally published in 1974,[4] numerous clinical prognostic scoring systems have been developed, the most prominent of which is the APACHE II score.[5] Although it is a widely validated instrument and clearly useful for research purposes, the APACHE II score has failed to gain widespread application in clinical practice as a result of its complexity. A simplified scoring system known as the Bedside Index of Severity in Acute Pancreatitis (BISAP) was developed based on data from 177 U.S hospitals and more than 17,000 cases of acute pancreatitis[6] (Table 1). This five-factor scoring system contains elements that are routinely available at the time of hospital admission and its use during the initial 24 hours of hospitalization has now been validated in several prospective cohort studies.[7,8] Two specific elements of the BISAP score warrant further discussion. First, blood urea nitrogen (BUN) has

The authors have no conflicts to disclose.
Department of Gastroeneterology, Kaiser Permanente Los Angeles Medical Center, 1526 North Edgemont Avenue, Los Angeles, CA 90027, USA
* Corresponding author.
E-mail address: Bechien.u.wu@kp.org

Gastroenterol Clin N Am 41 (2012) 1–8
doi:10.1016/j.gtc.2011.12.013
0889-8553/12/$ – see front matter © 2012 Elsevier Inc. All rights reserved.

Table 1		
BISAP score and its associated mortality		
Parameters	Value	If Present, Points Allocated
Serum BUN	>25	1
Mental status	Impaired	1
SIRS	Present	1
Age of the patient	>60 years	1
Pleural effusion	Present	1
	Total Score	Mortality (%)
	0	0.20
	1	0.60
	2	2
	3	5–8
	4	13–19
	5	22–27

received renewed interest as an early prognostic marker in acute pancreatitis. Either an elevated BUN at admission or early rise in BUN was found to be a strong risk factor for mortality in several retrospective and prospective cohort studies of acute pancreatitis.[9,10] Another component of the BISAP, the systemic inflammatory response syndrome (SIRS), has also been evaluated as a potential risk factor for severe acute pancreatitis (**Table 2**). Several prospective cohort studies of acute pancreatitis have shown that persistent SIRS,[11] lasting 48 hours or more, is associated with increased risk of necrosis, multiorgan failure, and death (**Fig. 1**).[12,13]

EARLY FLUID RESUSCITATION

Vigorous fluid resuscitation is a cornerstone of therapy during the early management of acute pancreatitis. However, recommendations on fluid resuscitation have been based primarily on expert opinion and data from animal models.[14] One retrospective study suggested that timing of fluid resuscitation may be more important than the total volume of fluid administered; in this study, patients receiving a greater proportion of their total fluid resuscitation during the initial 24 hours had reduced complications.[15] However, there are potential hazards associated with vigorous fluid resuscitation, such as pulmonary sequestration, as suggested by a prospective cohort study from Spain.[16] The data are difficult to interpret because fluid resuscitation parameters were driven by clinician judgment, and as such patients with more severe disease would most likely be those

Table 2	
SIRS criteria, defined by the presence of two or more	
Parameters	Value
Temperature	<36°C or >38°C
Heart rate	>90 per minute
Respiratory rate	>20 per minute or $Paco_2$ <32 mm Hg
White blood cell count	<4000 cells/mm^3 or >12,000 cells/mm^3 or 10% bands

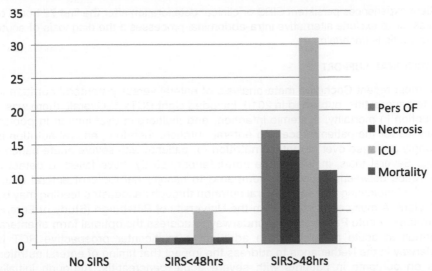

Fig. 1. Association of SIRS with Severe Acute Pancreatitis. Pers OF = persistant organ failure; Necrosis = pancreatic Necrosis; ICU = ICU admission; Mortality = Death.

receiving the more aggressive fluid resuscitation. An additional randomized controlled trial (RCT) from China showed that patients who were randomized to rapid hemodilution (targeting hematocrit <35%) received on average more than 10 L of fluid on the first hospital day and experienced greater frequency of sepsis and higher mortality.[17] Although these findings are difficult to generalize to Western populations because of variations in the underlying treatment of acute pancreatitis, these findings underscore the potential risks associated with very aggressive fluid resuscitation without hemodynamic monitoring. As a result of these potential concerns, a recent RCT evaluated the impact of a targeted approach to early fluid resuscitation in acute pancreatitis.[18] Although the study was underpowered to assess the effect of a goal-directed resuscitation algorithm because of a significant crossover effect, the study investigators found a reduction in SIRS based on the type of fluid used for initial resuscitation. Specifically, use of the more pH-balanced lactated Ringer's solution led to greater reduction in SIRS compared to the use of normal saline. In addition, there was no evidence of pulmonary sequestration among the 40 patients included in the trial.

APPROPRIATE USE OF RADIOGRAPHIC IMAGING IN THE EARLY PHASE OF ACUTE PANCREATITIS

Several studies have called attention to the increased use of cross-sectional imaging in the setting of acute pancreatitis, which has not been associated with either greater severity of disease or change in outcomes.[19,20] Based on several studies that have indicated a lack of sensitivity of early cross-sectional abdominal imaging to detect necrosis,[21] as well as the unlikely presence of infected necrosis within the first week of hospitalization,[22] current practice guidelines do not recommend computed tomography (CT) in the early phase of acute pancreatitis.[3,23] In contrast, transabdominal ultrasound is warranted to evaluate for the presence of possible gallstones as an etiology of pancreatitis. CT may be indicated if a patient experiences persistent SIRS or clinical deterioration after the first 72 hours of illness, or to exclude alternative intra-abdominal processes if the diagnosis of acute pancreatitis is uncertain.

NUTRITIONAL SUPPORT

The most recent Cochrane meta-analysis of enteral versus parenteral nutrition in acute pancreatitis, published in 2010, included eight RCTs.[24] Overall, there was a reduction in mortality, systemic infection, and multiorgan dysfunction in pooled analyses for the patients receiving enteral nutrition; therefore, enteral nutrition is strongly preferred over parenteral nutrition for patients with severe acute pancreatitis. Several trials, including one non-inferiority study, have failed to detect a difference between nasogastric compared to nasojejunal route of enteral nutrition,[25–27] indicating that early enteral nutrition through nasogastric feeding may be sufficient. A multicenter study from the University of Pittsburgh (Study of Enteral Nutrition in Acute Pancreatitis) is underway to address the optimal form of enteral nutrition in acute pancreatitis. In addition, a multicenter prospective RCT is underway in the Netherlands to address the impact that timing of enteral nutrition has on outcome in patients with severe acute pancreatitis. Although initially demonstrating promising results in small nonrandomized clinical trials, the addition of probiotics to enteral nutrition has been shown to be potentially detrimental in a large-scale RCT among patients with severe acute pancreatitis[28]; therefore, use of probitics is not recommended.

MANAGEMENT OF LOCAL COMPLICATIONS

Local complications from acute pancreatitis include pancreatic necrosis, acute fluid collections, and ductal disruption. Although previous small trials have suggested a benefit of prophylactic antibiotics in the setting of necrotizing pancreatitis, two more recent adequately powered double-blind RCTs[29,30] and the most recent Cochrane meta-analysis of seven RCTs, published in 2010,[31] did not demonstrate any impact on the incidence of infected necrosis or mortality with use of prophylactic antibiotics. At present, if infected necrosis is suspected, then the necrosis should be sampled by fine-needle aspiration. Once infected necrosis is confirmed, in addition to antibiotic treatment, a "step-up" approach can be pursued whereby percutaneous drainage is used as a temporizing maneuver, followed by minimally invasive retroperitoneal débridement if the patient fails to improve over the course of the next 72 hours. Such an approach has been shown to produce better overall outcome compared to traditional open débridement.[32] Overall, there has been a trend toward more conservative, less invasive approaches to management of necrosis, as well as infected necrosis, supported by observational studies that have demonstrated improved survival with delayed surgical intervention.[33]

Gallstone Pancreatitis and the Role of Endoscopic Retrograde Cholangiopancreatography

There are several clearly defined roles for endoscopic retrograde cholangiopancreatography (ERCP) in acute pancreatitis. Urgent ERCP—within 24 hours—is indicated in patients who have severe acute biliary pancreatitis with organ failure or cholangitis or both. Elective ERCP with sphincterotomy can be considered in patients with persistent or incipient biliary obstruction, those deemed to be poor candidates for cholecystectomy, and those in whom there is strong suspicion of bile duct stones after cholecystectomy. ERCP also is indicated for pancreatic ductal disruptions that occur as part of the inflammatory process and result in persistent peripancreatic fluid collections, pleural effusion, or ascites.

MANAGEMENT OF SYSTEMIC COMPLICATIONS

Systemic complications in acute pancreatitis include extrapancreatic infection, as well as distant organ failure.

Extrapancreatic Infection

Two large multicenter studies have called attention to the impact of extrapancreatic infection in acute pancreatitis. In a study from the Netherlands, more than 25% of patients with acute pancreatitis developed either bacteremia or pneumonia during their hospitalization.[22] The majority of these infections occurred within the first 2 weeks. By contrast, infected necrosis occurred on average 4 weeks after presentation. In a separate cohort study involving U.S. hospitals, hospital-acquired extrapancreatic infection was associated with a greater than twofold increased risk of mortality, even after adjusting for disease severity.[34] The clinical implication of these findings is that an extensive evaluation for potential sources of extrapancreatic infection should be undertaken and, if detected, these infections should be treated aggressively.

Respiratory failure is the most common form of organ dysfunction in acute pancreatitis.[35] Circulatory shock and renal insufficiency are also observed in severe cases. Although various measures of organ failure exist, the majority of recommendations define respiratory compromise as a room air oxygen saturation less than 90%, a systolic blood pressure less than 90 mm Hg, or a serum creatinine greater than 2.0 g/dL after initial fluid resuscitation.[36] Up to 20% of patients may have evidence of persistent organ failure 48 hours into their hospitalization. Patients with multiorgan dysfunction are at the greatest risk for mortality and should be managed in a critical care setting with a multidisciplinary care team. Recent data have suggested that centers with higher volume of acute pancreatitis cases achieve reduced mortality and costs.[37]

SECONDARY PREVENTION

The disease recurrence rate varies according to etiology of acute pancreatitis. Overall recurrence rates for acute pancreatitis range from 16.5% to 25%, with the majority of episodes occurring within the first several years of the initial attack. Continued alcohol consumption, smoking, and recurrent biliary complications are the major risk factors for disease recurrence. Prevention of disease recurrence is a major focus in acute pancreatitis. Appropriate prevention strategies vary according to etiology. Alcohol abstinence is the key to prevention of recurrence in the case of alcohol-associated pancreatitis. A RCT demonstrated that repeated alcohol cessation intervention at 6-month intervals was associated with reduced recurrence of acute pancreatitis compared to a one-time intervention session.[38]

Based on several retrospective and prospective observational cohort studies that demonstrate up to a 30% recurrence rate of gallstone pancreatitis, the recommendation for prevention of recurrent episodes of gallstone-associated pancreatitis is cholecystectomy. Although there is some variation in the recommended timing of cholecystectomy, most guidelines recommend operation before discharge whenever possible. In patients unable to undergo surgery, endoscopic sphincterotomy has been shown to reduce the risk of recurrent biliary pancreatitis, albeit to a lesser extent than cholecystectomy.[39]

ADDITIONAL ETIOLOGIES

Although less common, additional forms of acute pancreatitis such as medication-associated, hypertriglyceridemic-induced, and hypercalcemia-induced pancreatitis each require individualized strategies for prevention of recurrence. Discontinuation of any potentially offending medication is indicated in the case of suspected medication-associated pancreatitis.[40] Reduction of triglyceride levels through use of statin and fibrate medications is indicated in the case of acute pancreatitis secondary to hyperlipidemia.[41] Finally, treatment of the underlying cause of hypercalcemia is paramount for the prevention of acute pancreatitis due to hypercalcemia.

SUMMARY

There is a rising incidence of acute pancreatitis in the United States. Numerous clinical prognostic scoring systems have been developed, including the BISAP score. Vigorous fluid resuscitation remains a cornerstone of early management of acute pancreatitis. Cross-sectional imaging in the early phase of evaluation has not been associated with improvement of outcomes. There is no role for prophylactic antibiotics in early management. However, there is growing emphasis on the identification and treatment of extrapancreatic infections. Enteral nutrition in severe acute pancreatitis has reduced mortality, systemic infection, and multiorgan dysfunction compared to parenteral nutrition. Conservative management consisting of percutaneous drainage and delayed surgical intervention is now favored for local complications, such as infected necrosis. These developments have contributed to improved outcomes for patients with acute pancreatitis.

REFERENCES

1. Fagenholz PJ, Castillo CF, Harris NS, et al. Increasing United States hospital admissions for acute pancreatitis, 1988–2003. Ann Epidemiol 2007;17(7):491–7.
2. Fagenholz PJ, Fernandez-del Castillo C, Harris NS, et al. Direct medical costs of acute pancreatitis hospitalizations in the United States. Pancreas 2007;35(4):302–7.
3. Banks PA, Freeman ML. Practice guidelines in acute pancreatitis. Am J Gastroenterol 2006;101(10):2379–400.
4. Ranson JH, Rifkind KM, Roses DF, et al. Objective early identification of severe acute pancreatitis. Am J Gastroenterol 1974;61(6):443–51.
5. Larvin M, McMahon MJ. APACHE-II score for assessment and monitoring of acute pancreatitis. Lancet 1989;2(8656):201–5.
6. Wu BU, Johannes RS, Sun X, et al. The early prediction of mortality in acute pancreatitis: a large population-based study. Gut 2008;57(12):1698–703.
7. Papachristou GI, Muddana V, Yadav D, et al. Comparison of BISAP, Ranson's, APACHE-II, and CTSI scores in predicting organ failure, complications, and mortality in acute pancreatitis. Am J Gastroenterol 2010;105(2):435–41 [quiz: 42].
8. Singh VK, Wu BU, Bollen TL, et al. A prospective evaluation of the bedside index for severity in acute pancreatitis score in assessing mortality and intermediate markers of severity in acute pancreatitis. Am J Gastroenterol 2009;104(4):966–71.
9. Wu BU, Johannes RS, Sun X, et al. Early changes in blood urea nitrogen predict mortality in acute pancreatitis. Gastroenterology 2009;137(1):129–35.
10. Wu BU, Bakker OJ, Papachristou GI, et al. Blood urea nitrogen in the early assessment of acute pancreatitis: an international validation study. Arch Intern Med 2011; 171(7):669–76.
11. Bone RC, Sprung CL, Sibbald WJ. Definitions for sepsis and organ failure. Crit Care Med 1992;20(6):724–6.

12. Mofidi R, Duff MD, Wigmore SJ, et al. Association between early systemic inflammatory response, severity of multiorgan dysfunction and death in acute pancreatitis. Br J Surg 2006;93(6):738–44.
13. Singh VK, Wu BU, Bollen TL, et al. Early systemic inflammatory response syndrome is associated with severe acute pancreatitis. Clin Gastroenterol Hepatol 2009;7(11): 1247–51.
14. Gardner TB, Vege SS, Pearson RK, et al. Fluid resuscitation in acute pancreatitis. Clin Gastroenterol Hepatol 2008;6(10):1070–6.
15. Warndorf MG, Kurtzman JT, Bartel MJ, et al. Early fluid resuscitation reduces morbidity among patients with acute pancreatitis. Clin Gastroenterol Hepatol 2011; 9(8):705–9.
16. de-Madaria E, Soler-Sala G, Sanchez-Paya J, et al. Influence of fluid therapy on the prognosis of acute pancreatitis: a prospective cohort study. Am J Gastroenterol 2011;106(10):1843–50.
17. Mao EQ, Fei J, Peng YB, et al. Rapid hemodilution is associated with increased sepsis and mortality among patients with severe acute pancreatitis. Chin Med J [Engl] 2010;123(13):1639–44.
18. Wu BU, Hwang JQ, Gardner TH, et al. Lactated Ringer's solution reduces systemic inflammation compared with saline in patients with acute pancreatitis. Clin Gastroenterol Hepatol 2011;9(8):710–7, e1.
19. Mortele KJ, Ip IK, Wu BU, et al. Acute pancreatitis: imaging utilization practices in an urban teaching hospital—analysis of trends with assessment of independent predictors in correlation with patient outcomes. Radiology 2011;258(1):174–81.
20. Morgan DE, Ragheb CM, Lockhart ME, et al. Acute pancreatitis: computed tomography utilization and radiation exposure are related to severity but not patient age. Clin Gastroenterol Hepatol 2010;8(3):303–8 [quiz: e33].
21. Bollen TL, van Santvoort HC, Besselink MG, et al. Update on acute pancreatitis: ultrasound, computed tomography, and magnetic resonance imaging features. Semin Ultrasound CT MR 2007;28(5):371–83.
22. Besselink MG, van Santvoort HC, Boermeester MA, et al. Timing and impact of infections in acute pancreatitis. Br J Surg 2009;96(3):267–73.
23. Forsmark CE, Baillie J. AGA Institute technical review on acute pancreatitis. Gastroenterology 2007;132(5):2022–44.
24. Al-Omran M, Albalawi ZH, Tashkandi MF, et al. Enteral versus parenteral nutrition for acute pancreatitis. Cochrane Database Syst Rev 2010;1:CD002837.
25. Singh N, Sharma B, Sharma M, et al. Evaluation of early enteral feeding through nasogastric and nasojejunal tube in severe acute pancreatitis: a noninferiority randomized controlled trial. Pancreas 2012;41(1):153–9.
26. Eatock FC, Chong P, Menezes N, et al. A randomized study of early nasogastric versus nasojejunal feeding in severe acute pancreatitis. Am J Gastroenterol 2005; 100(2):432–9.
27. Kumar A, Singh N, Prakash S, et al. Early enteral nutrition in severe acute pancreatitis: a prospective randomized controlled trial comparing nasojejunal and nasogastric routes. J Clin Gastroenterol 2006;40(5):431–4.
28. Besselink MG, van Santvoort HC, Buskens E, et al. Probiotic prophylaxis in predicted severe acute pancreatitis: a randomised, double-blind, placebo-controlled trial. Lancet 2008;371(9613):651–9.
29. Dellinger EP, Tellado JM, Soto NE, et al. Early antibiotic treatment for severe acute necrotizing pancreatitis: a randomized, double-blind, placebo-controlled study. Ann Surg 2007;245(5):674–83.

30. Isenmann R, Runzi M, Kron M, et al. Prophylactic antibiotic treatment in patients with predicted severe acute pancreatitis: a placebo-controlled, double-blind trial. Gastroenterology 2004;126(4):997–1004.
31. Villatoro E, Mulla M, Larvin M. Antibiotic therapy for prophylaxis against infection of pancreatic necrosis in acute pancreatitis. Cochrane Database Syst Rev 2010;5: CD002941.
32. van Santvoort HC, Besselink MG, Bakker OJ, et al. A step-up approach or open necrosectomy for necrotizing pancreatitis. N Engl J Med 2010;362(16):1491–502.
33. van Santvoort HC, Bakker OJ, Bollen TL, et al. A conservative and minimally invasive approach to necrotizing pancreatitis improves outcome. Gastroenterology 2011; 141(4):1254–63.
34. Wu BU, Johannes RS, Kurtz S, et al. The impact of hospital-acquired infection on outcome in acute pancreatitis. Gastroenterology 2008;135(3):816–20.
35. Buter A, Imrie CW, Carter CR, et al. Dynamic nature of early organ dysfunction determines outcome in acute pancreatitis. Br J Surg 2002;89(3):298–302.
36. Bone RC. Why new definitions of sepsis and organ failure are needed. Am J Med 1993;95(4):348–50.
37. Singla A, Simons J, Li Y, et al. Admission volume determines outcome for patients with acute pancreatitis. Gastroenterology 2009;137(6):1995–2001.
38. Nordback I, Pelli H, Lappalainen-Lehto R, et al. The recurrence of acute alcohol-associated pancreatitis can be reduced: a randomized controlled trial. Gastroenterology 2009;136(3):848–55.
39. Bakker OJ, van Santvoort HC, Hagenaars JC, et al. Timing of cholecystectomy after mild biliary pancreatitis. Br J Surg 2011;98(10):1446–54.
40. Badalov N, Baradarian R, Iswara K, et al. Drug-induced acute pancreatitis: an evidence-based review. Clin Gastroenterol Hepatol 2007;5(6):648–61 [quiz: 4].
41. Tsuang W, Navaneethan U, Ruiz L, et al. Hypertriglyceridemic pancreatitis: presentation and management. Am J Gastroenterol 2009;104(4):984–91.

Diagnosis and Management of Autoimmune Pancreatitis

Aravind Sugumar, MD

KEYWORDS

- Pancreatic cancer • Idiopathic duct centric pancreatitis
- Lymphoplasmacytic sclerosing pancreatitis • IgG4

Autoimmune pancreatitis (AIP) is a unique form of corticosteroid responsive chronic pancreatitis. In recent years, a distinct clinical presentation, histology, serology, and subtypes of AIP have been identified. This rare form of chronic pancreatitis was probably first described by Henry Sarles in the 1960s.[1] He described a type of sclerosing pancreatitis associated with hypergammaglobulinemia, which is very similar to the present-day description of AIP. The term **autoimmune pancreatitis** was not used until 1995, when it was coined by Yoshida and colleagues to describe a type of chronic pancreatitis associated with Sjögren-like syndrome.[2] Early descriptions of the disease were mostly in the form of case reports.[3–5] Major milestones in the description of AIP include Hamano and colleagues' description of the association between serum IgG4 and AIP, Kamisawa and coworkers' explanation that AIP was a systemic disease affecting multiple organs, and Chari and colleagues' publication of the Histology, Imaging, Serology, Other organ involvement and Response to therapy (HISORt) criteria for the diagnosis of AIP.[6–9]

As with any new entity, a plethora of terms and synonyms were used to describe the same disease.[10–13] A major reason for this varied use of terms is that AIP is a heterogeneous disease. We now know that previously described entities such as lymphoplasmacytic sclerosing pancreatitis, idiopathic duct centric pancreatitis, IgG4-associated pancreatitis, and steroid-sensitive sclerosing pancreatitis are descriptions of the subtypes of AIP and not different diseases.[14,15] The use of these alternate terms hindered progress; therefore, it was recently agreed that AIP should be divided into type 1 and type 2 to facilitate international uniformity in description.[15,16]

SUBTYPES OF AIP

AIP is a heterogeneous disease with two distinct subtypes: type 1 and type 2, which are classified according to histology.[15,16] However, the clinical presentation can suggest a strong basis for suspecting one subtype from the other, as there are numerous

The author has nothing to disclose.
Division of Gastroenterology and Hepatology, University of Kansas Medical Center, 3901 Rainbow Boulevard, Kansas City, KS 66160, USA
E-mail address: asugumar@kumc.edu

Gastroenterol Clin N Am 41 (2012) 9–22
doi:10.1016/j.gtc.2011.12.008
0889-8553/12/$ – see front matter © 2012 Elsevier Inc. All rights reserved.

gastro.theclinics.com

Table 1 Differences between type 1 and type 2 AIP		
	Type 1 AIP	**Type 2 AIP**
Gender distribution	M > F	M = F
Histology		
• Lymphoplasmacytic infiltrate	Yes	Yes
• Storiform fibrosis	Present	Infrequent
• Obliterative phlebitis	Present	Infrequent
• IgG4 + cell infiltrate	Present	Scant\none
• Pancreatic duct destruction	Absent	Present
• GEL lesions	Absent	Present
Histologic confirmation need for diagnosis	Not in all cases	Yes
Serum IgG4 elevated	Mostly	No
Other organ involvement	Yes	No
Responds to steroids	Yes	Yes
Disease relapse	Present	Absent
Association with IBD	Some	Strong

Abbreviations: GEL, granulocyte epithelial lesion; IBD, inflammatory bowel disease.

differences between the two subtypes, along with a few similarities (**Table 1**). Most of the current literature on AIP is based on what we know about type 1 AIP.[16,17] We are still in the early stages of understanding and describing type 2 AIP. **In this article, unless explicitly stated, the generic term AIP pertains to type 1 AIP.**

Type 1 AIP is best described as the pancreatic manifestation of a systemic fibroinflammatory disease, which at its core has a unique histology and tissue infiltration of immunoglobulin G4 (IgG4)-positive inflammatory cells.[8,9,18] This systemic disease can affect many different organs in such a manner that the umbrella term "immunoglobulin G4–associated systemic diseases" is used to underscore the unique role played by IgG4.[8,9,19,20] All the organs afflicted by immunoglobulin G4–associated systemic diseases, including the pancreas, share a common, distinct, and discernible histology. Almost all of the early descriptions of type 1 AIP came from Asia, Japan in particular, and type 1 continues to be the predominant subtype seen there.[8,9,19,20] In addition to the established diagnostic criteria that exist for type 1 AIP, the clinical presentation is so distinctive that histologic confirmation is needed in a small proportion of patients.[16,17,21] Conversely, type 2 AIP, with its discernible histology, appears to exclusively affect the pancreas. Most of the literature describing this subtype comes from Europe and the United States.[11,22–25] As of now, although type 2 AIP can be clinically suspected, histologic confirmation is need in all cases to make a certain diagnosis. The differences between the two subtypes are illustrated in **Table 1**. It is important to note that the two subtypes are virtually indistinguishable on cross-sectional imaging, and both types are exquisitely sensitive to steroid therapy.[15–17,26]

PATHOPHYSIOLOGY

Because AIP is so responsive to steroid therapy, an autoimmune cause has been inferred.[8,27–29] The precise pathogenesis of AIP has not been elucidated; however, there are interesting genetic and immunologic associations, in addition to the possibility of molecular mimicry, surrounding AIP.[30–33] The most striking observation is the association between serum IgG4 and AIP.[7] IgG4 constitutes the smallest fraction of total IgG in humans.[34] IgG4 is involved in the activation of the classic pathway of complement.[35] Marked elevation in serum IgG4 is seen in only a limited number of autoimmune and parasitic diseases.[36-39] It is still unclear if IgG4 plays a direct pathogenic role in developing AIP or if it is an epiphenomenon.[40-42] Preliminary genetic studies from Japan have suggested that a specific human leukocyte antigen (HLA) type (DRB1*0405-DQB1*0401) is associated with AIP.[30] Molecular mimicry by microbial pathogen, which leads to a cross reaction with endogenous antigens, has been postulated as a cause of many autoimmune conditions including AIP. There is limited evidence pointing toward *Helicobacter pylori* as the punitive organism.[32,33] The theory suggests that exposure to *Helicobacter pylori* could lead to AIP in predisposed individuals.

HISTOLOGY

Both subtypes of autoimmune pancreatitis have common histologic features (periductal lymphoplasmacytic infiltrate and an inflammatory cellular stroma), which positively differentiate it from other types of chronic pancreatitis.[15-18] In addition, histology serves as the basis for distinguishing the two clinical phenotypes of AIP.[18] The histologic hallmark of type 1 AIP is a set of four features, which together are called lymphoplasmacytic sclerosing pancreatitis (LPSP). LPSP consists of a dense periductal lymphoplasmacytic infiltrate, storiform pancreatic fibrosis, presence of IgG4-positive cells (>10/high-power field), and obliterative phlebitis.[18] In addition, the pancreatic ductal architecture is often preserved and there are prominent lymphoid follicles. When most, if not all, of these features are present, they substantiate the diagnosis of type 1 AIP. In this context, it is important to point out that the presence of IgG4-positive cells is just one of the features of LPSP and that the histologic diagnosis of type 1 AIP should not be made or excluded solely on the presence or absence of this one feature alone. Features of LPSP are also seen in the histologic specimens of the other organs involved in type 1 AIP: salivary glands and lymph nodes.[19,43]

On histology, type 2 AIP also consists of a predominantly lymphoplasmacytic infiltrate but with a few key differences from type 1 AIP. There is a dense periductal inflammation with neutrophils leading to duct destruction in most cases. This characteristic lesion is called a granulocyte epithelial lesion. These lesions are pathognomonic of type 2 AIP.[18,23,25] There is no inflammation around the intra-pancreatic artery or vein and there are scant groups of IgG4-positive cells. In both forms of AIP, there is a striking absence of intraductal protein plugs, stones, and pseudocysts, which are seen in other types of chronic pancreatitis.[18]

CLINICAL CONTEXT

The true incidence of AIP is unknown. The best estimates so far come from studies of patients who were presumed to have pancreatic cancer and underwent resection, but the resection specimen showed AIP. AIP was the diagnosis in approximately 3% to 5% of such patients.[24,44] In Japan, the incidence of AIP was reported to be 0.82 per 100,000 people.[45] The clinical presentation of AIP can be best divided into the acute and the postacute phase. In the acute phase, the classic presentation of AIP is that of obstructive jaundice with abdominal imaging consistent with pancreatic enlargement.[6,15-17] Thus, in clinical practice it is imperative to differentiate AIP from pancreatic cancer. Less commonly, AIP presents with mild abdominal pain; elevated pancreatic enzymes, which may also signal acute pancreatitis; or jaundice with proximal bile duct involvement, which must be differentiated from cholangiocarcinoma. In the postacute phase, AIP can present with pancreatic atrophy and steatorrhea resembling chronic pancreatitis. A recent study from the Mayo Clinic concluded that fewer than 33% of patients with AIP have features of acute or chronic pancreatitis at presentation. More importantly, only 7 of 178 (3.9%) patients evaluated for etiology of suspected pancreatitis had AIP.[46] Although mild abdominal pain can be seen occasionally in patients with AIP, a feature conspicuous by its absence in AIP is severe unremitting abdominal pain requiring narcotic pain medications.[16] The presence of such severe pain should prompt a reevaluation of the diagnosis. Diabetes mellitus (DM) is seen in up to 50% of patients with AIP. Interestingly, this DM resolves in a proportion of patients with corticosteroid therapy.[47,48] After initial treatment with corticosteroids, the pancreas can undergo atrophy on cross-sectional imaging, which can be accompanied by significant steatorrhea (postacute phase presentation). Untreated AIP can also lead to pancreatic atrophy and fibrosis, which in its late stages can be indistinguishable from other forms of chronic pancreatitis.[49]

IMAGING

Pancreatic imaging is the cornerstone to the diagnosis of AIP. Pancreatic imaging can be subdivided into pancreatic parenchyma imaging and pancreatic ductal imaging. Pancreatic parenchymal imaging in the form of computed tomography (CT) or magnetic resonance imaging (MRI) is often performed as part of the initial testing for obstructive jaundice. A pancreas protocol abdominal CT is rapidly becoming the imaging modality of choice to diagnose AIP. Such a CT scan serves not only to diagnose AIP, but also to help rule in or rule out pancreatic cancer. There are three classic features of AIP on a pancreas protocol abdominal CT: a diffusely enlarged, sausage-shaped pancreas with featureless borders; a low-density rim surrounding the pancreas; and delayed enhancement of the pancreas in the late arterial phase.[16,50–53] (**Figs. 1** and **2**). The presence of a low-density mass, along with an abrupt cutoff of a dilated pancreatic duct and atrophy of the pancreas distal to the obstruction, are all signs of pancreatic cancer, which can be detected on CT/MRI[16,50,52,53] (**Fig. 3**). AIP can also present as a focal enlargement of the pancreas, in which case it can be very challenging to differentiate it from pancreatic cancer by imaging

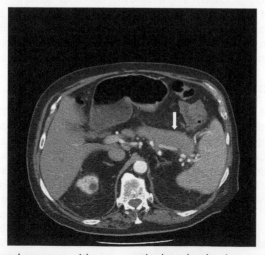

Fig. 1. Sausage-shaped pancreas with arrow at the low-density rim.

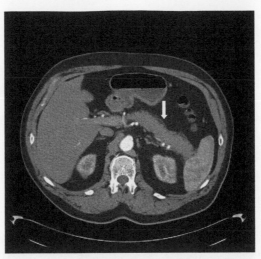

Fig. 2. Sausage-shaped pancreas with arrow showing a low-density rim.

alone. Although MRI of the abdomen is comparable to a CT scan, higher cost and decreased availably limit its use.[54–56] On MRI, T1-weighted images of the pancreas are often less intense than T2-weighted images when compared to the liver.[54–56] Endoscopic ultrasound (EUS) plays a very important adjunctive role in the workup of AIP. Although classic EUS features of AIP have been described (such as a diffusely hypoechoic gland), the greatest benefit of EUS is the access it provides to obtain pancreatic tissue by fine-needle aspiration (FNA) or a core biopsy.[57–59] Although an FNA is sufficient for diagnosing pancreatic cancer, it is not adequate for diagnosing AIP. For histologic confirmation of AIP a core biopsy of the pancreas is needed, and it can also help to establish the basis for the subtypes of AIP.[16,59,60] EUS-FNA is paramount in ruling out pancreatic cancer in patients with nonclassic CT imaging

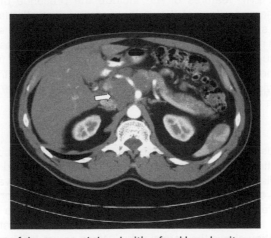

Fig. 3. Enlargement of the pancreatic head with a focal low-density mass (*arrow*) suggestive of pancreatic cancer.

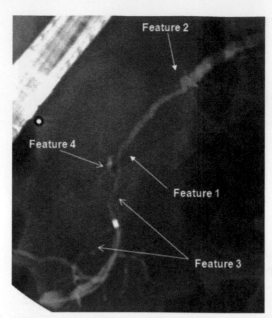

Fig. 4. ERP in AIP. *Feature 1*, Long narrow stricture greater than one third of the main pancreatic duct. *Feature 2*, Lack of upstream pancreatic duct dilatation from the stricture. *Feature 3*, Multiple noncontiguous strictures. *Feature 4*, Side branch duct arising from a stricture.

features. EUS elastography and positron emission tomography (PET) are exciting newer additions to the imaging armamentarium and hold much promise, but at present are not incorporated into the existing diagnostic criteria.[61–63]

Pancreatic duct imaging with endoscopic retrograde pancreatography (ERP) can be a useful adjunct in the diagnosis of AIP, especially in patients with nonclassic CT abdominal features for AIP, as well as for pancreatic cancer. A recently concluded study found that ERP features of AIP include the presence of a long narrow stricture (more than one third of the main pancreas duct), the lack of upstream dilation from the stricture, side branches arising from the strictured portion of the duct, and multiple noncontiguous strictures (**Figs. 4** and **5**). The presence of all these features is more suggestive of AIP than the presence of any one of them.[64] Although magnetic resonance cholangiopancreatography (MRCP) is an attractive minimally invasive way of visualizing the pancreatic duct, ERP and MRCP have not been compared to each other.

SEROLOGY

Although numerous autoimmune antibodies have been reported to be elevated in AIP, the latest international consensus diagnostic criteria recommend measuring only serum IgG4 for diagnosing AIP.[16] Initial studies showed that elevated IgG4 had a greater than 95% sensitivity and specificity in diagnosing AIP. More recent studies reveal a much lower sensitivity and specificity.[7,40,42] Because there is great variation in the way IgG4 is measured in different parts of the world, it is best to interpret it in terms of the elevation above the normal value. When serum IgG4 is at least twofold above the normal, the value is highly suggestive of AIP.[16,40] If all the typical features

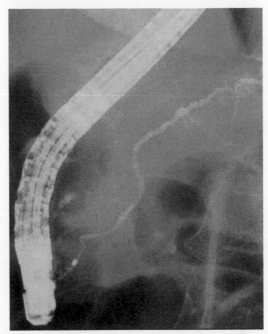

Fig. 5. Long narrow stricture greater than one third of the main pancreatic duct seen in AIP.

of AIP are seen on abdominal CT imaging, then any elevation in serum IgG4 is supportive of AIP (**Fig. 6**). In the absence of typical imaging features, the threshold for serum IgG4 to help diagnose AIP has been set to twofold of the upper limit of normal.[40] It is also important to note that some patients with type 1 AIP are seronegative for IgG4.[16] Therefore, it should not be assumed that patients who are seronegative have type 2 AIP. Also, up to 7% to 10% of patients with pancreatic cancer can have elevated IgG4 levels.[40,65] As helpful as serum IgG4 may be, elevated IgG4 level should never be considered the sole criterion for diagnosis of AIP, especially in the absence of abdominal imaging evidence. Likewise, during the treatment phase of AIP, serum IgG4 level should not be used as a marker to gauge response to therapy. IgG4 levels often fluctuate during corticosteroid therapy and do not correlate with disease activity.

OTHER ORGAN INVOLVEMENT

Type 1 AIP is the pancreatic manifestation of a multisystem disease. Thus, the well-described pattern of the multiple other organs involved is an important clue to the diagnosis.[14,16,66-69] The presence of other organ involvement can lead to characteristic symptoms, such as dry eyes and dry mouth (Sjögren-like syndrome), jaundice (bile duct involvement), and swelling in the groin (regional lymphadenopathy). Other organ involvement (OOI) that can also be seen on abdominal imaging includes retroperitoneal fibrosis, and renal involvement. Although not recommended as part of the routine workup of AIP, PET can be useful in picking up the other organs involved. When OOI is present, it not only strengthens the diagnosis of AIP, but it also allows for histologic confirmation of AIP, as tissue can be readily obtained if needed (eg, lymph node biopsy). The commonly described involvement of other organs includes

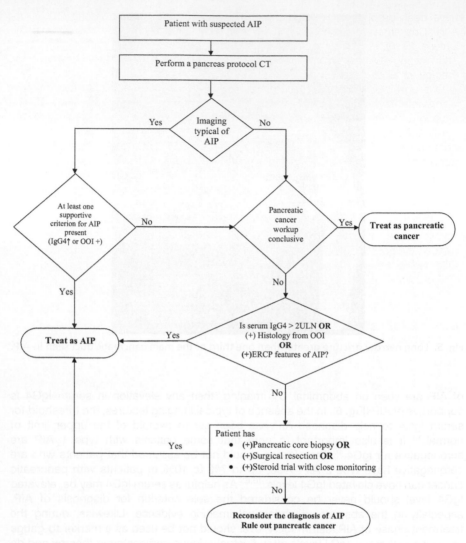

Fig. 6. Algorithm for distinguishing AIP from pancreatic cancer.

the proximal bile duct followed by salivary gland, retroperitoneum, orbits, ampulla of Vater, lymph nodes, and kidneys.[14,66–70] Less commonly, gallbladder and gastric involvement have also been described.[68,71] Symptoms related to OOI often improve with treatment and can serve as useful indicators of response to treatment.[17,72]

DIAGNOSIS

In clinical practice, diagnosing AIP can be quiet challenging. As the disease mimics pancreatic cancer, the price of misdiagnosis is often high. The Japan Pancreas Society (JPS) in 2002 devised the first diagnostic criteria for AIP. These criteria were later modified in 2006 (JPS 2006). Early on, the emphasis was to not miss pancreatic cancer, rather than to diagnose AIP. Since that time, a plethora of diagnostic criteria have been proposed, including the HISORt (2006), the Korean criteria (2007), the Asian Consensus criteria (2008), and the most recent International Consensus Diagnostic Criteria (2010).[6,16,73–76] All of these criteria, in some way, combine pancreatic imaging and histology with serology or other organ involvement or response to corticosteroid therapy, or all of these.

One possible algorithm to help diagnose AIP is illustrated in **Fig. 6**. More detailed algorithms have been published elsewhere.[16,50,53] When confronted with a clinical situation in which AIP is suspected, the gastroenterologist must remember two cardinal facts: first, AIP is a rare disease, and second, pancreatic cancer is far more common than AIP. Recent national and international consensus criteria agree that abdominal imaging in the form of CT/MRI should form the cornerstone to the diagnosis of AIP.[16,17] If imaging features typical of AIP are present, along with some collateral evidence in the form OOI or elevated serum IgG4 (any level), the patient can be started on corticosteroid therapy for AIP. In the absence of typical imaging features of AIP, a thorough workup to rule out pancreatic cancer needs to be done (EUS-FNA, carbohydrate antigen 19-9 [CA 19-9], etc). In this setting, despite ruling out pancreatic cancer, the bar for the collateral evidence for AIP has to be set high (ie, histology from OOI, twofold elevation of serum IgG4, or presence of ERP features of AIP). If the above highly suggestive pieces of collateral evidence for AIP are not present, then for these patients, a pancreatic core biopsy, a steroid trial, or surgical resection of the pancreas is required to make a diagnosis. These interventions, and especially the steroid trial (see later), should be limited to select situations and performed only by gastroenterologists with expertise in treating AIP.

TREATMENT

There are no prospective data from clinical trials to guide management of AIP; therefore, treatment regimens are based on retrospective analysis and expert opinion.[47,49] Both subtypes of AIP are exquisitely sensitive to corticosteroid therapy. This fact has been so well described that response to corticosteroid therapy can be both diagnostic and therapeutic. It is important to distinguish the two distinct roles corticosteroids play in AIP. When typical imaging features and collateral evidence for AIP are absent and pancreatic cancer has been reliably ruled out, a steroid trial of oral prednisone 40 mg (or 0.6 mg/kg) once a day for 2 weeks can be started. When performed by gastroenterologists experienced in treating AIP, a steroid trial can be used to diagnose AIP. Response to steroids is based on objective data such as radiologic evidence showing a dramatic decrease in the pancreatic mass or OOI, resolution of the obstructive jaundice without biliary stenting (or being able to remove preexisting biliary stent without the recurrence of the jaundice), and normalization of liver function test. If there is no such improvement or if the CA 19-9 level is rising, then the diagnosis of AIP should be reconsidered and further efforts to rule out pancreatic cancer should be pursued.[16,17,50] Subjective criteria, such as the patient reporting more energy or feeling better, or serum IgG4 levels normalizing, should not be considered a response to steroids.

Once the diagnosis of AIP has been established, the best initial treatment is oral prednisone 40 mg (or 0.6 mg/kg) for 4 weeks, including the 2-week steroid trial, if performed. Beginning at week 4, with continued objective response to therapy, the dose should be tapered by 5 mg per week. Thus, the total duration of initial corticosteroid therapy is 12 weeks (4 weeks of therapy plus 8 weeks of taper). Up to 40% of patients (mostly type 1 AIP) will have disease relapse after the first course of corticosteroid therapy.[72,77,78] Proximal bile duct involvement (away from common bile duct) can be a predictor of disease relapse. Disease relapse can be observed by radiologic (reappearance of the pancreatic mass), clinical (obstructive jaundice, recurrence of OOI, weight loss), or serologic (repeat elevation in serum IgG4) means. Most experts agree that an isolated serologic relapse can observed and does not need maintenance therapy. Clinical and radiologic relapses, on the other hand, require treatment.[72] Most patients with disease relapse will need a full course of oral prednisone similar to the initial 12-week treatment along with concomitant oral azathioprine (at 2–2.5 mg/kg).[26,79] These patients are advised to continue maintenance azathioprine (at 2–2.5 mg/kg) for at least 2 years. If there are no further relapses, maintenance therapy can be stopped. While the patient is on maintenance therapy, it is imperative to evaluate the complete blood counts and liver function test frequently. Early data for the use of Rituximab in patients with AIP who have relapsed on azathioprine or who cannot tolerate corticosteroids are encouraging.[80]

SUMMARY

- AIP is a heterogeneous disease with two distinct subtypes, now called type 1 and type 2. The proportions of these subtypes vary in their distribution worldwide.
- Pancreatic cancer is the leading differential diagnosis for AIP, although AIP can mimic any other major pancreatobiliary disease.
- Cross-sectional abdominal imaging CT/MRI should form the cornerstone to the diagnosis of AIP.
- Serum IgG4 provides collateral evidence for the diagnosis of AIP and should not be the sole basis for the diagnosis. False-positive elevation in serum IgG4 can be seen in up to 10% of patients with pancreatic cancer.
- A steroid trial should be performed only in select situations after ruling out pancreatic cancer and by gastroenterologists experienced in treating AIP.
- Disease recurrence can be seen in up to 40% of patients after initial steroid therapy.

REFERENCES

1. Sarles H, Sarles JC, Muratore R, et al. Chronic inflammatory sclerosis of the pancreas—an autonomous pancreatic disease? Am J Dig Dis 1961;6:688–98.
2. Yoshida K, Toki F, Takeuchi T, et al. Chronic pancreatitis caused by an autoimmune abnormality. Proposal of the concept of autoimmune pancreatitis. Dig Dis Sci 1995; 40(7):1561–8.
3. Chutaputti A, Burrell MI, Boyer JL. Pseudotumor of the pancreas associated with retroperitoneal fibrosis: a dramatic response to corticosteroid therapy. Am J Gastroenterol 1995;90(7):1155–8.
4. Sood S, Fossard DP, Shorrock K. Chronic sclerosing pancreatitis in Sjogren's syndrome: a case report. Pancreas 1995;10(4):419–21.
5. Horiuchi A, Kaneko T, Yamamura N, et al. Autoimmune chronic pancreatitis simulating pancreatic lymphoma. Am J Gastroenterol 1996;91(12):2607–9.
6. Chari ST, Smyrk TC, Levy MJ, et al. Diagnosis of autoimmune pancreatitis: the Mayo Clinic experience. Clin Gastroenterol Hepatol 2006;4(8):1010–6.
7. Hamano H, Kawa S, Horiuchi A, et al. High serum IgG4 concentrations in patients with sclerosing pancreatitis. N Engl J Med 2001;344(10):732–8.
8. Kamisawa T, Egawa N, Nakajima H. Autoimmune pancreatitis is a systemic autoimmune disease. Am J Gastroenterol 2003;98(12):2811–2.
9. Kamisawa T, Funata N, Hayashi Y. Lymphoplasmacytic sclerosing pancreatitis is a pancreatic lesion of IgG4-related systemic disease. Am J Surg Pathol 2004;28(8): 1114.

10. Kawaguchi K, Koike M, Tsuruta K, et al. Lymphoplasmacytic sclerosing pancreatitis with cholangitis: a variant of primary sclerosing cholangitis extensively involving pancreas. Hum Pathol 1991;22(4):387–95.
11. Ectors N, Maillet B, Aerts R, et al. Non-alcoholic duct destructive chronic pancreatitis. Gut 1997;41(2):263–8.
12. Kazumori H, Ashizawa N, Moriyama N, et al. Primary sclerosing pancreatitis and cholangitis. Int J Pancreatol 1998;24(2):123–7.
13. Petter LM, Martin JK Jr, Menke DM. Localized lymphoplasmacellular pancreatitis forming a pancreatic inflammatory pseudotumor. Mayo Clin Proc 1998;73(5):447–50.
14. Sugumar A, Chari S. Autoimmune pancreatitis: an update. Expert Rev Gastroenterol Hepatol 2009;3(2):197–204.
15. Sugumar A, Kloppel G, Chari ST. Autoimmune pancreatitis: pathologic subtypes and their implications for its diagnosis. Am J Gastroenterol 2009;104(9):2308–10 [quiz 11].
16. Shimosegawa T, Chari ST, Frulloni L, et al. International consensus diagnostic criteria for autoimmune pancreatitis: guidelines of the International Association of Pancreatology. Pancreas 40(3):352–8.
17. Chari ST, Kloeppel G, Zhang L, et al. Histopathologic and clinical subtypes of autoimmune pancreatitis: the Honolulu consensus document. Pancreas 2010;39(5):549–54.
18. Zhang L, Chari S, Smyrk TC, et al. Autoimmune pancreatitis (AIP) type 1 and type 2: an international consensus study on histopathologic diagnostic criteria. Pancreas 2011;40(8):1172–9.
19. Kamisawa T. IgG4-positive plasma cells specifically infiltrate various organs in autoimmune pancreatitis. Pancreas 2004;29(2):167–8.
20. Zen Y, Harada K, Sasaki M, et al. IgG4-related sclerosing cholangitis with and without hepatic inflammatory pseudotumor, and sclerosing pancreatitis-associated sclerosing cholangitis: do they belong to a spectrum of sclerosing pancreatitis? Am J Surg Pathol 2004;28(9):1193–203.
21. Okazaki K, Uchida K, Fukui T. Recent advances in autoimmune pancreatitis: concept, diagnosis, and pathogenesis. J Gastroenterol 2008;43(6):409–18.
22. Deshpande V, Chicano S, Finkelberg D, et al. Autoimmune pancreatitis: a systemic immune complex mediated disease. Am J Surg Pathol 2006;30(12):1537–45.
23. Kloppel G, Luttges J, Lohr M, et al. Autoimmune pancreatitis: pathological, clinical, and immunological features. Pancreas 2003;27(1):14–9.
24. Yadav D, Notahara K, Smyrk TC, et al. Idiopathic tumefactive chronic pancreatitis: clinical profile, histology, and natural history after resection. Clin Gastroenterol Hepatol 2003;1(2):129–35.
25. Zamboni G, Luttges J, Capelli P, et al. Histopathological features of diagnostic and clinical relevance in autoimmune pancreatitis: a study on 53 resection specimens and 9 biopsy specimens. Virchows Arch 2004;445(6):552–63.
26. Sugumar A, Chari ST. Autoimmune pancreatitis. J Gastroenterol Hepatol 2011;26(9):1368–73.
27. Kim KP, Kim MH, Song MH, et al. Autoimmune chronic pancreatitis. Am J Gastroenterol 2004;99(8):1605–16.
28. Kojima E, Kimura K, Noda Y, et al. Autoimmune pancreatitis and multiple bile duct strictures treated effectively with steroid. J Gastroenterol 2003;38(6):603–7.
29. Ito T, Nakano I, Koyanagi S, et al. Autoimmune pancreatitis as a new clinical entity. Three cases of autoimmune pancreatitis with effective steroid therapy. Dig Dis Sci 1997;42(7):1458–68.

30. Kawa S, Ota M, Yoshizawa K, et al. HLA DRB10405–DQB10401 haplotype is associated with autoimmune pancreatitis in the Japanese population. Gastroenterology 2002;122(5):1264–9.

31. Park do H, Kim MH, Oh HB, et al. Substitution of aspartic acid at position 57 of the DQbeta1 affects relapse of autoimmune pancreatitis. Gastroenterology 2008;134(2):440–6.

32. Kountouras J, Zavos C, Chatzopoulos D. A concept on the role of Helicobacter pylori infection in autoimmune pancreatitis. J Cell Mol Med 2005;9(1):196–207.

33. Kountouras J, Zavos C, Gavalas E, et al. Challenge in the pathogenesis of autoimmune pancreatitis: potential role of Helicobacter pylori infection via molecular mimicry. Gastroenterology 2007;133(1):368–9.

34. Vlug A, Nieuwenhuys EJ, van Eijk RV, et al. Nephelometric measurements of human IgG subclasses and their reference ranges. Ann Biol Clin [Paris] 1994;52(7–8):561–7.

35. van der Zee JS, van Swieten P, Aalberse RC. Inhibition of complement activation by IgG4 antibodies. Clin Exp Immunol 1986;64(2):415–22.

36. Aalberse RC, Van Milligen F, Tan KY, et al. Allergen-specific IgG4 in atopic disease. Allergy 1993;48(8):559–69.

37. Hussain R, Poindexter RW, Ottesen EA. Control of allergic reactivity in human filariasis. Predominant localization of blocking antibody to the IgG4 subclass. J Immunol 1992;148(9):2731–7.

38. Shirakata Y, Shiraishi S, Sayama K, et al. Subclass characteristics of IgG autoantibodies in bullous pemphigoid and pemphigus. J Dermatol 1990;17(11):661–6.

39. Ljungstrom I, Hammarstrom L, Kociecka W, et al. The sequential appearance of IgG subclasses and IgE during the course of Trichinella spiralis infection. Clin Exp Immunol 1988;74(2):230–5.

40. Ghazale A, Chari ST, Smyrk TC, et al. Value of serum IgG4 in the diagnosis of autoimmune pancreatitis and in distinguishing it from pancreatic cancer. Am J Gastroenterol 2007;102(8):1646–53.

41. Ghazale A, Chari ST, Zhang L, et al. Immunoglobulin G4-associated cholangitis: clinical profile and response to therapy. Gastroenterology 2008;134(3):706–15.

42. Raina A, Yadav D, Krasinskas AM, et al. Evaluation and management of autoimmune pancreatitis: experience at a large US center. Am J Gastroenterol 2009;104(9):2295–306.

43. Zhang L, Notohara K, Levy MJ, et al. IgG4-positive plasma cell infiltration in the diagnosis of autoimmune pancreatitis. Mod Pathol 2007;20(1):23–8.

44. Smith CD, Behrns KE, van Heerden JA, et al. Radical pancreatoduodenectomy for misdiagnosed pancreatic mass. Br J Surg 1994;81(4):585–9.

45. Nishimori I, Tamakoshi A, Otsuki M. Prevalence of autoimmune pancreatitis in Japan from a nationwide survey in 2002. J Gastroenterol 2007;42(Suppl 18):6–8.

46. Sah RP, Pannala R, Chari ST, et al. Prevalence, diagnosis, and profile of autoimmune pancreatitis presenting with features of acute or chronic pancreatitis. Clin Gastroenterol Hepatol 2010;8(1):91–6.

47. Kamisawa T, Shimosegawa T, Okazaki K, et al. Standard steroid treatment for autoimmune pancreatitis. Gut 2009;58(11):1504–7.

48. Nishimori I, Tamakoshi A, Kawa S, et al. Influence of steroid therapy on the course of diabetes mellitus in patients with autoimmune pancreatitis: findings from a nationwide survey in Japan. Pancreas 2006;32(3):244–8.

49. Kamisawa T, Yoshiike M, Egawa N, et al. Treating patients with autoimmune pancreatitis: results from a long-term follow-up study. Pancreatology 2005;5(2–3):234–8; discussion 8–40.

50. Chari ST, Takahashi N, Levy MJ, et al. A diagnostic strategy to distinguish autoimmune pancreatitis from pancreatic cancer. Clin Gastroenterol Hepatol 2009;7(10): 1097–103.
51. Irie H, Honda H, Baba S, et al. Autoimmune pancreatitis: CT and MR characteristics. AJR Am J Roentgenol 1998;170(5):1323–7.
52. Kamisawa T, Imai M, Yui Chen P, et al. Strategy for differentiating autoimmune pancreatitis from pancreatic cancer. Pancreas 2008;37(3):e62–7.
53. Sugumar A, Chari ST. Distinguishing pancreatic cancer from autoimmune pancreatitis: a comparison of two strategies. Clin Gastroenterol Hepatol 2009;7(11 Suppl): S59–62.
54. Mikami K, Itoh H. MR imaging of multifocal autoimmune pancreatitis in the pancreatic head and tail: a case report. Magn Reson Med Sci 2002;1(1):54–8.
55. Ito K, Koike S, Matsunaga N. MR imaging of pancreatic diseases. Eur J Radiol 2001;38(2):78–93.
56. Kamisawa T, Chen PY, Tu Y, et al. MRCP and MRI findings in 9 patients with autoimmune pancreatitis. World J Gastroenterol 2006;12(18):2919–22.
57. Kubota K, Kato S, Akiyama T, et al. A proposal for differentiation between early- and advanced-stage autoimmune pancreatitis by endoscopic ultrasonography. Dig Endosc 2009;21(3):162–9.
58. Hoki N, Mizuno N, Sawaki A, et al. Diagnosis of autoimmune pancreatitis using endoscopic ultrasonography. J Gastroenterol 2009;44(2):154–9.
59. Mizuno N, Bhatia V, Hosoda W, et al. Histological diagnosis of autoimmune pancreatitis using EUS-guided trucut biopsy: a comparison study with EUS-FNA. J Gastroenterol 2009;44(7):742–50.
60. Levy MJ, Smyrk TC, Takahashi N, et al. Idiopathic duct-centric pancreatitis: disease description and endoscopic ultrasonography-guided trucut biopsy diagnosis. Pancreatology 2011;11(1):76–80.
61. Dietrich CF, Hirche TO, Ott M, et al. Real-time tissue elastography in the diagnosis of autoimmune pancreatitis. Endoscopy 2009;41(8):718–20.
62. Itokawa F, Itoi T, Sofuni A, et al. EUS elastography combined with the strain ratio of tissue elasticity for diagnosis of solid pancreatic masses. J Gastroenterol 2011;46(6): 843–53.
63. Kamisawa T, Takum K, Anjiki H, et al. FDG-PET/CT findings of autoimmune pancreatitis. Hepatogastroenterology 2010;57(99–100):447–50.
64. Sugumar A, Levy MJ, Kamisawa T, et al. Endoscopic retrograde pancreatography criteria to diagnose autoimmune pancreatitis: an international multicentre study. Gut 60(5):666–70.
65. Raina A, Krasinskas AM, Greer JB, et al. Serum immunoglobulin G fraction 4 levels in pancreatic cancer: elevations not associated with autoimmune pancreatitis. Arch Pathol Lab Med 2008;132(1):48–53.
66. Fukukura Y, Fujiyoshi F, Nakamura F, et al. Autoimmune pancreatitis associated with idiopathic retroperitoneal fibrosis. AJR Am J Roentgenol 2003;181(4):993–5.
67. Eerens I, Vanbeckevoort D, Vansteenbergen W, et al. Autoimmune pancreatitis associated with primary sclerosing cholangitis: MR imaging findings. Eur Radiol 2001;11(8):1401–4.
68. Kamisawa T, Nakajima H, Egawa N, et al. Autoimmune pancreatitis can be confirmed with gastroscopy. Dig Dis Sci 2004;49(1):155–6.
69. Kamisawa T, Okamoto A. Autoimmune pancreatitis: proposal of IgG4-related sclerosing disease. J Gastroenterol 2006;41(7):613–25.
70. Kamisawa T, Tu Y, Egawa N, et al. A new diagnostic endoscopic tool for autoimmune pancreatitis. Gastrointest Endosc 2008;68(2):358–61.

71. Leise MD, Smyrk TC, Takahashi N, et al. IgG4-associated cholecystitis: another clue in the diagnosis of autoimmune pancreatitis. Dig Dis Sci 2011;56(5):1290–4.
72. Chari S, Murray JA. Autoimmune pancreatitis Part II: The relapse. Gastroenterology 2008.
73. Society MotCCfAPotJP. Diagnostic criteria for autoimmune pancreatitis by the Japan Pancreas Society. J Jpn Pancreas [Suizou] 2002;17:587.
74. Okazaki K, Kawa S, Kamisawa T, et al. Clinical diagnostic criteria of autoimmune pancreatitis: revised proposal. J Gastroenterol 2006;41(7):626–31.
75. Choi EK, Kim MH, Lee TY, et al. The sensitivity and specificity of serum immunoglobulin G and immunoglobulin G4 levels in the diagnosis of autoimmune chronic pancreatitis: Korean experience. Pancreas 2007;35(2):156–61.
76. Otsuki M, Chung JB, Okazaki K, et al. Asian diagnostic criteria for autoimmune pancreatitis: consensus of the Japan-Korea Symposium on Autoimmune Pancreatitis. J Gastroenterol 2008;43(6):403–8.
77. Gardner TB, Chari ST. Autoimmune pancreatitis. Gastroenterol Clin North Am 2008; 37(2):439–60, vii.
78. Ghazale A, Chari ST. Optimising corticosteroid treatment for autoimmune pancreatitis. Gut 2007;56(12):1650–2.
79. Sandanayake NS, Church NI, Chapman MH, et al. Presentation and management of post-treatment relapse in autoimmune pancreatitis/immunoglobulin G4-associated cholangitis. Clin Gastroenterol Hepatol 2009;7(10):1089–96.
80. Topazian M, Witzig TE, Smyrk TC, et al. Rituximab therapy for refractory biliary strictures in immunoglobulin G4-associated cholangitis. Clin Gastroenterol Hepatol 2008;6(3):364–6.

The Role of Endoscopic Retrograde Cholangiopancreatography in Patients with Pancreatic Disease

James Buxbaum, MD

KEYWORDS

- Endoscopic retrograde cholangiopancreatography
- Congenital abnormalities • Gallstones • Fistula

Since its introduction, endoscopic retrograde cholangiopancreatography (ERCP) has been an important tool for the confirmation and treatment of acute and chronic pancreatic disease. However, compared with other endoscopic procedures, ERCP carries the highest risk of complications, particularly pancreatitis, which may be fatal. As newer and less-invasive techniques have been introduced, it has evolved into a primarily therapeutic procedure and plays a core role in the management of biliary pancreatitis, idiopathic pancreatitis, chronic pancreatitis, and pancreatic duct leaks. These applications, as well as the important topic of post-ERCP pancreatitis, are explored in this article.

GALLSTONE PANCREATITIS

Biliary stones, along with excess alcohol consumption, account for more than 80% of cases of acute pancreatitis. Biliary pancreatitis is an absolute indication for chole-cystectomy, and clearance of persistent bile duct stones either by ERCP or surgery is requisite.[1] Stool analysis from patients with gallstone pancreatitis has led some investigators to propose that small stones that pass spontaneously are to blame for biliary pancreatitis.[2] Other researchers have proposed that obstructing distal bile duct stones may promote the evolution of interstitial pancreatitis to more serious necrotic forms.[3] The role of ERCP in the management of biliary pancreatitis has been the

The author has nothing to disclose.
Los Angeles County Hospital, Division of Gastroenterology and Liver Diseases, The University of Southern California, Keck School of Medicine, 2001 Zonal Avenue HMR 1201, Los Angeles, CA 90033, USA
E-mail address: jbuxbaum@usc.edu

Gastroenterol Clin N Am 41 (2012) 23–45
doi:10.1016/j.gtc.2011.12.010
0889-8553/12/$ – see front matter © 2012 Elsevier Inc. All rights reserved.

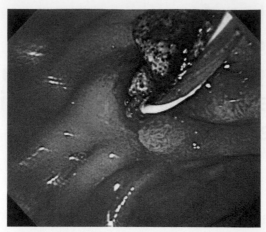

Fig. 1. Biliary sphinterotomy yields multiple stones in a patient with acute gallstone pancreatitis presenting with deep jaundice.

subject of several landmark trials. These publications suggest that early ERCP is primarily beneficial in patients with cholangitis or biliary obstruction (**Fig. 1**).

Neoptolemos and coworkers[4] randomly assigned 121 patients with gallstone pancreatitis to early ERCP, within 3 days of admission, versus conservative therapy. Patients with jaundice and cholangitis were enrolled in the study. After day 5, those in the conservative arm could undergo ERCP if needed. The researchers reported that fewer complications were seen in the early intervention group; although these findings were primarily found in patients with more severe disease.[4] In another study, Fan and colleagues[3] randomly assigned 195 patients with severe pancreatitis to emergency ERCP within 24 hours or to conservative therapy. Although the study was not limited to gallstone pancreatitis, the authors indicate that biliary pancreatitis was the prevalent form in their Hong Kong population. In the conservatively treated group, ERCP was performed for clinical deterioration. Although there was no significant difference in local or systemic complications of pancreatitis among the groups, no biliary sepsis developed in those treated with emergency ERCP, whereas 9% of those treated conservatively had sepsis. Additionally, the morality rate was somewhat lower in the early ERCP group, 5%, compared with 9% in the conservatively treated group.

The relationship between pancreatitis, cholangitis, and early ERCP was further explored by Folsch and colleagues[5] in a larger series of 238 patients. In this group, enrollment was restricted to patients with gallstone pancreatitis suggested by abnormal imaging or abnormal liver tests. Patients with biliary obstruction or cholangitis with a bilirubin level greater than or equal to 5mg/dL, fever, or persistent biliary pain were excluded. Urgent ERCP was performed in the intervention group within 3 days of admission. In the conservative group, ERCP was performed within the first 3 weeks for clinical deterioration, as defined by fever, an increase in bilirubin level of 3mg/dL, or persistent biliary pain. However, when a trend toward greater mortality was seen, the study was halted by the institutional review board. Fourteen patients in the treatment group died (10 from severe pancreatitis), compared with 7 deaths in the conservative treatment group (4 from severe pancreatitis). Although no overall difference was seen in complications between the groups, more serious complications were seen in the early ERCP group, including respiratory failure.

The explanation for the increased number of cases of severe pancreatitis and mortality in the early ERCP group in the study by Folsch and colleagues[5] is unclear. Worsening pancreatitis caused by ERCP was not measured but may have been a contributing factor. Fan and coworkers[3] noted increased amylase level, compared with amylase level at the time of admission, in 8% of those who underwent urgent ERCP, but in the setting of pancreatitis, interpretation of this information is not simple. The findings by Folsch and colleagues[3] run parallel to findings that both open and laparoscopic cholecystectomy, performed in the setting of moderately severe pancreatitis, are associated with more complications.[6,7]

IDIOPATHIC PANCREATITIS

Although most cases of acute pancreatitis result from gallstones and alcohol consumption, the origin in 10% to 30% of the cases remains unknown after a comprehensive noninvasive workup.[8]

During the last 2 decades, the optimization of minimally invasive imaging techniques, including magnetic resonance cholangiopancreatography, the advent of endoscopic ultrasound (EUS), and the universality of laparoscopic cholecystectomy have limited the role of ERCP to cases in which therapeutic intervention is needed. The biliary endoscopist has the responsibility to confirm that a comprehensive workup has been completed, including the appropriate history and noninvasive testing, as well as the consideration of EUS. ERCP may then be used appropriately to investigate and treat sources of pancreatitis that may be amenable to endoscopic therapy, including microlithiasis, sphincter of Oddi dysfunction (SOD), pancreas divisum, and other congenital abnormalities.

Initial Evaluation and Endoscopic Ultrasound

Before embarking on a course of interventional endoscopic evaluation, it is imperative to perform a detailed history to assess for alcohol consumption, previous surgery, trauma, toxins, and medications, as well as acquiring a family and past medical history.[9] Extensive family history of pancreatitis warrants testing for hereditary pancreatitis-associated mutations in the cationic trypsinogen, serine protease inhibitor Kazal type 1, and cystic fibrosis genes. In patients with a history of collagen vascular disease, autoimmune pancreatitis should be considered, and testing should include gamma globulin, ANA, and immunoglobulin-4 levels.[10] All patients should undergo transcutaneous sonography to assess for gallstones as well as assesment of calcium, lipid, and liver function. Fluctuating liver test levels, even in the absence of abnormal gallbladder imaging, warrant consideration of an empiric cholecystectomy.[11] A spiral computed tomography scan or magnetic resonance imaging of the pancreas is a consideration in older patients or if there is an increased risk of malignancy.[12]

Given the significant risk of procedure-induced pancreatitis, ERCP is not frequently recommended after a single episode of unexplained pancreatitis. EUS has a significant yield in the setting of both primary and recurrent idiopathic pancreatitis, with a diagnosis achieved in 51% to 92% of cases.[9,13–15] Studies suggest that, in patients who have not undergone a cholecystectomy, the most common etiologies are biliary stones or sludge.[9,13–15] Among those who have undergone gallbladder resection, the leading etiology is pancreas divisum.[9] Studies vary in their inclusion of chronic pancreatitis; however, it is a leading origin in patients both before and after cholecystectomy when included.[9,16] Using the yield of endoscopic sphincterotomy as a gold standard, Chak and colleagues reported that EUS has a superior accuracy (97%) to transabdominal ultrasound (83%) and diagnostic ERCP (89%) in the evaluation of bile duct stones.[17] EUS has an excellent correlation with ERCP and secretin testing in those with moderate or severe chronic pancreatitis and is fairly accurate for the diagnosis of pancreas divisum.[18,19] In their series of patients with idiopathic pancreatitis, Tandon and Topazian report that a diagnosis was confirmed in 68% of patients over a course of 16 months. ERCP was required in the 29% of the cases, and the EUS-based diagnosis changed in 13%.[15] Their findings suggest that patients with idiopathic pancreatitis should undergo EUS before ERCP, given the high yield of the former and potential morbidity of the latter.[15]

Microlithiasis

Microlithiasis and biliary sludge may trigger pancreatitis by occluding the pancreatic duct at the level of the papilla. In a prospective series of patients with idiopathic pancreatitis who had not undergone cholecystectomy or aspiration of bile at time of ERCP or via a duodenal feeding tube, demonstrated biliary sludge as the origin of pancreatitis in more than two-thirds of patients.[8] Biliary sludge and microlithiasis may be diagnosed by microscopy or imaging, and if confirmed, they both merit cholecystectomy.

Biliary sludge is a suspension of cellular debris and biliary crystals.[8] Microscopic analysis of bile is the gold standard for diagnosis of biliary sludge. Bile aspirated from the gallbladder theoretically has the highest yield, followed by bile obtained from the bile duct, and finally, that obtained from the duodenum.[20] In a recent trial using bedside microscopy at the time of ERCP in patients with idiopathic pancreatitis who had not undergone cholecystectomy, bile crystals were found in 50% of patients and were thought to be the primary etiology in 22%.[21] Nonetheless, duodenal bile aspirate at the time of EUS or duodenoscopy has a significant yield, and these procedures are less likely to be associated with complications.[9]

Biliary sludge, as well as microlithiasis, may also be detected radiographically at the time of ERCP. Microlithiasis is defined as bile duct stones that are smaller than 3 mm.[22] In a prospective study of ERCP in patients with recurrent idiopathic pancreatitis and intact gallbladder, 27.5% were found have cholangiographic evidence of microlithiasis.[23] Another approach has been the introduction of 20-MHz intraductal ultrasound probes at the time of ERCP.[24] In a study of the role of this probe in 31 patients with unremarkable diagnostic ERCP findings and idiopathic pancreatitis, intraductal ultrasound scan found a potential etiology in 42%, with most of these having biliary microlithiasis or sludge.[24] However, EUS has been demonstrated to have a 95% sensitivity and high negative predictive value for small gallbladder stones and sludge undetectable by transabdominal ultrasound scan but was not performed in this cohort (**Fig. 2**).[22,25]

ERCP may be used to diagnose microlithiasis and biliary sludge, but its use should be reserved for situations in which other testing, including sphincter of Oddi manometry (SOM), is being concurrently performed. Otherwise, less-invasive modalities, such as EUS, should be used. In centers where bedside microscopy is available during ERCP, sphincterotomy is performed on confirmation of biliary crystals.[21] Demonstration of microlithiasis or biliary sludge is an indication for cholecystectomy. Some experts, however, recommend cholecystectomy in patients with idiopathic recurrent pancreatitis and no other detectable etiologies, even if microlithiasis cannot be confirmed.[20]

Sphincter of Oddi Dysfunction and Papillary Stenosis

Among those with idiopathic pancreatitis who have undergone cholecystectomy, SOD is the most frequent diagnosis made after a comprehensive evaluation including ERCP is completed.[16,21,23,26] However, only in the cohort reported by Coyle and colleagues[16] was EUS routinely performed. Consistent with the other series, SOD was

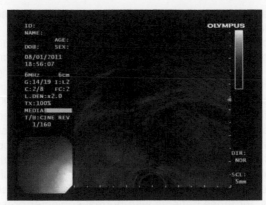

Fig. 2. EUS depicts layering gallbladder sludge in a patient with recurrent idiopathic pancreatitis.

the leading etiology confirmed in 31% of patients in this group.[16,21,23,26] It is proposed that dysfunction of the sphincter of Oddi may involve either a fibroinflammatory stenosis or a motility anomaly of the smooth muscle band that surrounds the distal common bile and pancreatic ducts as they pass through the ampulla of Vater.[27] SOD may be confirmed manometrically by measurement of the biliary sphincter, the pancreatic sphincter, or both. Similarly, treatment is sphincterotomy of either sphincter or both. The optimal evaluation and treatment strategies are the subject of several recent series.

SOD is clinically categorized as type 1 (definite) SOD in those with typical pancreaticobiliary pain, abnormal pancreatic or liver enzymes, or dilated or sluggishly emptying bile or pancreatic ducts. Patients with type 2 (probable) SOD have pain accompanied by either abnormal laboratory results or imaging, and type 3 (possible) have only pain. Papillary stenosis represents a subgroup of SOD thought to have a structural origin and is considered similar to SOD type 1 in studies of idiopathic pancreatitis.[21] By definition, those with symptomatic idiopathic pancreatitis have abnormal laboratory values and thus may have type 2 SOD if imaging shows normal ducts.

To confirm the diagnosis of SOD, measurements of the pressures in the distal bile or pancreatic ducts are taken with a manometry catheter. Studies have found that an increased basal pressure (>40 mm Hg) of the bile or pancreatic sphincters correlates best with clinical outcomes and is used to define SOD in most series.[28] Markers of biliary dyskinesia, including high-frequency contractions and preponderant retrograde contractions, are less reliable.[28] SOM has been found more likely to be abnormal in those with type 1 SOD (92.3%) than type 2 (58.2%) or type 3. Given the high correlation, manometry is generally deferred in those with type 1 SOD.[29] Additionally, studies have found nearly universal improvement in patients with type 1 SOD who undergo sphincterotomy, and negative manometry in this group may be misleading.[30]

To minimize intervention of the pancreatic duct, many endoscopists have historically measured only biliary pressures. Eversman and coworkers[30] reported that in a cohort of patients with idiopathic pancreatitis, 25.5% had only pancreatic sphincter abnormalities, 6.4% had only biliary sphincter abnormalities, and 40% had abnormalities of both.[30] It can be argued that if the first sphincter (pancreatic or biliary) exhibits normal manometry, it is then prudent to evaluate the remaining sphincter.

Given the invasive nature of ERCP with SOM, there have been a number of attempts to develop alternative modalities to assess for SOD.[27] Secretin causes temporary dilatation of the pancreatic duct; prolonged dilatation suggests an abnormal sphincter. Magnetic resonance cholangiopancreatography enhanced with secretin administration has been used to assess for SOD as the origin of idiopathic pancreatitis. Unfortunately, it was found to be insensitive, recognizing only 57.1% of patients who benefited from therapeutic ERCP, although it was 100% specific.[31]

Upon confirmation of SOD, endoscopic sphincterotomy is recommended. In 2 separate trials, patients with suspected SOD were randomly assigned to receive either a sphincterotomy or a sham sphincterotomy. All patients in both arms of each trial received ERCP and SOM. Pain levels were assessed at various points. In both series, patients with manometrically confirmed SOD benefited significantly more from the sphincterotomy compared with those receiving the sham procedure. Also, in both trials, for those patients with normal sphincter pressure, the results from sphincterotomy and sham procedures did not differ.[28,32] Nonetheless, patients with idiopathic pancreatitis were excluded from one of these trials, and both were primarily focused on those with suspected type 2 biliary SOD.[28,32] However, cohort studies suggest that at least 70% of those with idiopathic pancreatitis and confirmed SOD remained asymptomatic at a mean follow-up of at least 30 months after sphincterotomy.[21,26]

Studies suggest that treatment of both the pancreatic and biliary sphincters with dual sphincterotomy, may result in fewer recurrent symptoms and less reintervention for patients with elevated pancreatic sphincter pressure compared with the more historic approach of initiating treatment with a biliary sphincterotomy.[33] This concept also may apply to patients with idiopathic pancreatitis. Wehrmann and coworkers[34] recently reported that relapse occurred in only 29% of those who underwent dual sphincterotomy compared with 92% in those who initially underwent only a biliary or pancreatic sphincterotomy.

Pancreas Divisum and Other Structural Etiologies

Pancreas divisum is the most common congenital anomaly of the pancreas. Because of the failure of the dorsal and ventral pancreatic ducts to fuse during weeks 6 to 8 of gestation, it occurs in 5% to 10% of the population; however, less than 10% of those with pancreas divisum experience symptoms.[35] It is thought that recurrent pancreatitis is caused by increased intraductal pressure, which is caused by outlet obstruction at the level of the minor papilla. Minor papilla cannulation and ductal decompression may be technically challenging. Although decompression appears beneficial, particularly in those with recurrent pancreatitis, long-term treatment strategies are unclear. Additionally, a number of unusual congenital anomalies of the pancreas also present with recurrent pancreatitis and may be amenable to endoscopic therapy.

The primary aim of endoscopic treatment of pancreas divisum is decompression. Highly tapered and needle-tipped catheters often are used for pancreatic duct access, which is frequently difficult. Secretin may be administered to increase flow of bicarbonate as well as widen the pancreatic duct orifice to enhance its visibility.[36] In a double-blind trial, patients with difficult minor papilla cannulation were randomly assigned to receive either secretin or placebo during 2 discrete phases of the procedure.[37] Cannulation was achieved during the placebo phase in 8% versus 81% during the secretin phase. Methylene blue also can be used as a contrast agent to enhance visualization by spraying the minor papilla and by injecting the substance into the major papilla.[38]

Upon cannulation, endoscopic therapy, including papillotomy, stent placement, and balloon dilatation, may be performed (**Fig. 3**). Minor papillotomy may be

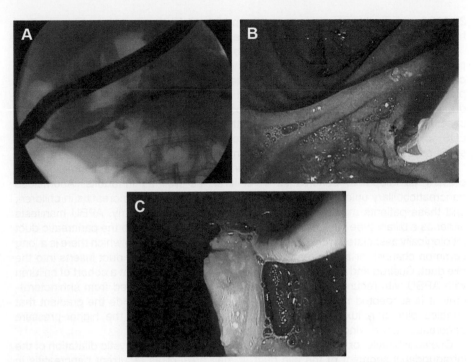

Fig. 3. Pancreas divisum therapy: Minor papilla cannulation and opacification shows pancreas divisum (*A*) in a patient with idiopathic recurrent pancreatitis. After minor papillotomy (*B*) balloon sweeps yield waxy debris (*C*). (*Courtesy of* Isaac Raijman, MD, Houston, TX.)

accomplished using a needle knife over a previously placed stent or by performing a pull-type sphincterotomy, with comparable success and complications.[39] Heyries and colleagues[40] treated 16 patients who had recurrent acute pancreatitis and pancreas divisum with stenting (most after papillotomy or papillectomy) for 8 months versus minor papillotomy alone in the remaining 8 patients. The results of this small series suggest that symptomatic recurrence occurred earlier in patients without stents. Another approach has been the placement of stents after balloon dilatation of the minor papilla without papillotomy.[41]

The most robust data regarding the efficacy of endotherapy for pancreas divisum are from the trial of Lans and coworkers.[42] Nineteen patients who had at least 2 episodes of documented pancreatitis in the previous 12 months were randomly assigned to receive either ERCP with placement of pancreatic stent through the minor papilla and stent exchange every 4 months for 1 year or clinical follow-up every 4 months but without therapy for 1 year. Among the 10 patients in the stent group, there were significantly fewer episodes of pancreatitis (1 episode) compared with 7 episodes among the 9 patients randomly assigned to clinical follow-up. In the studies by Heyries and coworkers[40] and Ertan and colleagues,[41] patients had significantly fewer episodes of pancreatitis in the 2 to 3 years after the course of treatment than the period before endoscopic therapy. Although endoscopic therapy has been performed in patients with chronic pancreatitis and abdominal pain, those with acute recurrent pancreatitis appear to have the greatest benefit. Lehman and colleagues[43] reported that at a mean follow-up of 1.7 years after minor papillotomy, the symptoms on patients with acute recurrent pancreatitis were markedly improved in 76.5% versus

27.3% for those with chronic pancreatitis and 26.1% for those with chronic pain. This has been corroborated by additional studies.[44]

Although stent placement may decrease the number of episodes of pancreatitis, particularly for patients with recurrent pancreatitis, it may result in adverse ductal changes. Kozarek and coworkers[45] reported that 36% of those who underwent stent placement for pancreas divisum, SOD, and other indications had de novo pancreatic ductal changes that resembled chronic pancreatitis that did not resolve in some cases. Sherman and colleagues[46] found that parenchymal changes were seen by EUS corresponding to ductal changes after pancreas stent placement and that, in some cases, these changes were persistent.

In addition to pancreas divisum, a number of rare congenital anomalies may present as idiopathic pancreatitis in children as well as in adults. Anomalous pancreaticobiliary union (APBU) is associated with recurrent pancreatitis in children, and these patients may benefit from ERCP with sphincterotomy. APBU manifests either as a biliary type in which the common bile duct inserts into the pancreatic duct (etiologically associated with choledochal cysts), a long-Y type in which there is a long common channel, or a pancreatic type in which the pancreatic duct inserts into the bile duct. Guelrud and colleagues[47] showed in a recent series that a cohort of children with APBU with recurrent pancreatitis all had SOD and benefited from sphincterotomy. It is suspected that the sphincter hypertension may provide the gradient that enables bile to reflux from the low-pressure bile duct into the higher-pressure pancreatic duct driving recurrent pancreatitis.[47]

Choledochocele, or type 3 choledochal cyst, manifests as a cystic dilatation of the intraduodenal segment of the bile duct. It may present as recurrent pancreatitis in adults and may be addressed with endoscopic sphincterotomy.[21] Annular pancreas is a very rare anomaly found in 1 of 20,000 individuals and is caused by faulty rotation of the ventral pancreas. It is associated with pancreas divisum in 30% of cases and most commonly presents with recurrent pancreatitis, although it may also present with bowel obstruction.[48] EUS results show an echogenic ring identical to the pancreatic parenchyma surrounding the duodenum, and ERCP findings often show a looping pancreas duct branch crossing the duodenum.[49] ERCP with pancreatic sphincterotomy may help patients with recurrent pancreatitis, whereas those with bowel obstruction will typically require surgery.[50]

Another anatomic cause of acute recurrent pancreatitis is cystic duct insertion at the papilla (Fig. 4). It is thought that greater reflux of bile into the pancreatic duct is a consequence of this anatomy, and the treatment is cholecystectomy.[51] It has been proposed that juxtapapillary diverticuli may predispose to recurrent pancreatitis. However, a matched-pair analysis of 350 cases found that although the diverticuli were correlated with bile duct stones, they were not correlated with acute or chronic pancreatitis.[52] Chronic pancreatitis with ductal strictures may also cause intermittent recurrent pancreatitis and is the topic of the next section.

CHRONIC PANCREATITIS

Chronic pancreatitis causes persistent abdominal pain as well as exocrine and endocrine dysfunction. Interventional endoscopic and surgical therapy may improve pain control but do not appear to enhance glandular function. It is hypothesized that strictures and stones lead to ductal hypertension and painful distension. Elevation in neurotransmitters caused by inflammation as well as sensitization of receptors due to perineural fibrosis may also contribute to pain.[53,54] Treatment with pancreatic enzymes is ineffective compared with placebo in the management of pain.[55] Evidence suggests that endoscopic therapy, which aims to decompress the main pancreatic

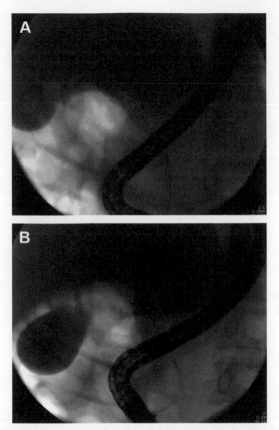

Fig. 4. Cystic duct insertion to the papilla. In a patient with recurrent pancreatitis, cannulation and opacification initially fill only the cystic duct and gallbladder (*A*), cannulation and injection at a slightly different region of the papilla fill the biliary tree (*B*).

duct, is relatively effective, although recent randomized work suggests that it may be inferior to surgery, particularly in severe cases. Nonetheless, contemporary techniques including multiple stent placement, extracorporeal shock wave lithotripsy (ESWL), and self-expandable metal stents (SEMS) may increase the efficacy of endoscopic therapy, which remains a tenable option, particularly for those concerned about the invasive nature of pancreatic surgery.

Well-established endoscopic therapy for chronic pancreatitis includes pancreatic sphincterotomy, balloon dilatation of strictures, stone removal, and long-term stent placement (**Fig. 5**). Several uncontrolled studies over the last 2 decades have reported long-term improvement in chronic pain in 67% to 85% of patients with chronic pancreatitis after treatment with these techniques.[56–58] However, the definition of success is variable, individual studies were small, and follow-up was incomplete. In the largest study of endoscopic therapy, Rosch and colleagues[59] present the prospective follow-up data of 1018 retrospectively identified patients. The prerequisite for endoscopic therapy was a dilated main pancreatic duct caused by an obstructing stone or stricture. Rosch and colleagues[59] found a significant overall improvement, which was defined as no pain or only mild symptoms in 85% of patients. Nonetheless, 238 patients eventually required surgery; thus, the final

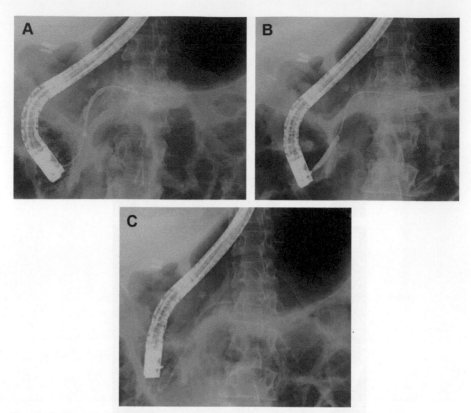

Fig. 5. Endoscopic treatment of symptomatic chronic pancreatitis. ERCP findings show chronic pancreatitis with distal stricture (*A*). After endoscopic sphincterotomy, a balloon dilatation is performed to improve drainage (*B*) and a pancreas stent is placed (*C*).

success rate was reported as 65%. Additionally, the impact of endoscopic management was not compared with either a surgically or medically managed group with chronic pancreatitis.

In the first published randomized study of endoscopic versus surgical therapy, Dite and coworkers[53] compared 36 patients treated with endoscopic therapy with 36 patients treated surgically. Both strategies initially appeared successful with 90% reporting complete or partial pain relief; however, at 5 years, only 61.4% of patients treated endoscopically, compared to 85.9% of those treated surgically, reported complete or partial relief.[53] However, the study was criticized because ESWL was not included in the treatment protocol, and those in whom recurrent symptoms developed after the initial treatment period did not undergo subsequent endoscopic therapy. The surgical treatment also primarily involved pancreatic resection, which may not be comparable to endoscopic decompression.

These clinically important concerns were addressed in a more recent randomized trial. Cahen and coworkers[60] randomly assigned 19 patients to endoscopic treatment and 20 to surgical decompression (18 underwent pancreaticojejunostomy). Endoscopic therapy involved the confirmation of a high-grade stenosis followed by balloon dilatation and stent placement. ESWL was performed if the stones were greater than 7 mm. The Izbicki pain score, which has been validated for chronic pancreatitis, was sequentially measured. At 2 years, complete or partial pain relief was achieved in 32% of the endoscopically treated patients, compared with 75% of those who underwent surgical drainage procedures. The Izbicki pain scores were also significantly better in the surgical group (25 ± 15) than in the endoscopically treated group (51 ± 23). Follow-up data of the cohort 6 years later shows that 67% of patients treated endoscopically eventually needed additional drainage versus 5% in the surgical group.[61] Additionally, 47% of those in the endoscopic group eventually underwent surgical drainage and overall required more procedures. Although there was a trend toward better Izbicki pain scores in the surgical group, (22 ± 31) versus (39 ± 28) in the endoscopy group, it was no longer significant, and there was no difference in quality-of-life scores.

While the Cahen study suggests that surgical therapy is more effective, there are several caveats. Technical success in stricture resolution in the endoscopic treatment arm was only 50%, which is much lower than what has been reported previously. Nearly all of the endoscopically treated patients had significant stone disease, and clearance was achieved in only 89% of patients. Thus, the endoscopic group represents severe chronic pancreatitis, unlike what has been represented in the previous studies. A reasonable conclusion is that patients with severe disease should go to surgery, and patients with mild to moderate pancreatic duct strictures and pain without extensive concretions may be eligible for endoscopy. Another consideration is that there was 1 major, albeit routine, surgical complication and 1 very unusual endoscopic complication. The small sample size might not allow a good comparison of the typical complications of these modalities.

Several recent technologic improvements may improve nonsurgical options. More powerful extracorporeal shock wave lithotripters have improved treatment of pancreatic stone disease. Kozarek and coworkers[62] reported that in a group of 40 patients with chronic calcific pancreatitis, stone obliteration was achieved by a single session in 88% of the group. Long-term follow up after combined ESWL and endotherapy show significant pain improvement, as well as reduction in pancreatic ductal diameter.[63] Interestingly, the results of a randomized trial show that for patients with calcifications obstructing the main pancreatic duct, the use of modern lithotripsy alone is comparable to ESWL combined with endoscopic therapy with regard to pain relief and ductal decompression.[54] However, among those in the ESWL group who relapsed, 80% required ERCP. Cholangioscopy-guided laser lithotripsy is another emerging therapy that may particularly benefit those patients who have stones that are not radiopaque and thus are not amenable to radiographically guided ESWL (**Figs. 6** and **7**).

To address refractory pancreatic duct strictures, investigators have also adopted the multistent strategy, which has proven efficacious for benign biliary strictures. Costamagna and coworkers[64] selected 19 patients with severe chronic pancreatitis who had unsuccessful treatment with placement of a single stent. They first dilated the stricture and then placed a maximal number of large diameter (8.5 to 11.5 French [F]) stents over a period of 7 months. Technical success was achieved in 95%. Three patients (16%) subsequently had recurrent strictures, but 2 were successfully retreated. In their randomized trial, Cahen and colleagues[60] utilized multiple stents in a minority of patients, but maximal therapy was not used as an initial approach to pancreatic duct strictures.

Another alternative strategy to manage pancreatic strictures has been the placement of self-expandable metal stents. Moon and colleagues[65] placed covered SEMS in 32 patients with recurrent pancreatic duct strictures, and pain relief, stricture resolution, and successful removal were achieved in 100%, although no long-term

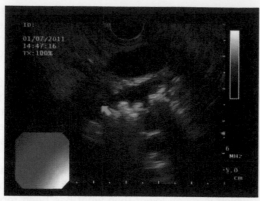

Fig. 6. Shadowing stones in the main pancreatic duct seen at EUS. ESWL was attempted but the stones were radiolucent, thus, radiographic visualization and lithotripsy were unsuccessful.

follow-up is yet available.[65] Sauer and coworkers[66] placed covered SEMS in 6 patients who did not respond to conventional stenting methods; however, 3 had recurrence. A potential problem with covered stents is that de novo proximal pancreatic strictures appear to develop in a minority of patients.[65] Another approach has been to perform sphincterotomy followed by serial balloon dilatation without stenting.[67] Theoretically, this may permit better drainage from side branches and prevent stent-associated stricture development.

PANCREATIC DUCT LEAKS

Pancreatic duct leaks occur most frequently in the setting of severe acute pancreatitis and chronic pancreatis.[68] They may also complicate pancreatic surgery, trauma, or malignancy **(Fig 8)**.[69] Conservative measures include treatment with pancreatic enzymes and somatostatin, along with limited oral intake. However, intervention is frequently necessary, with endoscopic therapy being a primary consideration. Success is most likely if a stent can be used to bridge the leak. Patients with complete duct disruption are unlikely to respond to endoscopic therapy and merit a multidisciplinary approach.

There are several important indications for ERCP in the setting of pancreatic duct leaks, including persistent pancreatic fistulas and ascites, symptomatic pseudocysts, and potentially unremitting severe pancreatitis. Costamagna and colleagues[70] report a series of 16 postsurgical patients who were unsuccessful with prolonged conservative therapy for pancreaticocutaneous fistula. ERCP with pancreatic duct decompression and prompt resolution was achieved in 69% with no recurrences at 2 years' follow-up. Comparably, Brachner and colleagues[71] reported a series of 8 patients with persistent high amylase ascites. ERCP with pancreatic stent placement led to resolution of ascites in 88% within 6 weeks. Additionally, among patients with symptomatic pancreatic pseudocyst requiring transmural ERCP drainage, greater treatment success was found in patients treated with the placement of a stent to bridge the pancreatic duct leak compared with patients not receiving the stent.[72]

Another possible role of ERCP is to evaluate for a pancreatic duct leak in patients with severe pancreatitis who did not respond to conservative therapy, particularly in the setting of an in-hospital exacerbation.[11] Lau and colleagues[73] describe a large

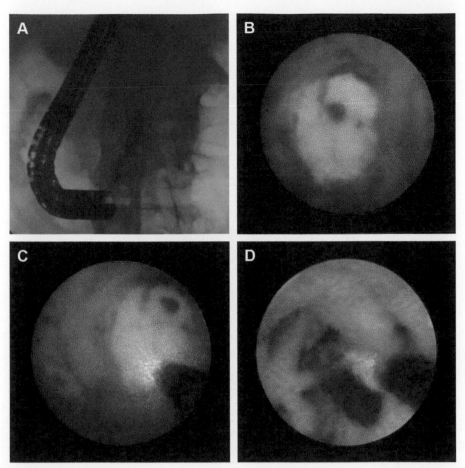

Fig. 7. Laser treatment of obstructed pancreatic duct. Cannulation of the pancreatic duct of a patient with persistent pain caused by chronic pancreatitis and pancreatic duct stones on EUS shows a cutoff of the pancreatogram (*A*). After endoscopic pancreatic sphincterotomy, a cholangioscope visualizes a concretion completely obstructing the duct (*B*). Using a holmium laser advanced through the choledochoscope (*C*), the obstructing stone is pulverized (*D*) and drainage improves. (*Courtesy of* Isaac Raijman, MD, Houston, TX.)

series of patients with severe necrotizing pancreatitis in whom leaks were identified in 37%. While those with leaks exhibited a 3.4-fold incidence of necrosis and 2.6-fold increase in prolonged hospitalization, they did not have increased mortality. ERCP was not associated with increased complications and potentially enabled key endoscopic, percutaneous, and surgical interventions in these patients. More prospective work is required to measure the role of ERCP in these patients before its use in this setting may be fully appraised.

Several technical factors have been identified that predict successful stenting of pancreatic duct extravasation. Telford and coworkers[74] analyzed 43 cases of pancreatic duct leak managed by ERCP and found that passage of a "bridging" stent that crossed the site of extravasation was associated with greater success than stents that merely crossed the papilla or were located in the region of the leak. A larger series

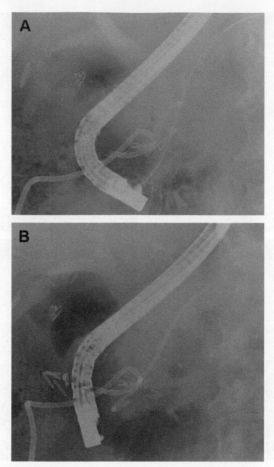

Fig. 8. Pancreatic duct leak. In a postoperative patient with persistent leakage from drain after pancreatic duct surgery, ERCP findings show a pancreatic duct leak (*A*). After bridging stent placement (*B*), the leakage ceased and the surgical drain was removed.

confirmed these findings and further demonstrated that pancreatic ducts with a partial disruption are more likely to respond to stenting than those with a complete disruption, largely because bridging stents could not be reliably placed in the latter group.[69] These studies suggest that, unlike the treatment of bile duct leaks, crossing the sphincter alone to lower intraductal pressure is not adequate to control pancreatic duct extravasation.

Patients with complete pancreatic duct disruption are at high risk of development of the disconnected duct syndrome, in which viable pancreatic tissue proximal to the disruption leaks digestive enzymes into surrounding tissue, causing necrosis, persistent fluid collections, and pseudocysts. Lawrence and coworkers[75] report a series of 29 patients who underwent endoscopic therapy for main pancreatic duct disruption complicated by pseudocysts. While success was initially achieved in 22 patients, within 37 months the majority had recurrent disease. Eventually, 63% required pancreatic surgery, 53% became diabetic mellitus, and 50% had left-sided portal hypertension. Endoscopic drainage may be a reasonable temporizing measure, but complete long-term response is seen in the minority of patients, and these patients benefit from comanagement with a pancreatic surgeon.[75]

Recently, several new endoscopic techniques to address pancreatic duct leaks have been proposed. Baron and colleagues[76] recently reported patients with a refractory leak from a pancreaticojejunostomy successfully treated with a covered SEMS. The authors suggest that, in the future, smaller covered SEMS with lateral fenestrations to allow for side branch drainage will be a consideration. Luthen and coworkers[77] recently reported a patient with a persistent pancreatic duct leak that did not respond to endoscopic therapy. ERCP was used to successfully place a coil designed for intravascular use, suggesting a future role for occlusive devices in this setting.

POST-ERCP PANCREATITIS

Although ERCP is a powerful tool to treat patients with gallstones, idiopathic pancreatitis, chronic pancreatitis, and pancreatic duct leaks, it is complicated by post-ERCP pancreatitis in up to 30% of cases, and severe pancreatitis occurs in approximately 1%.[78] Post-ERCP pancreatitis is diagnosed if 2 of 3 criterion are fulfilled: epigastric pain, amylase or lipase elevated to greater than 3 times the upper limit of normal, or cross-sectional imaging consistent with pancreatic inflammation (**Fig. 9**). It is categorized as mild if it is associated with a 2- to 3-day hospitalization, moderate if it requires 4 to 10 days of inpatient management, and severe if it results in a hospitalization of more than 10 days or if it requires a surgical or percutaneous procedure to drain a pseudocyst or phlegmon.[79] The biliary endoscopist must be cognizant of the risk factors associated with post-ERCP pancreatitis development, potential pharmacologic prevention options, as well as the endoscopic techniques that may be used to minimize the risk of the development and severity of post-ERCP pancreatitis.

Several investigators have identified risk factor associated with post-ERCP pancreatitis. Freeman and colleagues[80] analyzed 1463 consecutive ERCP and reported a 6.7% risk of pancreatitis. The strongest multivariate risk factors were previous ERCP-induced pancreatitis (odds Ratio [OR] = 5.4), biliary sphincter balloon dilatation (OR = 4.5), difficult cannulation (OR = 3.4), and pancreatic sphincterotomy (OR = 3.1). The reported risk of balloon dilatation of the sphincter was further demonstrated

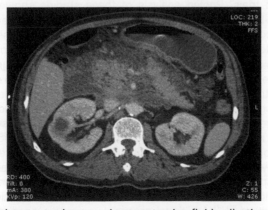

Fig. 9. A computed tomography scan shows extensive fluid collections in the setting of post-ERCP pancreatitis. The patient required necrosectomy.

by a randomized study of 117 cases in which balloon dilatation for the extraction of stones resulted in pancreatitis in 15.4% of cases compared with 0.8% of those treated with sphincterotomy.[81] Two of the cases in the balloon dilatation group were fatal.[81] Additional risk factors reported by Freeman and colleagues[80] included multiple injections of the pancreatic duct (OR = 2.7), suspected SOD (OR = 2.6), female sex (OR = 2.5), absence of chronic pancreatitis (OR = 1.9), and a normal bilirubin level (OR = 1.9). Additionally, the risk factors appeared to be cumulative. Patients with suspected SOD, difficult cannulation, and normal ducts had a risk of approximately 40%. Freeman and coworkers[80] emphasize that given the high risk associated with ERCP in patients with suspected SOD and otherwise normal findings, performing manometry does not add additional risk to the ERCP. Further, it is erroneous to assume that risk is minimized by not performing manometry when performing ERCP. A large case-control study further found that the risk of ERCP pancreatitis in patients with suspected SOD who underwent SOM is equivalent to those with SOD who did not undergo SOM (OR = 0.72: 95% confidence interval [CI], 0.08, 9.2).[82] In a large cohort of 1115 patients, Cheng and coworkers[83] identified several additional risk factors for post-ERCP pancreatitis, including trainee involvement (OR = 1.5) and minor papilla sphincterotomy (OR = 3.8).[83]

Pharmacologic prophylaxis of ERCP pancreatitis has been the subject of multiple studies with predominantly disappointing results. The aims of treatment are to decrease pancreatic inflammation, decrease exocrine activity, and lower sphincter of Oddi pressure.[84] Attempts to achieve the latter using botulinum, nifedipine, and nitrates administered by various routes have had mixed results.[84,85] Somatostatin and its synthetic variant, octreotide, have been used to promote pancreatic rest by inhibiting hormone secretion. Andriulli and colleagues[86] recently performed a meta-analysis of 9 high-quality, homogenous trials of somatostatin to prevent post-ERCP pancreatitis with a total enrollment of 2658 patients; overall, it did not appear effective (OR = 0.73; 95% CI, 0.5-1.0).[86]

Multiple trials have aimed to prevent post-ERCP pancreatitis by treating with anti-inflammatory medications. In a large 15-center trial, 1115 patients were randomly assigned to prednisone at 3 and 15 hours before ERCP or to placebo in a blinded fashion. There was no difference in the incidence of ERCP pancreatitis between the steroid group (16.6%) and the control group (13.6%).[78] Gabexate mesilate, a protease inhibitor that curbs the activity of neutrophil elastase and trypsin, has also been proposed as a preventive agent. Initial results were favorable, prompting 5 randomized trials. Pooled analysis of these studies showed no significant reduction in post-ERCP pancreatitis in those receiving gabexate mesilate (4.8%) versus (5.7%) of controls.[86]

Recently, nonsteroidal anti-inflammatory drugs (NSAIDs) have been used with more encouraging results. Murray and coworkers[87] randomly assigned 110 patients to receive either rectal diclofenac or placebo. Significantly less post-ERCP pancreatitis was seen in the diclofenac group (6%) compared with controls (16%). A recent meta-analysis using the study by Murray and 3 additional trials included a total of 912 patients and suggested that rectal NSAIDs were effective in preventing post-ERCP pancreatitis, with a pooled relative risk of 0.36 (95% CI, 0.22).[88] These findings prompted the European Society of Gastrointestinal Endoscopy to recommend rectal NSAIDs for prophylaxis.[89] Nonetheless, the meta-analysis excluded a randomized, double-blind prospective study that showed no benefit in administering NSAIDs because that particular study was an outlier and the drug was administered orally rather than per rectum.[89,90] Additional prospective work is needed to see whether NSAIDs are helpful in high-risk patients.

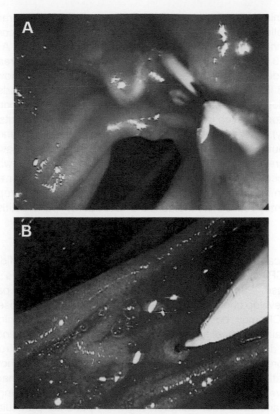

Fig. 10. Pancreatic stents are placed at the level of the (*A*) major papilla and (*B*) minor papilla after pancreatic endotherapy to minimize post-ERCP pancreatitis risk. (*Courtesy of* Isaac Raijman, MD, Houston, TX.)

Compared with pharmacologic therapy, several technical interventions, particularly pancreatic stents, have been shown to be more consistently beneficial (**Fig. 10**). A recent meta-analysis of 5 controlled trials of patients deemed to be at high risk suggested that pancreatic stents were effective in minimizing post-ERCP pancreatitis.[91] Among 481 patients at increased risk because of suspected SOD, difficult cannulation, ampullectomy, pancreatic therapy, and papillary balloon dilatation, 206 underwent pancreatic stent placement and 275 had no stent placed. There was significantly less pancreatitis among the group who underwent stent placement (5.8%) compared with the group who did not receive stents (15.5%). Furthermore, there were no episodes of severe pancreatitis in the stent group. A cost-effectiveness assessment using a Monte Carlo analysis suggests that pancreatic stents are more cost effective if used in high-risk patients.[92] Nonetheless, pancreatic stent placement can be associated with morbidity, such as pancreatic duct perforation and proximal migration; failed attempts may be correlated with increased pancreatitis.[93,94] Given these considerations and the focus of contemporary research on high-risk groups, the use of stents at this time is recommend primarily for those with increased risk of ERCP pancreatitis. Additionally, to avoid ductal changes, smaller 3- to 5-F stents are potentially advantagenous.[95]Another technical approach, which may reduce the risk of ERCP pancreatitis, is the use of wire-guided cannulation to avoid repeat contrast injections and minimize papillary trauma. In their meta-analysis of 5 randomized trials, Cennamo and colleagues[96] present that cannulation was more successful using the wire-guided technique (85.3%) than standard methods (74.9%). A pooling of the results from the 3 randomized trials that measured rates of pancreatitis suggested that the wire-guided technique was associated with significantly lower pancreatitis rates (OR = 0.23 [95% CI, 0.13-0.41]) than contrast-guided methods.[96]

After the development of pancreatitis, treatment is primarily supportive. The use of a structured protocol, which included admission of high-risk patients (SOD, pancreatic endotherapy), well-defined protocols for aggressive intravenous fluids, and optimization of nutrition, was associated with significantly fewer cases of moderate and severe pancreatitis (12.5%) compared with cases in patients who were treated outside the protocol (61.6%).[97] Recent data showing the benefit for early aggressive fluid resuscitation in pancreatitis raises the question of whether prophylactic use of increased fluids may reduce the incidence of post-ERCP pancreatitis.[98]

SUMMARY

Given the significant risk of pancreatitis and the advent of high-fidelity diagnostic techniques, ERCP is now reserved as a therapeutic procedure for those with pancreatic disease. Early ERCP benefits those with gallstone pancreatitis who present with or develop cholangitis or biliary obstruction. Among those with idiopathic pancreatitis, ERCP may be used to confirm and treat SOD, microlithiasis, and structural anomalies, including pancreas divisum. Pancreatic endotherapy is a consideration to decrease pain in those with pancreatic duct obstruction, although surgical decompression may be more durable, particularly in those with severe disease. Pancreatic duct leaks may respond to endoscopic drainage, but optimal therapy is achieved if a bridging stent can be placed. Finally, using a wire-guided technique and pancreatic duct stents in high-risk patients, particularly in cases of suspected SOD, may minimize the risk of post-ERCP pancreatitis.

REFERENCES

1. Rhodes M, Sussman L, Cohen L, et al. Randomised trial of laparoscopic exploration of common bile duct versus postoperative endoscopic retrograde cholangiography for common bile duct stones. Lancet 1998;351(9097):159–61.
2. Acosta JM, Ledesma CL. Gallstone migration as a cause of acute pancreatitis. N Engl J Med 1974;290(9):484–7.
3. Fan ST, Lai EC, Mok FP, et al. Early treatment of acute biliary pancreatitis by endoscopic papillotomy. N Engl J Med 1993;328(4):228–32.
4. Neoptolemos JP, Carr-Locke DL, London NJ, et al. Controlled trial of urgent endoscopic retrograde cholangiopancreatography and endoscopic sphincterotomy versus conservative treatment for acute pancreatitis due to gallstones. Lancet 1988; 2(8618):979–83.
5. Folsch UR, Nitsche R, Ludtke R, et al. Early ERCP and papillotomy compared with conservative treatment for acute biliary pancreatitis. The German Study Group on Acute Biliary Pancreatitis. N Engl J Med 1997;336(4):237–42.
6. Kelly TR, Wagner DS. Gallstone pancreatitis: a prospective randomized trial of the timing of surgery. Surgery 1988;104(4):600–5.
7. Tang E, Stain SC, Tang G, et al. Timing of laparoscopic surgery in gallstone pancreatitis. Arch Surg 1995;130(5):496–9; discussion 499–500.
8. Lee SP, Nicholls JF, Park HZ. Biliary sludge as a cause of acute pancreatitis. N Engl J Med 1992;326(9):589–93.

9. Yusoff IF, Raymond G, Sahai AV. A prospective comparison of the yield of EUS in primary vs. recurrent idiopathic acute pancreatitis. Gastrointest Endosc 2004;60(5): 673–8.

10. Okazaki K, Chiba T. Autoimmune related pancreatitis. Gut 2002;51(1):1–4.

11. Kozarek R. Role of ERCP in acute pancreatitis. Gastrointest Endosc 2002;56(6 Suppl):S231–6.

12. Wilcox CM, Varadarajulu S, Eloubeidi M. Role of endoscopic evaluation in idiopathic pancreatitis: a systematic review. Gastrointest Endosc 2006;63(7):1037–45.

13. Frossard JL, Sosa-Valencia L, Amouyal G, et al. Usefulness of endoscopic ultrasonography in patients with "idiopathic" acute pancreatitis. Am J Med 2000;109(3): 196–200.

14. Liu CL, Lo CM, Chan JK, et al. EUS for detection of occult cholelithiasis in patients with idiopathic pancreatitis. Gastrointest Endosc 2000;51(1):28–32.

15. Tandon M, Topazian M. Endoscopic ultrasound in idiopathic acute pancreatitis. Am J Gastroenterol 2001;96(3):705–9.

16. Coyle WJ, Pineau BC, Tarnasky PR, et al. Evaluation of unexplained acute and acute recurrent pancreatitis using endoscopic retrograde cholangiopancreatography, sphincter of Oddi manometry and endoscopic ultrasound. Endoscopy 2002;34(8): 617–23.

17. Chak A, Hawes RH, Cooper GS, et al. Prospective assessment of the utility of EUS in the evaluation of gallstone pancreatitis. Gastrointest Endosc 1999;49(5):599–604.

18. Catalano MF, Lahoti S, Geenen JE, et al. Prospective evaluation of endoscopic ultrasonography, endoscopic retrograde pancreatography, and secretin test in the diagnosis of chronic pancreatitis. Gastrointest Endosc 1998;48(1):11–7.

19. Lai R, Freeman ML, Cass OW, et al. Accurate diagnosis of pancreas divisum by linear-array endoscopic ultrasonography. Endoscopy 2004;36(8):705–9.

20. Levy MJ. The hunt for microlithiasis in idiopathic acute recurrent pancreatitis: should we abandon the search or intensify our efforts? Gastrointest Endosc 2002;55(2):286–93.

21. Kaw M, Brodmerkel GJ Jr. ERCP, biliary crystal analysis, and sphincter of Oddi manometry in idiopathic recurrent pancreatitis. Gastrointest Endosc 2002;55(2): 157–62.

22. Dahan P, Andant C, Levy P, et al. Prospective evaluation of endoscopic ultrasonography and microscopic examination of duodenal bile in the diagnosis of cholecystolithiasis in 45 patients with normal conventional ultrasonography. Gut 1996;38(2): 277–81.

23. Testoni PA, Caporuscio S, Bagnolo F, et al. Idiopathic recurrent pancreatitis: long-term results after ERCP, endoscopic sphincterotomy, or ursodeoxycholic acid treatment. Am J Gastroentero. 2000;95(7):1702–7.

24. Kim HS, Moon JH, Choi HJ, et al. The role of intraductal US in the management of idiopathic recurrent pancreatitis without a definite cause on ERCP. Gastrointest Endosc 2011;73(6):1148–54.

25. Rashdan A, Fogel E, McHenry L Jr, et al. Frequency of biliary crystals in patients with suspected sphincter of Oddi dysfunction. Gastrointest Endosc 2003;58(6):875–8.

26. Venu RP, Geenen JE, Hogan W, et al. Idiopathic recurrent pancreatitis. An approach to diagnosis and treatment. Dig Dis Sci 1989;34(1):56–60.

27. Frulloni L, Cavallini G. Acute recurrent pancreatitis and dysfunction of the sphincter of Oddi: comparison between invasive and non-invasive techniques. JOP. 2001;2(6): 406–13.

28. Toouli J, Roberts-Thomson IC, Kellow J, et al. Manometry based randomised trial of endoscopic sphincterotomy for sphincter of Oddi dysfunction. Gut 2000;46(1):98–102.

29. Sherman S, Troiano FP, Hawes RH, et al. Frequency of abnormal sphincter of Oddi manometry compared with the clinical suspicion of sphincter of Oddi dysfunction. Am J Gastroenterol 1991;86(5):586–90.

30. Eversman D, Fogel EL, Rusche M, et al. Frequency of abnormal pancreatic and biliary sphincter manometry compared with clinical suspicion of sphincter of Oddi dysfunction. Gastrointest Endosc 1999;50(5):637–41.

31. Testoni PA, Mariani A, Curioni S, et al. MRCP-secretin test-guided management of idiopathic recurrent pancreatitis: long-term outcomes. Gastrointest Endosc 2008; 67(7):1028–34.

32. Geenen JE, Hogan WJ, Dodds WJ, et al. The efficacy of endoscopic sphincterotomy after cholecystectomy in patients with sphincter-of-Oddi dysfunction. N Engl J Med 1989;320(2):82–7.

33. Park SH, Watkins JL, Fogel EL, et al. Long-term outcome of endoscopic dual pancreatobiliary sphincterotomy in patients with manometry-documented sphincter of Oddi dysfunction and normal pancreatogram. Gastrointest Endosc 2003;57(4): 483–91.

34. Wehrmann T. Long-term results (>/= 10 years) of endoscopic therapy for sphincter of Oddi dysfunction in patients with acute recurrent pancreatitis. Endoscopy 2011; 43(3):202–7.

35. Saltzman JR. Endoscopic treatment of pancreas divisum: why, when, and how? Gastrointest Endosc 2006;64(5):712–5.

36. Devereaux BM, Lehman GA, Fein S, et al. Facilitation of pancreatic duct cannulation using a new synthetic porcine secretin. Am J Gastroenterol 2002;97(9):2279–81.

37. Devereaux BM, Fein S, Purich E, et al. A new synthetic porcine secretin for facilitation of cannulation of the dorsal pancreatic duct at ERCP in patients with pancreas divisum: a multicenter, randomized, double-blind comparative study. Gastrointest Endosc 2003;57(6):643–7.

38. Park SH, de Bellis M, McHenry L, et al. Use of methylene blue to identify the minor papilla or its orifice in patients with pancreas divisum. Gastrointest Endosc 2003; 57(3):358–63.

39. Attwell A, Borak G, Hawes R, et al. Endoscopic pancreatic sphincterotomy for pancreas divisum by using a needle-knife or standard pull-type technique: safety and reintervention rates. Gastrointest Endosc 2006;64(5):705–11.

40. Heyries L, Barthet M, Delvasto C, et al. Long-term results of endoscopic management of pancreas divisum with recurrent acute pancreatitis. Gastrointest Endosc 2002; 55(3):376–81.

41. Ertan A. Long-term results after endoscopic pancreatic stent placement without pancreatic papillotomy in acute recurrent pancreatitis due to pancreas divisum. Gastrointest Endosc 2000;52(1):9–14.

42. Lans JI, Geenen JE, Johanson JF, et al. Endoscopic therapy in patients with pancreas divisum and acute pancreatitis: a prospective, randomized, controlled clinical trial. Gastrointest Endosc 1992;38(4):430–4.

43. Lehman GA, Sherman S, Nisi R, et al. Pancreas divisum: results of minor papilla sphincterotomy. Gastrointest Endosc 1993;39(1):1–8.

44. Chacko LN, Chen YK, Shah RJ. Clinical outcomes and nonendoscopic interventions after minor papilla endotherapy in patients with symptomatic pancreas divisum. Gastrointest Endosc 2008;68(4):667–73.

45. Kozarek RA. Pancreatic stents can induce ductal changes consistent with chronic pancreatitis. Gastrointest Endosc 1990;36(2):93–5.
46. Sherman S, Hawes RH, Savides TJ, et al. Stent-induced pancreatic ductal and parenchymal changes: correlation of endoscopic ultrasound with ERCP. Gastrointest Endosc 1996;44(3):276–82.
47. Guelrud M, Morera C, Rodriguez M, et al. Sphincter of Oddi dysfunction in children with recurrent pancreatitis and anomalous pancreaticobiliary union: an etiologic concept. Gastrointest Endosc 1999;50(2):194–9.
48. Gress F, Yiengpruksawan A, Sherman S, et al. Diagnosis of annular pancreas by endoscopic ultrasound. Gastrointest Endosc 1996;44(4):485–9.
49. Bhasin DK, Rana SS, Nanda M, et al. Ansa pancreatica type of ductal anatomy in a patient with idiopathic acute pancreatitis. JOP 2006;7(3):315–20.
50. Hwang SS, Paik CN, Lee KM, et al. Recurrent acute pancreatitis caused by an annular pancreas in a child. Gastrointest Endosc 2010;72(4):848–9.
51. Dodda G, Brown RD, O'Neil HK, et al. Cystic duct insertion at ampulla as a cause for acute recurrent pancreatitis. Gastrointest Endosc 1998;47(2):181–3.
52. Zoepf T, Zoepf DS, Arnold JC, et al. The relationship between juxtapapillary duodenal diverticula and disorders of the biliopancreatic system: analysis of 350 patients. Gastrointest Endosc 2001;54(1):56–61.
53. Dite P, Ruzicka M, Zboril V, et al. A prospective, randomized trial comparing endoscopic and surgical therapy for chronic pancreatitis. Endoscopy 2003;35(7):553–8.
54. Dumonceau JM, Costamagna G, Tringali A, et al. Treatment for painful calcified chronic pancreatitis: extracorporeal shock wave lithotripsy versus endoscopic treatment: a randomised controlled trial. Gut 2007;56(4):545–52.
55. Mossner J, Secknus R, Meyer J, et al. Treatment of pain with pancreatic extracts in chronic pancreatitis: results of a prospective placebo-controlled multicenter trial. Digestion 1992;53(1–2):54–66.
56. Delhaye M, Arvanitakis M, Verset G, et al. Long-term clinical outcome after endoscopic pancreatic ductal drainage for patients with painful chronic pancreatitis. Clin Gastroenterol Hepatol 2004;2(12):1096–106.
57. Smits ME, Badiga SM, Rauws EA, et al. Long-term results of pancreatic stents in chronic pancreatitis. Gastrointest Endosc 1995;42(5):461–7.
58. Eleftherladis N, Dinu F, Delhaye M, et al. Long-term outcome after pancreatic stenting in severe chronic pancreatitis. Endoscopy 2005;37(3):223–30.
59. Rosch T, Daniel S, Scholz M, et al. Endoscopic treatment of chronic pancreatitis: a multicenter study of 1000 patients with long-term follow-up. Endoscopy 2002;34(10):765–71.
60. Cahen DL, Gouma DJ, Nio Y, et al. Endoscopic versus surgical drainage of the pancreatic duct in chronic pancreatitis. N Engl J Med 2007;356(7):676–84.
61. Cahen DL, Gouma DJ, Laramee P, et al. Long-term outcomes of endoscopic versus surgical drainage of the pancreatic duct in patients with chronic pancreatitis. Gastroenterology 2011;141(5):1690–5.
62. Kozarek RA, Brandabur JJ, Ball TJ, et al. Clinical outcomes in patients who undergo extracorporeal shock wave lithotripsy for chronic calcific pancreatitis. Gastrointest Endosc 2002;56(4):496–500.
63. Brand B, Kahl M, Sidhu S, et al. Prospective evaluation of morphology, function, and quality of life after extracorporeal shockwave lithotripsy and endoscopic treatment of chronic calcific pancreatitis. Am J Gastroenterol 2000;95(12):3428–38.
64. Costamagna G, Bulajic M, Tringali A, et al. Multiple stenting of refractory pancreatic duct strictures in severe chronic pancreatitis: long-term results. Endoscopy 2006;38(3):254–9.

65. Moon SH, Kim MH, Park do H, et al. Modified fully covered self-expandable metal stents with antimigration features for benign pancreatic-duct strictures in advanced chronic pancreatitis, with a focus on the safety profile and reducing migration. Gastrointest Endosc 2010;72(1):86–91.

66. Sauer B, Talreja J, Ellen K, et al. Temporary placement of a fully covered self-expandable metal stent in the pancreatic duct for management of symptomatic refractory chronic pancreatitis: preliminary data (with videos). Gastrointest Endosc 2008;68(6):1173–8.

67. Ostroff JW. Pain and chronic pancreatitis: are we really ready for metal in the pancreatic duct? Gastrointest Endosc 2008;68(6):1179–81.

68. Deviere J, Bueso H, Baize M, et al. Complete disruption of the main pancreatic duct: endoscopic management. Gastrointest Endosc 1995;42(5):445–51.

69. Varadarajulu S, Noone TC, Tutuian R, et al. Predictors of outcome in pancreatic duct disruption managed by endoscopic transpapillary stent placement. Gastrointest Endosc 2005;61(4):568–75.

70. Costamagna G, Mutignani M, Ingrosso M, et al. Endoscopic treatment of postsurgical external pancreatic fistulas. Endoscopy 2001;33(4):317–22.

71. Bracher GA, Manocha AP, DeBanto JR, et al. Endoscopic pancreatic duct stenting to treat pancreatic ascites. Gastrointest Endosc 1999;49(6):710–5.

72. Trevino JM, Tamhane A, Varadarajulu S. Successful stenting in ductal disruption favorably impacts treatment outcomes in patients undergoing transmural drainage of peripancreatic fluid collections. J Gastroenterol Hepatol 2010;25(3):526–31.

73. Lau ST, Simchuk EJ, Kozarek RA, et al. A pancreatic ductal leak should be sought to direct treatment in patients with acute pancreatitis. Am J Surg 2001;181(5):411–5.

74. Telford JJ, Farrell JJ, Saltzman JR, et al. Pancreatic stent placement for duct disruption. Gastrointest Endosc 2002;56(1):18–24.

75. Lawrence C, Howell DA, Stefan AM, et al. Disconnected pancreatic tail syndrome: potential for endoscopic therapy and results of long-term follow-up. Gastrointest Endosc 2008;67(4):673–9.

76. Baron TH, Ferreira LE. Covered expandable metal stent placement for treatment of a refractory pancreatic duct leak. Gastrointest Endosc 2007;66(6):1239–41.

77. Luthen R, Jaklin P, Cohnen M. Permanent closure of a pancreatic duct leak by endoscopic coiling. Endoscopy 2007;39 (Suppl 1):E21–22.

78. Sherman S, Blaut U, Watkins JL, et al. Does prophylactic administration of corticosteroid reduce the risk and severity of post-ERCP pancreatitis: a randomized, prospective, multicenter study. Gastrointest Endosc 2003;58(1):23–9.

79. Cotton PB, Lehman G, Vennes J, et al. Endoscopic sphincterotomy complications and their management: an attempt at consensus. Gastrointest Endosc 1991;37(3):383–93.

80. Freeman ML, DiSario JA, Nelson DB, et al. Risk factors for post-ERCP pancreatitis: a prospective, multicenter study. Gastrointest Endosc 2001;54(4):425–34.

81. Disario JA, Freeman ML, Bjorkman DJ, et al. Endoscopic balloon dilation compared with sphincterotomy for extraction of bile duct stones. Gastroenterology 2004;127(5):1291–9.

82. Singh P, Gurudu SR, Davidoff S, et al. Sphincter of Oddi manometry does not predispose to post-ERCP acute pancreatitis. Gastrointest Endosc 2004;59(4):499–505.

83. Cheng CL, Sherman S, Watkins JL, et al. Risk factors for post-ERCP pancreatitis: a prospective multicenter study. Am J Gastroenterol 2006;101(1):139–47.

84. Badalov N, Tenner S, Baillie J. The Prevention, recognition and treatment of post-ERCP pancreatitis. JOP 2009;10(2):88–97.

85. Shao LM, Chen QY, Chen MY, et al. Nitroglycerin in the prevention of post-ERCP pancreatitis: a meta-analysis. Dig Dis Sci 2010;55(1):1–7.
86. Andriulli A, Leandro G, Federici T, et al. Prophylactic administration of somatostatin or gabexate does not prevent pancreatitis after ERCP: an updated meta-analysis. Gastrointest Endosc 2007;65(4):624–32.
87. Murray B, Carter R, Imrie C, et al. Diclofenac reduces the incidence of acute pancreatitis after endoscopic retrograde cholangiopancreatography. Gastroenterology 2003;124(7):1786–91.
88. Elmunzer BJ, Waljee AK, Elta GH, et al. A meta-analysis of rectal NSAIDs in the prevention of post-ERCP pancreatitis. Gut 2008;57(9):1262–7.
89. Dumonceau JM, Andriulli A, Deviere J, et al. European Society of Gastrointestinal Endoscopy (ESGE) Guideline: prophylaxis of post-ERCP pancreatitis. Endoscopy 2010;42(6):503–15.
90. Cheon YK, Cho KB, Watkins JL, et al. Efficacy of diclofenac in the prevention of post-ERCP pancreatitis in predominantly high-risk patients: a randomized double-blind prospective trial. Gastrointest Endosc 2007;66(6):1126–32.
91. Singh P, Das A, Isenberg G, et al. Does prophylactic pancreatic stent placement reduce the risk of post-ERCP acute pancreatitis? A meta-analysis of controlled trials. Gastrointest Endosc 2004;60(4):544–50.
92. Das A, Singh P, Sivak MV Jr, et al. Pancreatic-stent placement for prevention of post-ERCP pancreatitis: a cost-effectiveness analysis. Gastrointest Endosc 2007; 65(7):960–8.
93. Tarnasky PR, Palesch YY, Cunningham JT, et al. Pancreatic stenting prevents pancreatitis after biliary sphincterotomy in patients with sphincter of Oddi dysfunction. Gastroenterology 1998;115(6):1518–24.
94. Freeman ML, Overby C, Qi D. Pancreatic stent insertion: consequences of failure and results of a modified technique to maximize success. Gastrointest Endosc 2004; 59(1):8–14.
95. Neuhaus H. Therapeutic pancreatic endoscopy. Endoscopy 2004;36(1):8–16.
96. Cennamo V, Fuccio L, Zagari RM, et al. Can a wire-guided cannulation technique increase bile duct cannulation rate and prevent post-ERCP pancreatitis?: a meta-analysis of randomized controlled trials. Am J Gastroenterol 2009;104(9):2343–50.
97. Reddy N, Wilcox CM, Tamhane A, et al. Protocol-based medical management of post-ERCP pancreatitis. J Gastroenterol Hepatol 2008;23(3):385–92.
98. Warndorf MG, Kurtzman JT, Bartel MJ, et al. Early fluid resuscitation reduces morbidity among patients with acute pancreatitis. Clin Gastroenterol Hepatol 2011; 9(8):705–9.

Endoscopic Management of Pancreatic Pseudocysts

Andrew L. Samuelson, MD[a], Raj J. Shah, MD[b],*

KEYWORDS

- Endoscopic necrosectomy
- Endoscopic retrograde cholangiopancreatography • EUS
- Pancreatic pseudocyst • Pancreatic stents
- Pseudocyst drainage

Pseudocysts are common lesions of the pancreas that arise from pancreatic ductal disruption. They range from simple, self-resolving cysts to complex, life-threatening cysts that present challenging management decisions. The Atlanta International Symposium on Acute Pancreatitis defined pancreatic pseudocysts as fluid collections more than 4 weeks old that are surrounded by a nonepithelial wall of fibrous or granulation tissue arising as a consequence of acute pancreatitis, chronic pancreatitis, or pancreatic trauma.[1] Pseudocysts complicate 10% to 26% of acute pancreatitis cases and 20% to 40% of chronic pancreatitis cases; they are typically round or ovoid on imaging and nonpalpable on physical examination. Because of the disruption of the pancreatic duct, they are rich in pancreatic enzymes such as amylase.[2–5] Acute fluid collections complicate more than 50% of cases of acute pancreatitis and are distinct from pseudocysts because acute fluid collections are irregular in shape and lack a well-defined wall.[1,5,6] In the absence of infection, acute fluid collections are managed expectantly, because most resolve spontaneously, whereas the management of pseudocysts more often requires endoscopic, percutaneous, or surgical drainage.[3,5,6]

DISTINGUISHING PSEUDOCYSTS FROM PANCREATIC CYSTIC NEOPLASMS

Careful exclusion of a pancreatic cystic neoplasm is mandatory before considering draining pseudocysts. Pseudocysts account for at least 75% of all pancreas cysts, but they can be difficult to distinguish from pancreatic cystic neoplasms, retention cysts, and congenital cysts, especially in patients without a clear history of pancreatitis.[5,7] Retention cysts are nonneoplastic localized areas of dilation of the pancreatic

Disclosure: Raj J. Shah is a consultant and has a royalty agreement (patent pending) with Cook Endoscopy. He has received unrestricted educational grants from Boston Scientific, Cook, and Olympus, and a research grant from Xlumena, Inc.
[a] University of Colorado Anschutz Medical Campus, Aurora, CO, USA
[b] University of Colorado School of Medicine, 1635 Aurora Ct. AIP Rm 2.031, Aurora, CO 80045, USA
* Corresponding author.
E-mail address: raj.shah@ucdenver.edu

Gastroenterol Clin N Am 41 (2012) 47–62
doi:10.1016/j.gtc.2011.12.007   gastro.theclinics.com
0889-8553/12/$ – see front matter © 2012 Elsevier Inc. All rights reserved.

duct owing to a ductal obstruction from an obstructing neoplasm, stricture, or stone. Like pseudocysts, retention cysts are common complications of chronic pancreatitis. Pancreatic cystic neoplasms include those with malignant potential such as mucinous cystic neoplasms, intraductal papillary mucinous neoplasms, solid pseudopapillary neoplasms with cystic components, pancreatic adenocarcinoma, or neuroendocrine tumors with cystic degeneration, and benign serous cystadenoma.[8,9] Many malignant pancreatic cysts are well treated with surgical resection; however, intervention to drain a cystic neoplasm mistakenly diagnosed as a pseudocyst can compromise any subsequent attempt at operative resection.[5,7]

A careful clinical history of preceding pancreatitis of a known origin or established chronic pancreatitis can assist in distinguishing between pseudocysts and potential cystic neoplasms.[10] However, this may not be helpful in all cases. Warshaw and colleagues[7] reported on 12 years of experience with pancreatic cystic neoplasms and noted that 37% of lesions had been misdiagnosed as pseudocysts before operation. They found that clinical factors such as abdominal pain and pancreatitis were unhelpful in distinguishing between the two lesions, because both patients with cystic neoplasms and pseudocysts commonly experienced these symptoms. Warshaw and others also found cyst diameter to be a poor distinguishing factor as the mean size of neoplastic cysts is frequently similar to that of pseudocysts.[7,11] Computed tomography (CT) and magnetic resonance imaging may be helpful in identifying dependent debris within the lesion, suggestive of a pseudocyst, or rim calcification, indicative of neoplasia.[7] External microlobulated morphology and internal septae were more common in neoplasms than in pseudocysts, but neither of these findings attained significance in one study utilizing magnetic resonance imaging.[12] Further, Chalian and colleagues[11] found that CT attenuation was significantly higher in pseudocysts than in mucin-containing cysts (mean of 18.9 HU for pseudocysts, 13.0 HU for mucinous cystic neoplasms, and 11.4 for intraductal papillary mucinous neoplasms), further helping to distinguish these lesions noninvasively.[11]

Endoscopic ultrasonography (EUS) permits visualization of cystic lesions that are within close proximity to the gastrointestinal (GI) lumen and offers the ability for tissue sampling and cyst fluid analysis before pursuing drainage of a potential pseudocyst.[9,13] Van der Waaij and colleagues[14] analyzed 12 different studies comprising data from 450 patients with pancreatic cyst fluid analysis and found that an amylase level of less than 250 U/L had 98% specificity for serous cystadenoma, mucinous cystadenoma, or mucinous cystadenocarcinoma and virtually excluded the diagnosis of pseudocyst. Carcinoembryonic antigen less than 5 ng/mL showed a specificity of 95% for pseudocyst and serous cystadenoma as did carbohydrate-associate antigen 19 (CA 19-9) concentration less than 37 U/mL with a specificity of 98%. All of these cyst fluid biomarkers showed sensitivities of 50% or less; therefore, these tests are most helpful when the measured value falls below the stated thresholds (ie, the negative predictive value). There are several promising new candidates for cyst fluid biomarkers, such as glycosolation variants of mucins and carcinoembryonic antigen cell adhesion molecules.[15] It would seem that these diagnostic difficulties would favor surgical drainage over percutaneous or endoscopic drainage of cystic lesions, because surgery affords a more generous cyst wall biopsy; however, the magnitude of this benefit is questionable. In one study, the epithelial lining of cystic lesions was partially (5%–98%) missing in 40% to 72% of all major tumor types, implying that even biopsy of a cyst during surgical cystenterostomy can lead to a missed diagnosis of a neoplasm.[7] Currently, no single test can rule out a pancreatic cystic neoplasm; rather, a careful assessment including a detailed clinical history, radiologic studies, and EUS-guided cyst fluid analysis is the most reliable method for distinction.

INDICATIONS FOR DRAINAGE OF PANCREATIC PSEUDOCYSTS

The natural history of pseudocysts and the complications associated with conservative management by observation have traditionally demanded intervention to drain pseudocysts. This is largely based on the work of Bradley and colleagues,[3] who followed patients with pseudocysts until cyst resolution or the occurrence of complications such as rupture, abscess, jaundice, or hemorrhage. During the observation period, 41% of their patients experienced complications with cyst resolution occurring in 20%. They also demonstrated that observation past 7 weeks had more risk than operative management.[3] Their work contributed to an oft-quoted guideline recommending that physicians actively drain all pseudocysts that persisted longer than 6 weeks. More recent work suggests that longer periods of observation are safe and effective in permitting spontaneous resolution in up to 86% of patients with a 3% to 9% rate of serious complications developing during an average of 1-year expectant follow-up.[16–18]

Further, traditional guidelines have held that pseudocysts greater than 6 cm in diameter should be drained because they showed lower rates of spontaneous resolution and exposed patients to greater risks of complications than smaller pseudocysts.[19] Although data regarding pseudocyst size and outcome are mixed, a smaller size (<4 cm) is an important predictor of spontaneous resolution.[2,20,21] One study of 36 patients with asymptomatic pseudocysts found that 67% of pseudocysts greater than 6 cm in diameter and 40% of pseudocysts less than 6 cm required surgical treatment.[17] Cheruvu and colleagues[18] had differing results, finding that the median pseudocyst size of those requiring intervention was similar (8 cm) to those successfully managed conservatively (7 cm), arguing that pseudocyst size is a less important factor in the eventual outcome. Nguyen and colleagues[22] similarly found that size greater than or less than 6 cm had no effect on rates of spontaneous resolution, need for operative management, complications, recurrence, or mortality. The heterogeneity of findings regarding outcomes and pseudocyst size highlight that criteria for pseudocyst drainage based on cyst size are not appropriate. Rather, persistent pain, gastric or duodenal obstruction, biliary obstruction, ascites, pleural effusion, enlarging size on serial imaging, signs of pseudocyst infection or bleeding, or the possibility of a pancreatic cystic malignancy are more important factors in considering interventions for pseudocyst drainage.

DRAINAGE TECHNIQUES

The method of drainage is based primarily on local expertise with the endoscopic approach being favored for simple pseudocysts that are in close proximity to the gastric or duodenal wall. It is considered to be the first-line approach.[23,24] A percutaneous approach is reserved for those collections that do not communicate with the pancreatic duct or are not adjacent to the GI lumen, or in patients who are not optimal candidates for surgery. If regional expertise in endoscopy is not available, then surgical drainage for complex pseudocysts and walled-off organized pancreatic necrosis is preferred.[23–25] There are many advantages to endoscopic drainage of pseudocysts: The ability to place multiple internal drains, irrigation via a nasocystic catheter, treating downstream pancreatic ductal obstruction via endoscopic retrograde cholangiopancreatography, direct endoscopic necrosectomy, and the lack of known sequelae if a persistent fistula develops at the site of the cystenterostomy. Indeed, the latter may help to reduce the risk of pseudocyst recurrence by promoting drainage of pancreatic juices in the case of a "disconnected tail syndrome."[26]

Percutaneous and surgical options for drainage are indeed associated with greater morbidity.[27–29]

Transmural endoscopic drainage is generally performed when the pseudocyst is within 1 cm of the gastric or duodenal lumen. Smaller, symptomatic pseudocysts more than 1 cm from the GI lumen may be appropriate for transpapillary drainage if communication is evident on pancreatography.[29] In our experience, a combined transmural or transpapillary approach is not generally required for successful resolution of most pseudocysts. Periprocedural prophylactic antibiotics with a fluoroquinolone or other broad-spectrum antibiotic is recommended to reduce the incidence of pseudocyst infection. Antibiotics can be continued for 3 to 5 days after the procedure.[30]

Techniques of Endoscopic Drainage

Transpapillary drainage

In general, transpapillary stenting is the sole means of drainage if the pseudocyst is smaller than 6 cm and there is communication with the main pancreatic duct,[31,32] or if transmural drainage is not feasible owing to distance (eg, >1 cm from the GI lumen) or is contraindicated (eg, significant coagulopathy). Ancillary interventions include major or minor papilla pancreatic sphincterotomy, judicious dilation of downstream pancreatic duct strictures, and placement of a large-bore pancreatic duct stent preferably across any ductal disruption or into the pseudocyst cavity (**Fig. 1**).

Transmural

EUS or non–EUS-guided techniques may be utilized. Non–EUS-guided transmural drainage requires not only close proximity of the pseudocyst to the GI lumen, but also an endoscopically visible bulge.

Non–EUS-guided transmural drainage

Endoscopic needle localization (ENL) of the point of maximal endoscopic bulge aims to confirm an appropriate location before cystenterostomy tract dilation and stent placement (**Fig. 2**). The two methods of ENL that have been well-described are diathermic puncture and the Seldinger technique.[33,34] Diathermic puncture involves inserting a 22-gauge, precurved biliary aspiration needle mounted in a 7-Fr catheter (HBAN22, Cook Endoscopy, Winston-Salem, NC, USA) or a Cystotome (Cook Endoscopy, Inc.) that is a 10-Fr catheter with a diathermic ring and a 5-Fr inner catheter housing a low-profile, 0.38-inch needle knife to facilitate close apposition of the pseudocyst to the gut lumen. For initial puncture, the needle knife should be directed perpendicularly to the axis of maximal endoscopic bulge with pure cutting current recommended by some authorities. The return of blood upon needle puncture is concerning for entry into either a vascular structure, such as a pseudoaneurysm, or a blood vessel in the wall of the pseudocyst. Repuncture at a different site with bloody return warrants consideration for terminating the procedure and reevaluating for a pseudoaneurysm or portal hypertension with perigastric varices. Stroking of the needle knife is not recommended because a cut of even a few millimeters on the cyst bulge can enter an adjacent gastric vessel wall. Electrocautery should be discontinued immediately upon entry of the needle knife into the cyst cavity to avoid thermal injuries to surrounding structures. Once a site is found with suitable fluid return, limited contrast is injected under fluoroscopic guidance to confirm position within the pseudocyst.[33]

The Seldinger technique for entry involves creating an initial puncture with an 18-gauge needle and then a 0.035-mm guidewire is placed through the needle, which

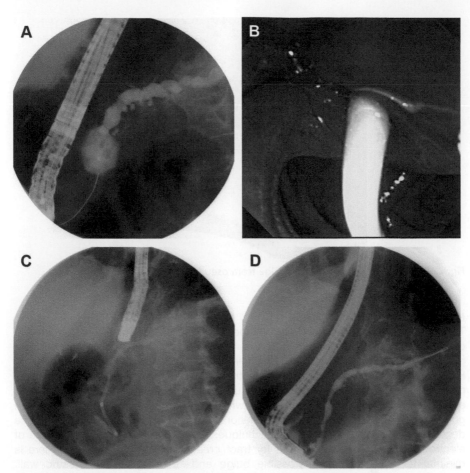

Fig. 1. (*A*) Pancreatography showing pancreatic head pseudocyst before transpapillary drainage. (*B, C*) Endoscopic and fluoroscopic views of transpapillary stent. (*D*) Pancreatography showing resolution of pancreatic head pseudocyst after transpapillary drainage.

allows an 8- to 10-mm balloon tract dilation over the guidewire before stent placement. This technique was studied in 94 consecutive patients with comparable efficacy to needle-knife entry (95% vs 92%, respectively), although it showed a significantly lower bleeding complication rate of 4.6% compared with 15.7% with diathermic puncture.[34]

Following deep access with a guidewire and 2 to 3 curls of the wire within the pseudocyst cavity, the needle or catheter is exchanged for an 8- or 10-mm dilating balloon. Inflation is done under fluoroscopic guidance making sure to visualize the waist between the gut lumen and pseudocyst to ensure adequate cystenterostomy tract dilation. Many endoscopists prefer double pigtail stents to reduce migration, and they place 2 or more 10-Fr stents of differing lengths and angles of insertion, especially in large cysts, to ensure drainage of the most dependent and distal portions (**Fig. 3**). Stents are removed at the time of pseudocyst resolution, which is generally 4 to 6 weeks. Undrained segments related to internal debris or septations may lead to nonresolution.

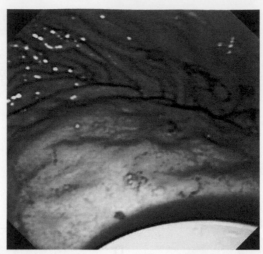

Fig. 2. Endoscopically visible gastric bulge from pseudocyst.

EUS-guided transmural drainage

Traditionally, lack of a pseudocyst bulge into the GI lumen was considered a contraindication to endoscopic drainage. EUS may be utilized to mark a site for duodenoscopic drainage and to assist in excluding perigastric varices (**Fig. 4**). However, a single-step approach is currently the most commonly utilized method and permits pseudocyst puncture under direct ultrasound guidance.[35] After puncture with a 19-gauge needle, the stylet is withdrawn followed by placement of a .035-inch guidewire. The cystenterostomy, tract dilation, and stent insertion are similar to those described for the non–EUS-guided technique. Passage dilators without the use of electrocautery can also be utilized for tract creation, but in cases where there is minimal to no endoscopically visible bulge and "thinning" of the gastric wall, electrocautery is still required (authors' personal observation).

A nonrandomized, prospective study comparing conventional duodenoscopic with EUS-guided drainage by Kahaleh and colleagues[36] showed equivalent rates of efficacy (93% vs 94%) and complications (84% vs 91%) with EUS and non–EUS-guided procedures, respectively. However, only patients with an endoscopically visible bulge were treated with non–EUS-guided procedures and all patients with portal hypertension were treated with EUS guidance.[36] Several studies have shown that predrainage EUS alters management by identifying mucinous cystic neoplasms and relative contraindications to endoscopic drainage, such as distance greater than 1 cm and normal intervening pancreatic parenchyma.[37,38] Because of its oblique view, EUS promotes a more tangential puncture, which could theoretically be less efficacious and associated with higher complication rates than the perpendicular puncture afforded by the side-viewing duodenoscope; however, success rates and complications with the echoendoscope have not validated this concern.

A device for single-step drainage using a system (NAVIX, XLUMENA, Inc., San Francisco, CA, USA) that permits needle puncture with a 3-mm retractable blade to create the cystenterostomy does not utilize cautery.[39] It has an anchoring and dilating balloon, as well as 2 guidewire ports to permit double wire advancement with the same puncture for sequential stent placement. However, because of the limits of currently available echoendoscope working channels, a 10-Fr stent cannot be

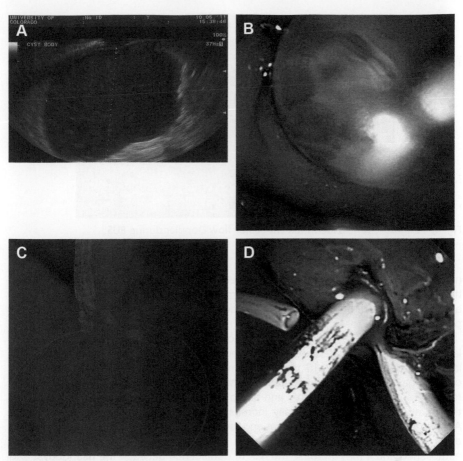

Fig. 3. (*A*) EUS of pseudocyst before drainage. (*B*) Cystgastrostomy tract balloon dilation. (*C*) Guidewire curled in the pseudocyst cavity and a fluoroscopic "waist" noted on dilating balloon. (*D*) Transgastric stents in place.

advanced coaxially alongside an 0.035-inch guidewire. Therefore, the system requires placement first of a 7-Fr and then a 10-Fr stent.[39] The off-label use of covered metal stents for drainage has been limited because of stent migration[40]; however, a novel "dumbbell"-shaped, coated metal stent (AXIOS, XLUMENA, Inc.) is currently available in Europe and undergoing clinical trials in the United States. Whether larger internal diameter expandable metal stents will permit enhanced drainage and resolution of pseudocysts remains to be seen.

Pseudocysts with internal necrotic debris

Residual necrosis has been found to be the most important factor influencing inferior treatment outcome, especially as compared with simple pseudocyst and pancreatic abscess.[41,42] As such, if the draining cyst fluid is thick or contains debris, the endoscopist should take further measures to lower the risk of infection, including additional large-bore stents and placement of nasocystic tubes. Nasocystic tubes can be lavaged every 3 to 4 hours or flushed continuously with IV line setups with

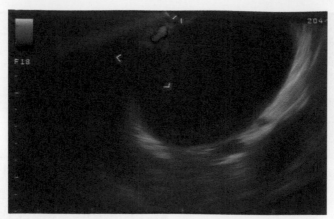

Fig. 4. Perigastric varices identified with color flow Doppler during EUS.

normal sterile saline for several days to weeks, depending on patient tolerance and the amount of debris (**Fig. 5**). For longer term irrigation, especially if nasocystic tubes are not well-tolerated, percutaneous endoscopic gastrostomy with the catheter placed in the cyst fossa is possible.

Direct endoscopic necrosectomy, although often tedious, utilizes pseudocyst lavage and mechanical debridement in select patients. During repeat endoscopy and large balloon dilation (12–15 mm, 15–18 mm, or larger), diagnostic or therapeutic channel gastroscopes are advanced into the cavity for debridement (**Fig. 6**). Devices for necrosectomy include snares and polyp retrieval devices, followed by upsizing of the number of stents to gradually increase the diameter of the cystenterostomy. Although it has been reported, direct endoscopic necrosectomy does not need to be done at the time of the index drainage procedure once temporary drainage is established and it may increase the risk of dehiscence between the pseudocyst and GI lumen. Subsequent debridement can be performed through a mature tract (2–4 weeks minimum). Gardner and associates[43] reported a direct endoscopic necrosectomy success rate of 91% in a multicenter series of 104 patients with a mean time to resolution of 4.1 months, whereas Voermans and colleageus[44] reported a 93% success rate with no mortality in 25 patients who underwent the procedure.

For complex organized necrosis, a technique of creating 2 or more transluminal drainage sites to permit irrigation and drainage has been described in a small series. A cystenterostomy followed by 7-Fr double pigtail stent is performed. A second transmural drainage site as maximally distant from the initial site is identified by EUS-guidance and then balloon dilated to 15 mm followed by placement of multiple (2–4) double pigtail stents. A nasocystic catheter is placed through the initial transmural site with 200 mL of saline irrigated every 4 hours combined with patient position changes. This technique resulted in successful resolution in 11 of 12 (91%) patients.[45]

Efficacy

A study of 116 patients who underwent endoscopic drainage of pancreatic fluid collections by either transmural stenting alone, transpapillary stenting alone, or combined transmural and transpapillary stenting found no difference in efficacy between the 3 methods, although complications were higher in the transmural and

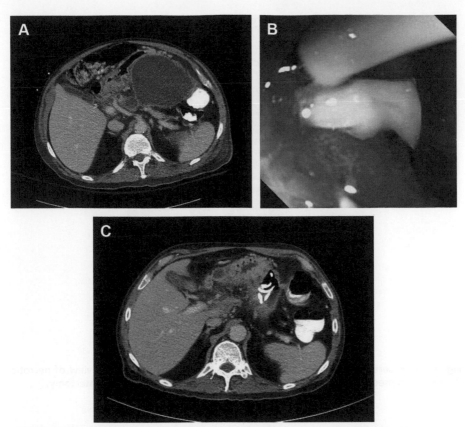

Fig. 5. (*A*) Mature pancreatic pseudocyst on CT before endoscopic drainage. (*B*) Purulent drainage after stent placement. (*C*) Nearly resolved pseudocyst after 3 days of transmural drainage and nasocystic flushing.

combined groups (10% and 17%, respectively). The authors reported a higher rate of recurrence with the combined approach compared with transpapillary or transmural drainage alone and suggested that the lack of maturation of a transenteric fistula in the setting of transpapillary stenting may explain the recurrence.[29] In this study, a transpapillary approach was used when the collection was less than 7 cm in diameter, if pancreatic duct obstruction such as a stricture or a stone was evident, and there was communication between the pancreatic duct and the cyst shown on pancreatography or preprocedural magnetic resonance cholangiopancreatography.[29] Limited data on treating pancreatic abscess by transpapillary saline irrigation have been reported.[46] The technique entails introduction of a 6-Fr catheter into the pseudocyst after pancreatography and saline irrigation until clearance of pus and contrast material is achieved, followed by 10-Fr stent placement into the abscess. In a small series of 15 patients, an average of 2.2 ERCPs per patient yielded resolution in 74% of the patients, which was comparable with the 76% in a similar cohort who underwent surgical drainage.[46]

For transmural drainage, our group prospectively reported that single-step EUS guidance was successful in 94% of pseudocysts despite 48% of the pseudocysts not displaying a visible endoscopic bulge.[35] Portal hypertension with gastric varices was

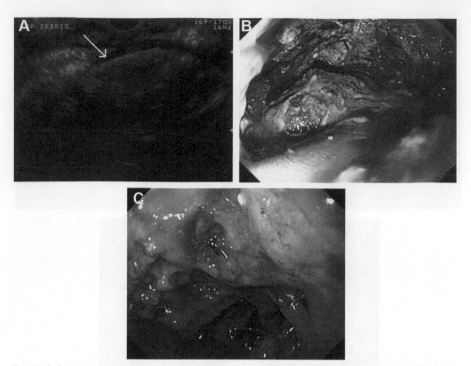

Fig. 6. (*A*) Hyperechoic necrotic debris within pseudocyst. (*B*) Endoscopic view of necrotic debris within pseudocyst. (*C*) Partial clearance of necrotic debris after necrosectomy.

also traditionally a contraindication for endoscopic drainage; however, 24% of our patients had perigastric varices.[35] Other groups have reported a similar ability to perform transenteric drainage in the setting of portal hypertension and intervening perigastric vessels.[47] Overall, endoscopic drainage has been found to be a good first-line therapy for drainage of pancreatic pseudocysts with complete resolution of pseudocysts in 71% to 95% of cases, complication rates of 0% to 37%, and procedure-related mortality rates of 0% to 1%, with most series reporting no procedural mortality.[23,24,29,31,32,36,48-52] Pseudocysts that arise in the setting of acute pancreatitis tend to respond better to endoscopic drainage than those arising in patients with chronic pancreatitis; however, in 1 study, higher success rates were actually seen in those patients with chronic pancreatitis (92% vs 74%), with the difference potentially related to timing of drainage in the acute pancreatitis group.[23,48,53]

It is well-recognized that fluid collections with necrosis have lower rates of success (25%–72%) and higher complication rates.[29,48] Drainage procedures in the group reporting the lowest success rate were performed an average of 23 days after the onset of disease and may reflect a more acutely ill population because of infection or deterioration of patient clinical condition, thus underscoring the importance of patient selection.[29] The presence of necrosis is further associated with pseudocyst recurrence, which may be as high as 29%, whereas pseudocysts related to chronic pancreatitis and acute pancreatitis without organized necrosis recur at a lower rate (12% and 9%, respectively).[31] An additional study of 92 patients found a 16% recurrence rate and multivariate analysis showed a significantly better outcome in those with stent duration longer than 6 weeks.[49] It seems that longer-term drainage is beneficial, probably because this allows the formation and continued maturation of the cystenterostomy, which permits ongoing drainage after stent removal.

SURGICAL DRAINAGE

Surgical management may include cystenterostomy, partial pancreatic resection, and combined laparoscopic–endoscopic interventions, depending on the extent of disease and local expertise.[19,54] Laparoscopic techniques, compared with conventional open surgery, offer lower morbidity, such as the anterior transgastric cystgastrostomy or the more common lesser sac posterior cystgastrostomy. Both may produce less bleeding and create a larger diameter anastomosis, thereby decreasing the incidence of occlusion and recurrence.[19,54] A compilation of studies covering 89 patients undergoing laparoscopic pseudocyst drainage (10% conversion rate to open) showed success in 95% of cases with 1% mortality and a 12% complication rate, results that are comparable with open surgical drainage procedures.[19] Similarly, Melman and colleagues[27] retrospectively compared outcomes of 83 patients who underwent cystgastrostomy from 1999 to 2007 by either open (n = 22), laparoscopic (n = 16), or endoscopic (n = 45) approaches and found comparable overall success rates of 94% for the laparoscopic transgastric approach and 91% for open cystgastrostomy, with no difference in complication rates between the open and laparoscopic groups.

Comparison of Endoscopic and Surgical Therapy

Several authors have directly compared the success and complication rates of endoscopic drainage with those of surgical therapy and have found them to be comparable.[23,24,27] Melman and colleagues[27] found that laparoscopic and open surgery had higher rates of primary success (88% and 81%, respectively), but their index endoscopic therapy success was unusually poor (51%), thus limiting its interpretation.[27] Several studies have found lesser rates of complications with endoscopic therapy as compared with surgery.[27,28,41] Additionally, in a tertiary referral center study of patients with simple pseudocysts (no abscess or necrosis) and matched comorbidities, Varadarajulu and colleagues[24] found that a lower mean postprocedural hospital stay (2.65 vs 6.5 days) and estimated direct cost savings per case of $5,738 were seen in the EUS-directed drainage group. This was evident despite the costs associated with patients in the EUS arm undergoing repeat CT for assessment of response to therapy and an additional endoscopy session for stent removal.[24] In complex pancreatic pseudocysts with manifestation of duodenal or biliary compression, endoscopic therapy may be employed, but surgical therapy can be considered first-line in appropriate patients.[23]

Percutaneous pseudocyst drainage

Percutaneous catheter drainage (PCD) of pancreatic fluid collections involves ultrasound- or CT-guided placement of a drainage catheter that may be used for frequent irrigation to maintain patency. The catheter is kept in place until the daily flow decreases to 5 to 10 mL with repeat CT to confirm that the catheter tip remains in the pseudocyst cavity. Percutaneous transgastric internal drainage has also been performed; however, it is less well-studied.[5]

Studies comparing PCD with surgical management are somewhat difficult to interpret, because they are predominately retrospective and few clearly define treatment failure. They show poor success rates (42% vs 74%) with unacceptably high complication (16% vs 74%) and mortality rates (0% vs 16%); most conclude that surgical therapy is preferred.[25,53,55–58] One study found PCD as effective as surgical management, but noted a mean duration of catheter drainage of 42 days with 48% of patients experiencing catheter tract infection requiring antibiotic therapy.[58] Other authors have suggested that operative management was superior to PCD because many patients with unsuccessful PCD required urgent operative pancreatic debridement because of sepsis or clinical deterioration.[56] PCD is less effective in multiple/loculated pseudocysts; if ductal communication is present, then prolonged drainage time may occur, which increases the risk for developing pancreaticocutaneous fistula.[5,56–58] PCD has not been directly compared with endoscopic therapy, but it seems that in patients who are at high risk for operative or endoscopic procedures, PCD is a reasonable choice.

Complications

The major complications of endoscopic pseudocyst drainage include immediate or delayed infection (0%–8%), bleeding (0%–9%), retroperitoneal perforation (0%–5%), and lack of resolution (6%–14%).[29,32,34,36,49,52,59] Infection is the most common complication and is caused by contamination of an incompletely drained pseudocyst from premature stent occlusion or uneven collapse. We emphasize that associated pancreatic necrosis is a major risk factor for infection and failure of endoscopic pseudocyst drainage.[44,48,60] Intensive endotherapy, if warranted based on index imaging, is required to successfully treat infectious complications that arise from retained debris.

Bleeding from transmural drainage represents the greatest risk of mortality, and transpapillary stenting has higher rates of postprocedural pancreatitis.[5,31,32] It is critical to avoid puncturing a pseudoaneurysm, because it can cause severe, life-threatening bleeding. All patients should undergo a careful search for pseudoaneurysms with dynamic bolus high-resolution CT scanning before attempted drainage. If equivocal, predrainage Doppler ultrasonography or angiography is required. Use of EUS guidance with Doppler imaging can also decrease the risk of inadvertent vascular puncture. For non-EUS approaches, bleeding from the gastric or duodenal wall after puncture can be minimized by keeping steady position during ENL and avoiding a "stroking" motion during needle-knife puncture. If bleeding does occur, it can generally be managed with endoscopic injection of 1:10,000 epinephrine, endoscopic electrocautery, and hemostatic clips.

Retroperitoneal perforation is another serious complication that has been reduced with the use of ENL and EUS guidance. If the pseudocyst wall is poorly defined or has a distance of more than 1 cm from the intestinal lumen, the risk of perforation and leakage of pseudocyst contents into the peritoneum are greater, and puncture should be avoided.

SUMMARY

Techniques of endoscopic pseudocyst management continue to evolve, but the principles of proper patient selection and careful consideration of the available therapeutic options remain unchanged. Endoscopic management is considered first-line therapy in the treatment of symptomatic pseudocysts. Clinicians should be vigilant in the evaluation of all peripancreatic fluid collections to exclude the presence of a pancreatic cystic neoplasm and avoid draining an immature collection. Expectant management with periodic observation should be considered for the minimally symptomatic patients, even after the traditional 6 weeks of maturation. Further, symptoms, complications, and expansion on serial imaging should prompt intervention by endoscopic, surgical, or percutaneous methods.

Pseudocysts should only be punctured when the wall has had sufficient time to mature and after pseudoaneurysm has been ruled out by careful imaging. Small to moderately sized pseudocysts (<4–6 cm) that communicate with the pancreatic duct are good candidates for endoscopic transpapillary stenting. For larger lesions requiring transmural drainage, EUS guidance is preferable, but good results can be achieved with ENL. EUS may be particularly useful in permitting drainage in patients with suspected perigastric varices or if an endoscopically visible bulge is not apparent. Necrosis is a significant factor for a worse outcome; aggressive debridement with nasocystic or percutaneous endoscopic gastrostomy–cystic catheter lavage plus manual endoscopic techniques for clearing debris should be used. Endoscopic failure, especially in cases with significant necrosis, should be managed operatively. Percutaneous drainage is a good option for immature infected pseudocysts or in patients who are not optimal candidates for other procedures. Close cooperation between endoscopists, surgeons, interventional radiologists, and other healthcare providers is paramount in successfully managing these patients.

REFERENCES

1. Bradley EL III. A clinically based classification system for acute pancreatitis. Summary of the International Symposium on Acute Pancreatitis. Arch Surg 1993;128:586–90.
2. O'Malley VP, Cannon JP, Postier RG. Pancreatic pseudocysts: cause, therapy, and results. Am J Surg 1985;150:680–2.
3. Bradley EL III, Clements JL Jr, Gonzalez AC. The natural history of pancreatic pseudocysts: a unified concept of management. Am J Surg 1979;137:135–41.
4. Grace P, Williamson R. Modern management of pancreatic pseudocysts. Br J Surg 1993;80:573–81.
5. Pitchumoni CS, Agarwal N. Pancreatic pseudocysts. When and how should drainage be performed? Gastroenterol Clin North Am 1999;28:615–39.
6. Bradley EL III, Gonzalez AC, Clements JL Jr. Acute pancreatic pseudocysts: incidence and implications. Ann Surg 1976;184:734–7.
7. Warshaw AL, Compton CC, Lewandrowski, et al. Cystic tumors of the pancreas. Ann Surg 1990;212:432–43.
8. Turner BG, Brugge WR. Pancreatic cystic lesions: when to watch, when to operate, and when to ignore. Curr Gastroenterol Rep 2010;12:98–105.
9. Ahmad NA, Kochman ML, Lewis JD, et al. Can EUS alone differentiate between malignant and benign cystic lesions of the pancreas? Am J Gastroenterol 2001;96:3295–300.
10. Sand JA, Hyoty AK, Mattlla J, el al. Clinical assessment compared with cyst fluid analysis in the differential diagnosis of cystic lesions of the pancreas. Surgery 1996;119:275–80.
11. Chalian H, Tore HG, Miller FH, et al. CT attenuation of unilocular pancreatic cystic lesions to differentiate pseudocysts from mucin-containing cysts. JOP 2011;12:384–8.
12. Macari M, Finn ME, Bennett GL, et al. Differentiating pancreatic cystic neoplasms from pancreatic pseudocysts at MR imaging: value of perceived internal debris. Radiology 2009;251:77–84.
13. Brugge WR, Lewandrowski K, Lee-Lewandrowski E, et al. Diagnosis of pancreatic cystic neoplasms: a report of the cooperative pancreatic cyst study. Gastroenterology 2004;126:1330–6.

14. Van der Waaij LA, van Dulleman HM, Porte RJ. Cyst fluid analysis in the differential diagnosis of pancreatic cystic lesions: a pooled analysis. Gastrointest Endosc 2005; 62:383–9.

15. Haab BB, Porter A, Yue T, et al. Glycosylation variants of mucins and CEACAMs as candidate biomarkers for the diagnosis of pancreatic cystic neoplasms. Ann Surg 2010;251:937–45.

16. Vitas GJ, Sarr MG. Selected management of pancreatic pseudocysts: operative versus expectant management. Surgery 1992;111:123–30.

17. Yeo CJ, Bastidas JA, Lynch-Nyham A, et al. The natural history of pancreatic pseudocysts documented by computed tomography. Surg Gynecol Obstet 1990; 170:411–7.

18. Cheruvu CVN, Clarke MG, Prentice M, et al. Conservative treatment as an option in the management of pancreatic pseudocyst. Ann R Coll Surg Engl 2003;85:313–6.

19. Bergman S, Melvin WS. Operative and nonoperative management of pancreatic pseudocysts. Surg Clin North Am 2007;87:1447–60.

20. Beebe DS, Bubrick MP, Onstad GR, et al. Management of pancreatic pseudocysts. Surg Gynecol Obstet 1984;159:562–4.

21. Gouyon B, Levy P, Ruszniewski P, et al. Predictive factors in the outcome of pseudocysts complicating alcoholic chronic pancreatitis. Gut 1997;41:821–5.

22. Nguyen BL, Thompson JS, Edney JA, et al. Influence of the etiology of pancreatitis on the natural history of pancreatic pseudocysts. Am J Surg 1991;162:527–30.

23. Johnson MD, Walsh RM, Henerson JM, et al. Surgical versus non-surgical management of pancreatic pseudocysts. J Clin Gastroenterol 2009;43:586–90.

24. Varadarajulu S, Lopes TL, Wilcox CM, et al. EUS versus surgical cyst-gastrostomy for management of pancreatic pseudocysts. Gastrointest Endosc 2008;68:649–55.

25. Andersson B, Nilsson E, Willner J, et al. Treatment and outcome in pancreatic pseudocysts. Scand J Gastroenterol 2006;6:751–6.

26. Lawrence C, Howell DA, Stefan AM, et al. Disconnected pancreatic tail syndrome: potential for endoscopic therapy and results of long term follow-up. Gastrointest Endosc 2008;67:673–9.

27. Melman L, Azar R, Beddow K, et al. Primary and overall success rates for clinical outcomes after laparoscopic, endoscopic, and open pancreatic cystsgastrostomy for pancreatic pseudocysts. Surg Endosc 2009;23:267–71.

28. Rosso E, Alexakis N, Ghaneh P, et al. Pancreatic pseudocyst in chronic pancreatitis: endoscopic and surgical treatment. Dig Surg 2003;397–406.

29. Hookey LC, Debroux S, Delhaye M, et al. Endoscopic drainage of pancreatic-fluid collections in 116 patients: a comparison of etiologies, drainage techniques, and outcomes. Gastrointest Endosc 2006;63:635–43.

30. American Society for Gastrointestinal Endoscopy. Guidelines for antibiotic prophylaxis for GI endoscopy. Gastrointest Endosc 2008;67:791–7.

31. Catalano MF, Geenen JE, Schmalz MJ, et al. Treatment of pancreatic pseudocysts with ductal communication by transpapillary pancreatic duct endoprosthesis. Gastrointest Endosc 1995;42:214–8.

32. Binmoeller KF, Seifert H, Walter A, et al. Transpapillary and transmural drainage of pancreatic pseudocysts. Gastrointest Endosc 1995;42:219–24.

33. Howell DA, Holbrook RF, Bosco JJ et al. Endoscopic needle localization of pancreatic pseudocysts before transmural drainage. Gastrointest Endosc 1993;39:693–8.

34. Mönkemüller KE, Baron TH, Morgan DE. Transmural drainage of pancreatic fluid collections without electrocautery using the Seldinger technique. Gastrointest Endosc 1998;48:195–200.

35. Antillon MR, Shah RJ, Stiegmann G, et al. Single-step EUS-guided transmural drainage of simple and complicated pancreatic pseudocysts. Gastrointest Endosc 2006;63:797–803.
36. Kahaleh M, Shami VM, Conaway MR, et al. Endoscopic ultrasound drainage of pancreatic pseudocyst: a prospective comparison with conventional endoscopic drainage. Endoscopy 2006;38:355–9.
37. Varadarajulu S, Wilcox CM, Tamhane A, et al. Role of EUS in drainage of peripancreatic fluid collections not amenable for endoscopic transmural drainage. Gastrointest Endosc 2007;66:1107–19.
38. Fockens P, Johnson TG, van Dullemen HM, et al. Endosonographic imaging of pancreatic pseudocysts before endoscopic transmural drainage. Gastrointest Endosc 1997;46:412–6.
39. Binmoeller KF, Weilert F, Marson F, et al. EUS-Guided transluminal drainage of pancreatic pseudocysts using the NAVIX access device and two plastic stents: initial clinical experience. Gastrointest Endosc 2011;73:AB331.
40. Talreja JP, Shami VM, Ku J, et al. Transenteric drainage of pancreatic–fluid collections with fully covered self-expanding metal stents. Gastrointest Endosc 2008;68:1199–203.
41. Soliani P, Franzini C, Ziegler S, et al. Pancreatic pseudocysts following acute pancreatitis: risk factors influencing therapeutic outcomes. JOP 2004;5:338–47.
42. Varadarajulu S, Bang JY, Phadnis MA, et al. Endoscopic transmural drainage of peripancreatic fluid collections: outcomes and predictors of treatment success in 211 consecutive patients. J Gastrointest Surg 2011;15:2080–8.
43. Gardner TB, Coelho-Prabhun N, Gordon SR, et al. Direct endoscopic necrosectomy for the treatment of walled-off pancreatic necrosis: results from a multicenter U.S. series. Gastrointest Endosc 2011;73:718–26.
44. Voermans RP, Veldkamp MC, Rauws EA, et al. Endoscopic transmural debridement of symptomatic organized pancreatic necrosis. Gastrointest Endosc 2007;66:909–16.
45. Varadarajulu S, Phadnis MA, Christein JD, et al. Multiple transluminal gateway technique for EUS-guided drainage of symptomatic walled-off pancreatic necrosis. Gastrointest Endosc 2011;74:74–80.
46. Venu RP, Brown RD, Marrero JA, et al. Endoscopic transpapillary drainage of pancreatic abscess: technique and results. Gastrointest Endosc 2000;51:391–5.
47. Sriram PVJ, Kaffes AJ, Rao GV, et al. Endoscopic ultrasound-guided drainage of pancreatic pseudocysts complicated by portal hypertension or by intervening vessels. Endoscopy 2005;37:231–5.
48. Baron TH, Harewood GC, Morgan DE, et al. Outcome differences after endoscopic drainage of pancreatic necrosis, acute pancreatic pseudocysts, and chronic pancreatic pseudocysts. Gastrointest Endosc 2002;56:7–17.
49. Cahen D, Rauws E, Fockens P, et al. Endoscopic drainage of pancreatic pseudocysts: long-term outcome and procedural factors associated with safe and successful treatment. Endoscopy 2005;37:977–83.
50. Giovannini M, Pesenti C, Rolland AL, et al. Endoscopic ultrasound-guided drainage of pancreatic pseudocysts or pancreatic abscesses using a therapeutic echo endoscope. Endoscopy 2001;33:473–7.
51. Barthet M, Sahel J, Bodiou-Bertei C, et al. Endoscopic transpapillary drainage of pancreatic pseudocysts. Gastrointest Endosc 1995;42:208–13.
52. Weckman L, Kylanpaa ML, Puolakkainen P, et al. Endoscopic treatment of pancreatic pseudocysts. Surg Endosc 2006;20:603–7.

53. Morton JM, Brown A, Galanko JA, et al. A national comparison of surgical versus percutaneous drainage of pancreatic pseudocysts: 1997-2001. J Gastrointest Surg 2004;9:15–20.

54. Park AE, Heniford BT. Therapeutic laparoscopy of the pancreas. Ann Surg 2002;236: 149–58.

55. Heider R, Meyer AA, Galanko JA, et al. Percutaneous drainage of pancreatic pseudo-cysts is associated with a higher failure rate than surgical treatment in unselected patients. Ann Surg 1999;229:781–9.

56. Spivak H, Galloway JR, Amerson JR, et al. Management of pancreatic pseudocysts. J Am Coll Surg 1998;186:507–11.

57. Nealon WH, Walser E. Main pancreatic ductal anatomy can direct choice of modality for treating pancreatic pseudocysts (surgery versus percutaneous drainage). Ann Surg 2002;235:751–8.

58. Adams DB, Anderson MC. Percutaneous catheter drainage compared with internal drainage in the management of pancreatic pseudocyst. Ann Surg 1992;215:571–8.

59. Kruger M, Schneider AS, Manns MP, et al. Endoscopic management of pancreatic pseudocysts or abscesses after an EUS-guided 1-step procedure for initial access. Gastrointest Endosc 2006;63:409–16.

60. Hariri M, Slivka A, Carr-Locke DL, et al. Pseudocyst drainage predisposes to infection when pancreatic necrosis is unrecognized. Am J Gastroenterol 1989;10:1781–4.

Modern Treatment of Patients with Chronic Pancreatitis

Guru Trikudanathan, MD[a], Udayakumar Navaneethan, MD[b],
Santhi Swaroop Vege, MD[c],*

KEYWORDS

- Chronic pancreatitis • Pain relief • Exocrine insufficiency
- Pancreatogenic diabetes

Chronic pancreatitis (CP) is a progressive fibroinflammatory process of the pancreas in which the pancreatic secretory parenchyma is damaged and replaced by fibrous tissue, resulting in morphologic changes of the ducts and parenchyma. This process eventually culminates in permanent impairment of the pancreas's exocrine and endocrine function. The reported incidence of CP in industrialized countries has been estimated at 3.5 to 10 per 100,000 person-years.[1] Two forms of CP are recognized: a large-duct type and a small-duct variant both with or without calcification. Approximately 40 to 50% of patients with CP develop chronic exocrine pancreatic insufficiency resulting in maldigestion and malabsorption, which are characterized by diarrhea, steatorrhea, and weight loss.

Despite the evolution of new medications and emergence of novel techniques, a clear consensus on the optimal management of CP still eludes us. In this review, the authors focus on the modern management of CP and its resultant complications, including chronic abdominal pain, pancreatic exocrine insufficiency, malabsorption, malnutrition, pancreatic endocrine insufficiency, diabetes mellitus, and labile glycemic control.

PAIN MANAGEMENT

Chronic disabling pain, which poses a major detriment to the quality of life, is present in nearly 80% to 90% of patients with CP and is the inciting symptom in nearly 93% of admissions.[1] This high incidence of pain has resulted in an inordinate utilization of health care resources, with the financial burden estimated to be in excess of $638

All authors contributed equally to the manuscript.
The authors declare no conflict of interest.
The authors confirm that there is no financial arrangement with anybody or any institution.
[a] Department of Internal Medicine, University of Connecticut Medical Center, Farmington, CT, USA
[b] Digestive Disease Institute, The Cleveland Clinic, 9500 Euclid Avenue, Cleveland, OH 44195, USA
[c] Division of Gastroenterology, Mayo Clinic, Rochester, MN, USA
* Corresponding author.
E-mail address: vege.santhi@mayo.edu

million annually.[2] The expression of pain ranges from a conspicuous absence to very severe. In the two well differentiated patterns that are typical, one pattern consists of repeated flare-ups of pancreatitis separated by pain-free interval. The other pattern consists of prolonged periods of persistent pain with exacerbations, with relatively few days of pain-free days in between. A recently reported large multicentric prospective study suggested that patients who experience constant pain have significantly lower quality of life and greater rates of disability and resource utilization than patients who experience intermittent pain.[3]

Previously, it was thought that pancreatic pain decreases in intensity and frequency as the disease evolves, and a spontaneous resolution of pain occurs with the eventual "burnout."[4] It is now firmly established that repeated inflammation and insult to the pancreas progress to irreversible damage for which the management of pain becomes less effective. It is therefore critical to intervene as early as possible to halt or even reverse progression.[5] The pathobiology of pain still remains enigmatic, but putative pathogenetic factors include perineural inflammation, fibrotic encasement of sensory nerves, increased pressure within the ductal system and parenchyma, recurrent ischemia of the parenchyma, and abnormal feedback mechanisms. Other hypotheses include proliferation of unmyelinated nerve fiber and upregulation of pain mediators such as substance P and calcitonin gene-related peptide and nerve growth factor–dependent nociceptors.[6] In addition, local complications, such as acute pseudocyst, bile duct entrapment and duodenal stenosis, could exacerbate the pain.[7,8] Last, patients with CP have a high incidence of dysmotility, which can become aggravated with concomitant narcotic use.[9]

Recognizing the underlying cause of CP is paramount, because identifying possible interventions to reduce the progressive pancreatic damage is the first step in alleviating pain. Alcohol abuse has been recognized as the most common cause of CP; therefore, cessation of alcohol consumption can slow the progression of disease and have some beneficial effect on pain.[10–12] A few studies, however, have refuted this association, reporting that continued use of alcohol has no effect on pain severity.[3,4] Heavy alcohol abuse is associated with constant pain patterns, whereas abstinence from alcohol is associated with intermittent pain patterns. Recently, smoking has been independently implicated in CP, progression to calcifications, and functional impairment.[13–15] Hence, smoking cessation has been strongly encouraged. Further studies have demonstrated that being proactive in addressing abstinence is more efficacious than simple office-based advice.[16]

Further, it is imperative to systematically look for disease states or complications related to CP that could potentiate this pain. These factors include conditions such as gastroparesis and pancreatic cancer, as well as complications such as pseudocyst and duodenal or biliary obstruction. The distinction between large-duct and small-duct CP has important implications for guiding therapeutic choices. In general, all patients may benefit from medical therapy, endoscopy or surgery is needed for large-duct disease and surgery for small duct disease.

Nonspecific Supportive Therapy

Analgesic medications are still the most commonly adopted method for pain relief. Although the reluctance to use narcotics is understandable, the primary focus should be on the relief of pain and not the risk of dependence. All management guidelines for pain in CP follow the World Health Organization's three-step ladder for the treatment of chronic pain. The treatment should be initiated with monotherapy, either acetaminophen or nonsteroidal antiinflammatory drug, or both. If there is insufficient effect, a combination therapy—peripherally acting medication with centrally acting medication—is considered. A nonopioid analgesic is combined with a weak opioid, such as tramadol. A simple pain diary with a 10-cm visual analog scale is useful, both as a baseline quality-of-life assessment and for titration of the analgesics. Analgesics are coupled with a neuroleptic antidepressant for concurrent depression. In this regard, tricyclic antidepressants, selective serotonin reuptake inhibitors, and combined serotonin and norepinephrine reuptake inhibitors (duloxetine) are definitely worth a therapeutic trial. In a recent placebo-controlled trial, pregabalin was shown to be an effective adjuvant therapy for pain in patients with CP.[17,18]

A recent pilot study evaluated the utility of intrathecal narcotic infusion pumps as an alternative to aggressive surgical interventions such as total pancreatectomy. In this study, pumps were offered to 13 patients who were deemed to have intractable pain characterized by persistent severe pain (median duration of 6 years) despite high-dose narcotics, frequent hospitalization, jejunal feedings, and endoscopic retrograde cholangiopancreatography sphincter therapy. Overall, 10 of 13 (76.9%) had a 1-year decline in pain score from 8.3 to 2.7 and median narcotic usage from 337.5 to 40 mg per day. Although the infusion pump carries risk, the potential benefits of bringing relief to these patients with intractable painful CP cannot be ignored.[19]

Enzyme Supplementation

The suspected mechanism for pain relief after administration of oral pancreatic enzymes is through negative feedback inhibition to the pancreas. In CP, consequent to damage to the acinar cells, there is a diminished secretion of pancreatic trypsin and hence, insufficient denaturing of the cholecystokinin-releasing peptide. This mechanism leads to uninterrupted potentiation of cholecystokinin (CCK), which causes hyperstimulation of the pancreas and leads to basolateral secretion rather than apical secretion of pancreatic enzymes, or both. Increased pressure in the setting of pancreatic ductal obstruction causes pain. By supplementing active proteases to the feedback-sensitive portion of the small bowel (duodenum), CCK secretion, and hence pancreatic secretion, is reduced.[20] To date, there are six randomized trials wherein two studies using a nonenteric-coated enzyme preparation reported benefit,[21,22] and the other four studies using an enteric-coated capsule showed no effect on pain in CP.[23-26] The enteric-coated preparations are not active in the duodenum and therefore cannot degrade CCK-releasing factor. The nonenteric-coated preparations should be administered along with acid suppressants such as a proton pump inhibitor or H_2 receptor blocker, because they are otherwise susceptible to degradation in the stomach by gastric acids before they reach the duodenum. A metaanalysis of the six randomized double- blind placebo-controlled trials involving both enteric-coated and nonenteric-coated preparations for the treatment of CP showed no real benefit of either preparation.[27] Nevertheless, the role of pancreatic enzymes in mitigating pain still remains unclear. However, experts recommend a 6-week trial of nonenteric pancreatic enzyme for small-duct disease.[5] If patients respond, they should continue until a 6-month pain-free interval has been achieved, because nearly 50% of patients relapse upon withdrawal of the supplements.

Octreotide

Octreotide, a synthetic long-acting somatostatin analogue, inhibits pancreatic secretions directly and also indirectly by blocking CCK and secretin release. In experimental models it has been shown to have antiinflammatory properties and to alter the cytokine milieu; it may also protect pancreatic cells. Octreotide is known to lower the intraductal pressure in pancreatic ductal obstruction and decrease proteolysis. A more recent pilot study showed that a once-monthly long-acting octreotide depo preparation is a useful substitute for the three times daily short-acting octreotide in the management of pain in CP.[28] Experts, however, have warned of the increased risk of hypoglycemia or poorer glucose control in persons with diabetes. Since octreotide predisposes to biliary stasis, patients need to be closely monitored for biliary stones.[5] Overall, octreotide therapy has not been accepted widely due to the above reasons and because its effectiveness could not be demonstrated consistently.[29,30]

Antioxidant Therapy

Free radicals and oxidative stress have been implicated in the pathogenesis of CP.[31] A decreased plasma concentration of antioxidants due to reduced micronutrient intake (vitamin E, riboflavin, choline, magnesium, copper, manganese and sulfur) has been demonstrated in an Indian study.[32] This result was attributed to the dietary modifications secondary to pain as well as to reduced caloric intake, thereby contributing to oxidative stress both in alcoholic and nonalcoholic pancreatitis. A modest improvement in pain with an antioxidant cocktail (L-methionine, β-carotene, vitamin C, vitamin E, and organic selenium) has been demonstrated in a randomized controlled study.[33] The benefit of combined antioxidant therapy for 20 weeks was also reported by a different group.[34] Allopurinol, which reduces the formation of oxygen radicals by inhibiting xanthine oxidase, was investigated in a crossover double-blind study and was found to be effective.[35] Another study in which allopurinol was combined with intramuscular pethidine showed a significantly superior effect as compared with pethidine alone.[36] However, due to lack of other effective therapies and at least one good randomized control trial, antioxidants are currently administered to most patients with CP.

Nerve Block for Pain Relief

Unfortunately, a substantial group of patients have CP that is refractory to conventional treatment, and other forms of pain relief have been explored. In this regard, celiac plexus blockade (CPB) and celiac plexus neurolysis (CPN) are used to disrupt the signaling of the pancreatic nociceptive afferent to the spinal cord in an effort to diminish pancreatic-induced abdominal pain. CPN refers to permanent ablation of the celiac plexus, often achieved with alcohol or phenol administered with local anesthetic such as bupivacaine. However, CPN is restricted to control of refractory pain for malignant indications, given the potential risk of retroperitoneal fibrosis. CPB, on the other hand, refers to the temporary inhibition of celiac plexus achieved with a corticosteroid in combination with bupivacaine for a more sustained analgesic effect.

Before the advent of widespread use of computed tomography (CT) and endoscopic ultrasound (EUS), CPB was performed through a posterior (blind translumbar) approach, with a risk of serious complications including paraplegia and pneumothorax in 1% of cases. This risk led to the emergence of the anterior approach under the guidance of transcutaneous, CT-guided, or EUS-guided techniques. EUS-guided CPB has been shown to be superior to fluoroscopic-guided percutaneous technique. Better localization of the celiac plexus and targeted injection into the celiac plexus allows substantial pain relief for a greater duration of time.[37] In a small random prospective comparison of 22 patients managed with either EUS-guided CPB or CT-guided CPB, EUS-guided CPB provided more initial (50% compared with 25%) and persistent (30% compared with 12%) pain relief than CT-guided CPB.[38] In a follow-up prospective study of 90 patients with refractory CP pain, all of whom received EUS-guided CPB, the same investigators reported that pain reduction was achieved in 55% patients at a mean follow-up of 8 weeks, whereas 10% experienced persistent relief at 24 weeks. However, EUS-guided CPB is less effective in younger patients as well as in those with previous pancreatic surgery.[39] This result was further corroborated by a recent metaanalysis of six studies of EUS-guided CPB (n = 221 patients), which reported relief of pain by CPB in 51.5%.

From these studies, it was felt that EUS-guided CPB, a relatively effective outpatient procedure, for CP pain.[38,39] CPB may provide temporary respite from pain for patients and also allow some temporary downward titration of dose and potency of narcotic analgesics.[5] A recent prospective randomized trial comparing bilateral (two injections) to central (one injection) EUS-guided CPB did not show a difference in duration or time to onset of pain relief between the two arms of the trial.[40] Identification of predictors for response to CPB is essential for appropriate selection of patients. Until then, EUS-guided CPB should be restricted to treating flares of chronic pain in patients with otherwise limited therapeutic options as it can be rarely associated with major complications.

Thoracoscopic-directed sectioning of splanchnic nerves (either unilateral or bilateral approach) is another neurolysis technique that has been explored. Previous opioid use, which is common in this group of patients, is known to impact analgesia after splanchnicectomy.[41] Splanchnicectomy may not be feasible in all patients and, because of its poor long-term efficacy, it is used rarely and as a last resort.[41,42]

Endoscopic Therapy for Pain

Elevated pressure in the main pancreatic duct allegedly causes changes in parenchymal blood flow and pH, resulting in tissue ischemia and pain.[43] There is an inconsistent relationship between pancreatic anatomy and pain severity. The aim of endoscopic therapy is to relieve the obstruction of the pancreatic duct and to reduce pressure in the pancreatic duct and pancreas. Pancreatic duct decompression via endoscopic retrograde cholangiopancreatography includes the dilatation and stenting of pancreatic duct strictures, which is usually preceded by pancreatic sphincterotomy, and removal of obstructing pancreatic duct stones. Endoscopic therapy is most appropriate in the presence of a single obstructing lesion (stricture or stone), with ductal dilation upstream from the site of obstruction, and preferably with the stone smaller than 1 cm that is located in the main pancreatic duct, not too numerous or tightly impacted, and easily amenable to endoscopic manipulation.[5] Other indications for endoscopy include drainage of pseudocyst, treatment of a benign stricture of the distal bile duct due to compression from the fibrotic process in the head of the pancreas, or treatment of pancreatic duct disruption.

In one of the largest series consisting of 1018 retrospectively identified patients followed for 5 years, endoscopic intervention (pancreatic stricture dilatation, stone extraction, or pancreatic duct sphincterotomy) resulted in pain relief in 86% in the entire group but only 65% in an intention-to-treat analysis. Over this same time, one-quarter of the patients required surgery because of failure of endoscopic therapy.[44] The pain secondary to tropical pancreatitis seems to respond better to endoscopic therapy than does pain from alcoholic pancreatitis.[45]

Extracorporeal shockwave lithotripsy (ESWL) is useful for rapid fragmentation of pancreatic ductal stones to facilitate endoscopic extraction. A metaanalysis of 17 studies concluded that ESWL is effective for the relief of main pancreatic duct obstruction and amelioration of pain in chronic calcific pancreatitis in combination with endoscopic therapy.[46] A more recent randomized trial that compared ESWL alone to ESWL followed by endoscopic removal of stones found equal efficacy in pain relief between the two arms of the study in patients with chronic calcific pancreatitis. The duration of hospital stay was shorter and the need for subsequent invasive procedures was smaller in ESWL alone, resulting in better cost effectiveness (three times lower cost in the ESWL-alone group). The investigators speculated that ESWL may have a "stunning" effect on nociceptive neurons or some other mechanisms of pain in addition to the obvious dissolution of stone. They also commented that patients with calcifications confined to the head of the pancreas are most likely to benefit from this treatment.[47]

Intraductal lithotripsy, although extremely popular for the management of difficult common bile duct stone, is rarely used for managing pancreatic calcifications. The success rate is less than 10% for pancreatic ductal stones.[48] A larger multicentric trial reported a complication rate of nearly 12%, which is three times the complication rate for biliary lithotripsy.[49] Therefore, intraductal lithotripsy is used as a second-line option in cases in which ESWL fails to fragment the obstructive stones.

An alternative to ESWL involves the use of endoprostheses or stents placed in the pancreatic duct endoscopically. Three large retrospective studies have established the utility of stents in pain relief.[50–52] The latest study with a longer follow-up period concluded that 70% of patients with severe CP who respond to pancreatic stenting maintain this response after definitive stent removal. However, a significantly higher restenting rate was observed in patients with CP and pancreas divisum.[51] The benefit of placing multiple sequential stents has been recently evaluated. During a mean follow-up of 38 months, 84% of patients with multiple stents (median of three stents) were asymptomatic, and only 11% experienced a symptomatic recurrence.[53] Thus, endoscopic multiple stenting of a dominant pancreatic duct stricture seems to be feasible and promising.

Endoscopic therapy can be technically demanding with results that are highly operator-dependent; therefore, reports from expert centers cannot be easily extrapolated to centers with smaller volume or less experience.

Surgery

For patients who do not respond to medical therapy, surgical therapy is emerging as a viable option, particularly for patients with a clear correctible anatomic abnormality. Goals of surgery are to decompress the obstructed ducts (to eradicate pain) and to preserve pancreatic tissue and adjacent organs (to preserve function). The modified Puestow procedure, or lateral pancreaticojejunostomy, is a relatively simple procedure that is commonly performed. Ductal strictures are incised, allowing any ductal stones to be removed. Short-term pain relief is seen in about 80% of patients; however, long-term relief drops to 50% in about 5 years.

The classic Whipple procedure is also used for the excision of the inflammatory pancreatic head masses. It is curative, with complete resolution of symptoms in groove pancreatitis, and is also considered if there is a duodenal obstruction or if cancer cannot be excluded preoperatively.[54] However, the Whipple procedure sacrifices an extensive portion of the functional pancreatic parenchyma. There have been many modifications to this procedure, such as the duodenum-preserving pancreatic head resection (Beger's procedure) and the Frey procedure, which aim to preserve the duodenum and pylorus. Both procedures are associated with low morbidity and mortality and demonstrate a high rate of sustained pain relief and return to productivity, in spite of the difference in the amount of pancreas excised.[55,56] Randomized trials comparing these two procedures found equal efficacy although beger's procedure is technically more demanding.[57] In general, although the immediate pain relief is similar in patients receiving the modified Puestow procedure, long-term relief seems to be superior at the expense of more perioperative and postoperative complications.[5] A recent analysis of mortality after pancreatectomy for

CP showed that proximal pancreatectomy was associated with a 2.5-fold increased risk of death compared with distal pancreatectomy.[58]

Recently, randomized trials have compared endotherapy to surgery for the treatment of painful large-duct CP. A prospective randomized controlled trial concluded that at 1 year, pain relief was similar in both groups. At 5 years, however, more patients who underwent surgery had complete absence of pain and greater weight gain than patients who underwent endotherapy (34% vs 15% and 47 vs 29%, respectively).[59] In this study, surgery encompassed more than just a drainage procedure, and endoscopic therapy did not include lithotripsy, which is currently the cornerstone of endoscopic drainage. But these findings were corroborated more recently by the Amsterdam group in a randomized trial comparing endoscopic lithotripsy to surgical drainage of pancreatic duct. In this study, although the rate of complications, length of stay, and changes in pancreatic function were similar in both groups, patients receiving endoscopic treatment required more procedures than the patients treated surgically (a median of 8 compared with 3 surgeries). At the end of the 24-month follow-up period, complete or partial pain relief was achieved in 32% of patients assigned to endoscopic drainage, as compared with 75% of patients assigned to the surgery group.[60] The same investigators published their latest 5-year outcome in a recent study, which further confirmed that surgery at the time of initial presentation was superior to lithotripsy and stenting, not only in terms of pain relief but also in terms of complications and required reinterventions, without being associated with higher costs.[61] These randomized trials, although criticized for methodological flaws, suggest that surgical therapy is superior and more durable compared with endoscopic therapy for selected CP patients with dilated pancreatic duct.

To summarize, operative approaches have dramatically evolved over the last few years, in that the head of the pancreas has been universally accepted as the nidus of chronic inflammation. The final choice of the appropriate procedure, however, should be guided by the experience of the individual surgeon and the center.

Total Pancreatectomy and Autologous Islet Cell Transplantation

The final surgical option is a total pancreatectomy in conjunction with harvesting islet cells and reinfusing these isolated cells through the portal vein into the liver, a procedure that is available in very few highly specialized pancreatic centers in the world.[62,63] This procedure is an attractive option for patients with hereditary pancreatitis, for prevention of pancreatic cancer that can be associated with CP, for the preservation of some endocrine function when eventual glandular depletion is inevitable, and as a last resort for treatment of refractory pain.[64] Currently, the procedure is being performed in patients with painful refractory small-duct disease (pancreatic duct is not dilated). Some experts consider this aggressive life-changing intervention as a trade of chronic refractory pain for lifelong brittle diabetes with all its inherent downstream complications.[64] In adults, 60% to 80% of patients who have undergone total pancreatectomy and autologous islet cell transplantation (TP/AICT) have a marked reduction in narcotic use.[62,63,65] Insulin independence is achieved in 40% of patients.[63] Previous pancreatic surgeries adversely affect the total yield and reduce the rate of postoperative insulin independence.[63,66] A recent study concluded that more severe histopathology staging of CP is associated with lower islet yield. Therefore, the investigators advocate that TP/AICT should not be delayed in patients with painful CP; otherwise, progressive damage to the pancreas may limit islet yield and increase the risk of diabetes.[67] If results are further improved, TP/AICT may become a promising option for those with small-duct diffuse inflammatory disease and at the present time more studies from other centers are needed to see if the results can be duplicated.

Other Modalities of Pain Relief

Yoga resulted in reduced pain, reduced use of analgesics, increased weight gain, and an improvement in quality of life in a study comparing patients with CP who were randomized to usual care by their physicians or to usual care plus yoga three times per week for a 12-week period.[68,69]

Among new medications, CCK-receptor antagonists seem to be promising. Proglumide, a nonspecific CCK-receptor antagonist, was noted to not only reverse tolerance to morphine and potentiate its effects but also to ameliorate pain on its own.[70] A few years later the therapeutic efficacy of loxiglumide, a CCK-A antagonist, was reaffirmed by multicenter dose response study in Japan.[71]

The antiinflammatory effects of radiotherapy were recognized nearly 5 decades ago in a Russian study showing sustained good response after 2 years in 66% of the 56 patients with CP who were treated with radiation.[72] A more recent prospective pilot trial of 15 consecutive patients treated with a single 8 Gy dose of radiation applied to the pancreatic area demonstrated that a single low dose of radiation was effective in preventing new flare-ups, in addition to alleviating pancreatic pain and improving quality of life in severely symptomatic patients, without significant side effects.[73]

PANCREATIC EXOCRINE INSUFFICIENCY

Clinicians, when focusing intently on pain, should not overlook the management of exocrine and endocrine insufficiency. A majority of patients with CP will develop pancreatic insufficiency at some point secondary to loss of pancreatic parenchyma. Pancreatic lipase secretion is lost faster than other secretions. It is believed that steatorrhea develops because of decreased luminal hydrolysis of dietary fat only when the lipase levels reach less than 10%. Traditionally, supplementing pancreatic enzymes is indicated in patients with steatorrhea (fecal fat greater than 15 g/d) and weight loss.[74] However, in clinical practice, measurement of fecal fat is seldom performed, and the decision for enzyme replacement is based on clinical assessment. A recent study showed that even patients with less than 15 g/d of steatorrhea benefit from enzyme substitution, assuring an adequate nutrition status.[75] Overall, enzyme supplementation improves coefficient of fat absorption as compared with placebo but may not clearly abolish steatorrhea and weight loss.[76,77] To prevent steatorrhoea in these patients, enzyme preparations should be able to deliver at least 30,000 IU of active lipase and preferably 48000 IU into the duodenum with meals; however, absorption is hindered by factors such as gastric acid secretion and nonparallel gastric emptying of nutrients and enzyme preparation.[78] To mimic the postprandial physiologic secretion of pancreatic enzymes in terms of amount and secretion pattern, a minimum dose of 40,000 to 50,000 U of lipase per meal is required.[74] Currently available data do not confirm if escalating dosage of pancreatic enzyme supplementation is routinely effective in decreasing fat malabsorption. However, a single well-designed placebo-controlled randomized control trial suggests that higher doses of enzyme supplements are better at reducing fat malabsorption.[79] Enzymes are most commonly derived from porcine pancreas, although bacterial lipases have been shown to be more stable than those derived from porcine sources.[80] Because oral lipases are rapidly degraded by gastric acid, the modern pancreatin preparations are engineered as acid-resistant pH-sensitive microspheres to allow mixing with food in the stomach. In cases of insufficient response, inhibition of gastric acid secretion with concomitant use of proton pump inhibitor is to be considered. One has to also advise about proper way of administration like taking them in between the meal and compliance as they are expensive. If there is no improvement with higher doses and PPI administration, then other causes like bacterial overgrowth need to be ruled out.

Nutrition in Chronic Pancreatitis

There is no specific diet for patients with pancreatitis. Traditionally, fat restriction has been recommended in the setting of CP. However, curtailing fat intake has been associated with insufficient intake of fat-soluble vitamins, which are inherently malabsorbed in CP.[74] Hence, fat restriction is no longer recommended. Consuming frequent small meals and avoiding food difficult to digest such as legumes are recommended. Although a fiber-rich diet seems to increase pancreatic secretion, it also inhibits pancreatic lipase secretion by more than 50%.[81] In patients with weight loss, medium-chain triglycerides, which are directly absorbed by the intestinal mucosa, may be useful for providing extra calories in patients with weight loss and for reducing steatorrhea in patients who are not responding adequately to pancreatic enzyme supplementation. Fat-soluble vitamins (A, D, E, and K), vitamin B_{12}, and micronutrients, including antioxidants, should be replaced as clinically indicated. Calcium and vitamin D supplements are indicated for vitamin D deficiency, even in the setting of pancreatic calcifications.

PANCREATIC ENDOCRINE INSUFFICIENCY

Pancreatogenic diabetes due to CP ranges in severity from mild to extreme. Although the predominant cause is relative or absolute insulin deficiency, other hormone deficiencies contribute to this form of diabetes. Pancreatic endocrine insufficiency secondary to CP is difficult to manage because of brittle fluctuations of hyperglycemia and hypoglycemia, particularly in patients with total or subtotal pancreatectomy.[82]

A variety of medications can be used in the management of diabetes, including sulfonylureas, metformin, and insulin; the initial choice depends on the clinical presentation. Patients with severe hyperglycemia with catabolic symptoms may require insulin as the preferred initial treatment, whereas patients with mild hyperglycemia without many symptoms can be treated initially with metformin.[82] Metformin is the initial drug of choice when oral treatment is warranted because of its insulin-lowering effects on glucose metabolism and also because of its specific antineoplastic actions on cellular mediators of replication and protein synthesis.[83]

Patients with persistent hyperglycemia can be treated initially with a different class of drug such as a thiazolidinedione or an alpha-glucosidase inhibitor. In patients with poor glycemic control despite maximum oral therapy, adjunctive treatment with insulin is required.

SUMMARY

CP remains a challenging disease. Endoscopic and surgical management, along with antioxidants, have helped in reducing chronic pain. Management of exocrine and endocrine insufficiency forms the cornerstone for improving nutrition in these patients. Newer therapeutic targets that will transcend the management of CP beyond just pain control and enzyme supplementation are required in the future.

REFERENCES

1. Thuluvath PJ, Imperio D, Nair S, et al. Chronic pancreatitis. Long-term pain relief with or without surgery, cancer risk, and mortality. J Clin Gastroenterol 2003; 36(2):159–65.

2. Everhart JE, Ruhl CE. Burden of digestive diseases in the United States Part III: liver, biliary tract, and pancreas. Gastroenterology 2009;136(4):1134–44.

3. Mullady DK, Yadav D, Amann ST, et al. Type of pain, pain-associated complications, quality of life, disability and resource utilisation in chronic pancreatitis: a prospective cohort study. Gut 2011;60(1):77–84.

4. Ammann RW, Muellhaupt B. The natural history of pain in alcoholic chronic pancreatitis. Gastroenterology 1999;116(5):1132–40.

5. Lieb JG 2nd, Forsmark CE. Pain and chronic pancreatitis. Aliment Pharmacol Ther 2009;29(7):706–19.

6. Di Sebastiano P, di Mola FF, Buchler MW, et al. Pathogenesis of pain in chronic pancreatitis. Dig Dis 2004;22(3):267–72.

7. Bradley EL 3rd. Pancreatic duct pressure in chronic pancreatitis. Am J Surg 1982; 144(3):313–6.

8. Makrauer FL, Antonioli DA, Banks PA. Duodenal stenosis in chronic pancreatitis: clinicopathological correlations. Dig Dis Sci 1982;27(6):525–32.

9. Gupta V, Toskes PP. Diagnosis and management of chronic pancreatitis. Postgrad Med J 2005;81(958):491–7.

10. de las Heras G, de la Peña J, López Arias MJ, et al. Drinking habits and pain in chronic pancreatitis. J Clin Gastroenterol 1995;20(1):33–6.

11. Strum WB. Abstinence in alcoholic chronic pancreatitis. Effect on pain and outcome. J Clin Gastroenterol 1995;20(1):37–41.

12. Hayakawa T, Kondo T, Shibata T, Sugimoto Y, Kitagawa M. Chronic alcoholism and evolution of pain and prognosis in chronic pancreatitis. Dig Dis Sci 1989;34(1):33–8.

13. Andriulli A, Botteri E, Almasio PL, et al. Smoking as a cofactor for causation of chronic pancreatitis: a meta-analysis. Pancreas 2010;39(8):1205–10.

14. Coté GA, Yadav D, Slivka A, et al. Alcohol and smoking as risk factors in an epidemiology study of patients with chronic pancreatitis. Clin Gastroenterol Hepatol 2011;9(3):266–73 [quiz: e27].

15. Law R, Parsi M, Lopez R, et al. Cigarette smoking is independently associated with chronic pancreatitis. Pancreatology 2010;10(1):54–9.

16. Nordback I, Pelli H, Lappalainen-Lehto R, et al. The recurrence of acute alcohol-associated pancreatitis can be reduced: a randomized controlled trial. Gastroenterology 2009;136(3):848–55.

17. Olesen SS, Bouwense SA, Wilder-Smith OH, et al. Pregabalin reduces pain in patients with chronic pancreatitis in a randomized, controlled trial. Gastroenterology 2011; 141(2):536–43.

18. Olesen SS, Graversen C, Olesen AE, et al. Randomised clinical trial: pregabalin attenuates experimental visceral pain through sub-cortical mechanisms in patients with painful chronic pancreatitis. Aliment Pharmacol Ther 2011;34(8):878–87.

19. Kongkam P, Wagner DL, Sherman S, et al. Intrathecal narcotic infusion pumps for intractable pain of chronic pancreatitis: a pilot series. Am J Gastroenterol 2009;104(5): 1249–55.

20. Owyang C, Louie DS, Tatum D. Feedback regulation of pancreatic enzyme secretion. Suppression of cholecystokinin release by trypsin. J Clin Invest 1986;77(6):2042–7.

21. Slaff J, Jacobson D, Tillman CR, et al. Protease-specific suppression of pancreatic exocrine secretion. Gastroenterology 1984;87(1):44–52.

22. Isaksson G, Ihse I. Pain reduction by an oral pancreatic enzyme preparation in chronic pancreatitis. Dig Dis Sci 1983;28(2):97–102.

23. Malesci A, Gaia E, Fioretta A, et al. No effect of long-term treatment with pancreatic extract on recurrent abdominal pain in patients with chronic pancreatitis. Scand J Gastroenterol 1995;30(4):392–8.

24. Halgreen H, Pedersen NT, Worning H. Symptomatic effect of pancreatic enzyme therapy in patients with chronic pancreatitis. Scand J Gastroenterol 1986;21(1): 104–8.
25. Mössner J, Secknus R, Meyer J, et al. Treatment of pain with pancreatic extracts in chronic pancreatitis: results of a prospective placebo-controlled multicenter trial. Digestion 1992;53(1–2):54–66.
26. Vecht J, Symersky T, Lamers CB, et al. Efficacy of lower than standard doses of pancreatic enzyme supplementation therapy during acid inhibition in patients with pancreatic exocrine insufficiency. J Clin Gastroenterol 2006;40(8):721–5.
27. Brown A, Hughes M, Tenner S, et al. Does pancreatic enzyme supplementation reduce pain in patients with chronic pancreatitis: a meta-analysis. Am J Gastroenterol 1997;92(11):2032–5.
28. Lieb JG 2nd, Shuster JJ, Theriaque D, et al. A pilot study of Octreotide LAR vs. octreotide tid for pain and quality of life in chronic pancreatitis. JOP 2009;10(5): 518–22.
29. Malfertheiner P, Mayer D, Büchler M, et al. Treatment of pain in chronic pancreatitis by inhibition of pancreatic secretion with octreotide. Gut 1995;36(3):450–4.
30. Uhl W, Anghelacopoulos SE, Friess H, et al. The role of octreotide and somatostatin in acute and chronic pancreatitis. Digestion 1999;60(Suppl 2):23–31.
31. Verlaan M, Roelofs HM, van-Schaik A, et al. Assessment of oxidative stress in chronic pancreatitis patients. World J Gastroenterol 2006;12(35):5705–10.
32. Bhardwaj P, Thareja S, Prakash S, et al. Micronutrient antioxidant intake in patients with chronic pancreatitis. Trop Gastroenterol 2004;25(2):69–72.
33. Bhardwaj P, Garg PK, Maulik SK, et al. A randomized controlled trial of antioxidant supplementation for pain relief in patients with chronic pancreatitis. Gastroenterology 2009;136(1):149–59.e2.
34. Kirk GR, White JS, McKie L, et al. Combined antioxidant therapy reduces pain and improves quality of life in chronic pancreatitis. J Gastrointest Surg 2006;10(4):499–503.
35. Banks PA, Hughes M, Ferrante M, et al. Does allopurinol reduce pain of chronic pancreatitis? Int J Pancreatol 1997;22(3):171–6.
36. McCloy R. Chronic pancreatitis at Manchester, UK. Focus on antioxidant therapy. Digestion 1998;59(Suppl 4):36–48.
37. Santosh D, Lakhtakia S, Gupta R, et al. Clinical trial: a randomized trial comparing fluoroscopy guided percutaneous technique vs. endoscopic ultrasound guided technique of coeliac plexus block for treatment of pain in chronic pancreatitis. Aliment Pharmacol Ther 2009;29(9):979–84.
38. Gress F, Schmitt C, Sherman S, Ikenberry S, Lehman G. A prospective randomized comparison of endoscopic ultrasound- and computed tomography-guided celiac plexus block for managing chronic pancreatitis pain. Am J Gastroenterol 1999;94(4): 900–5.
39. Gress F, Schmitt C, Sherman S, et al. Endoscopic ultrasound-guided celiac plexus block for managing abdominal pain associated with chronic pancreatitis: a prospective single center experience. Am J Gastroenterol 2001;96(2):409–16.
40. Leblanc JK, Dewitt JM, Symms M, et al. EUS-guided celiac plexus block (CPB) for chronic pancreatitis pain: a randomized trial of 1 versus 2 injections. Gastrointest Endosc 2007;65(5):AB206.
41. Buscher HC, Schipper EE, Wilder-Smith OH, et al. Limited effect of thoracoscopic splanchnicectomy in the treatment of severe chronic pancreatitis pain: a prospective long-term analysis of 75 cases. Surgery 2008;143(6):715–22.

42. Baghdadi S, Abbas MH, Albouz F, et al. Systematic review of the role of thoraco-scopic splanchnicectomy in palliating the pain of patients with chronic pancreatitis. Surg Endosc 2008;22(3):580–8.

43. Reber PU, Patel AG, Toyama MT, et al. Feline model of chronic obstructive pancreatitis: effects of acute pancreatic duct decompression on blood flow and interstitial pH. Scand J Gastroenterol 1999;34(4):439–44.

44. Rösch T, Daniel S, Scholz M, et al. Endoscopic treatment of chronic pancreatitis: a multicenter study of 1000 patients with long-term follow-up. Endoscopy 2002;34(10): 765–71.

45. Pai CG, Alvares JF. Endoscopic pancreatic-stent placement and sphincterotomy for relief of pain in tropical pancreatitis: results of a 1-year follow-up. Gastrointest Endosc 2007;66(1):70–5.

46. Guda NM, Partington S, Freeman ML. Extracorporeal shock wave lithotripsy in the management of chronic calcific pancreatitis: a meta-analysis. JOP 2005;6(1):6–12.

47. Dumonceau J-M, Costamagna G, Tringali A, et al. Treatment for painful calcified chronic pancreatitis: extracorporeal shock wave lithotripsy versus endoscopic treatment: a randomised controlled trial. Gut 2007;56(4):545–52.

48. Farnbacher MJ, Schoen C, Rabenstein T, et al. Pancreatic duct stones in chronic pancreatitis: criteria for treatment intensity and success. Gastrointest Endosc 2002; 56(4):501–6.

49. Thomas M, Howell DA, Carr-Locke D, et al. Mechanical lithotripsy of pancreatic and biliary stones: complications and available treatment options collected from expert centers. Am J Gastroenterol 2007;102(9):1896–902.

50. Binmoeller KF, Jue P, Seifert H, et al. Endoscopic pancreatic stent drainage in chronic pancreatitis and a dominant stricture: long-term results. Endoscopy 1995;27(9):638–44.

51. Eleftherladis N, Dinu F, Delhaye M, et al. Long-term outcome after pancreatic stenting in severe chronic pancreatitis. Endoscopy 2005;37(3):223–30.

52. Ponchon T, Bory RM, Hedelius F, et al. Endoscopic stenting for pain relief in chronic pancreatitis: results of a standardized protocol. Gastrointest Endosc 1995;42(5): 452–6.

53. Costamagna G, Bulajic M, Tringali A, et al. Multiple stenting of refractory pancreatic duct strictures in severe chronic pancreatitis: long-term results. Endoscopy 2006; 38(3):254–9.

54. Manzelli A, Petrou A, Lazzaro A, et al. Groove pancreatitis. A mini-series report and review of the literature. JOP 2011;12(3):230–3.

55. Beger HG, Büchler M, Bittner RR, et al. Duodenum-preserving resection of the head of the pancreas in severe chronic pancreatitis. Early and late results. Ann Surg 1989;209(3):273–8.

56. Frey CF, Smith GJ. Description and rationale of a new operation for chronic pancreatitis. Pancreas 1987;2(6):701–7.

57. McClaine RJ, Lowy AM, Matthews JB, et al. A comparison of pancreaticoduodenectomy and duodenum- preserving head resection for the treatment of chronic pancreatitis. HPB (Oxford) 2009;11(8):677–83.

58. Hill JS, McPhee JT, Whalen GF, et al. In-hospital mortality after pancreatic resection for chronic pancreatitis: population-based estimates from the nationwide inpatient sample. J Am Coll Surg 2009;209(4):468–76.

59. Díte P, Ruzicka M, Zboril V, et al. A prospective, randomized trial comparing endoscopic and surgical therapy for chronic pancreatitis. Endoscopy 2003;35(7):553–8.

60. Cahen DL, Gouma DJ, Nio Y, et al. Endoscopic versus surgical drainage of the pancreatic duct in chronic pancreatitis. N Engl J Med 2007;356(7):676–84.

61. Cahen DL, Gouma DJ, Laramée P, et al. Long-term outcomes of endoscopic vs surgical drainage of the pancreatic duct in patients with chronic pancreatitis. Gastroenterology 2011. Available at: http://www.ncbi.nlm.nih.gov/pubmed/21843494. Accessed August 23, 2011.

62. Garcea G, Weaver J, Phillips J, et al. Total pancreatectomy with and without islet cell transplantation for chronic pancreatitis: a series of 85 consecutive patients. Pancreas 2009;38(1):1–7.

63. Ahmad SA, Lowy AM, Wray CJ, et al. Factors associated with insulin and narcotic independence after islet autotransplantation in patients with severe chronic pancreatitis. J Am Coll Surg 2005;201(5):680–7.

64. Schmulewitz N. Total pancreatectomy with autologous islet cell transplantation in children: making a difference. Clin Gastroenterol Hepatol 2011;9(9):725–6.

65. Argo JL, Contreras JL, Wesley MM, et al. Pancreatic resection with islet cell autotransplant for the treatment of severe chronic pancreatitis. Am Surg 2008;74(6):530–6 [discussion: 536–7].

66. Nath DS, Kellogg TA, Sutherland DER. Total pancreatectomy with intraportal auto-islet transplantation using a temporarily exteriorized omental vein. J Am Coll Surg 2004;199(6):994–5.

67. Kobayashi T, Manivel JC, Carlson AM, et al. Correlation of histopathology, islet yield, and islet graft function after islet autotransplantation in chronic pancreatitis. Pancreas 2011;40(2):193–9.

68. Sareen S, Kumari V, Gajebasia K-S, et al. Yoga: a tool for improving the quality of life in chronic pancreatitis. World J Gastroenterol 2007;13(3):391–7.

69. Sareen S, Kumari V. Yoga for rehabilitation in chronic pancreatitis. Gut 2006;55(7):1051.

70. McCleane GJ. The cholecystokinin antagonist proglumide has an analgesic effect in chronic pancreatitis. Pancreas 2000;21(3):324–5.

71. Shiratori K, Takeuchi T, Satake K, et al. Clinical evaluation of oral administration of a cholecystokinin-A receptor antagonist (loxiglumide) to patients with acute, painful attacks of chronic pancreatitis: a multicenter dose-response study in Japan. Pancreas 2002;25(1):e1–5.

72. Volkova LP, Sharova LA. [Experience with radiotherapy of chronic painful recurrent pancreatitis]. Ter Arkh 1964;36:21–4 [in Russian].

73. Guarner L, Navalpotro B, Molero X, et al. Management of painful chronic pancreatitis with single-dose radiotherapy. Am J Gastroenterol 2009;104(2):349–55.

74. Domínguez-Muñoz JE. Chronic pancreatitis and persistent steatorrhea: what is the correct dose of enzymes? Clin Gastroenterol Hepatol 2011;9(7):541–6.

75. Domínguez-Muñoz JE, Iglesias-García J. Oral pancreatic enzyme substitution therapy in chronic pancreatitis: is clinical response an appropriate marker for evaluation of therapeutic efficacy? JOP 2010;11(2):158–62.

76. Waljee AK, Dimagno MJ, Wu BU, et al. Systematic review: pancreatic enzyme treatment of malabsorption associated with chronic pancreatitis. Aliment Pharmacol Ther 2009;29(3):235–46.

77. Taylor JR, Gardner TB, Waljee AK, et al. Systematic review: efficacy and safety of pancreatic enzyme supplements for exocrine pancreatic insufficiency. Aliment Pharmacol Ther 2010;31(1):57–72.

78. DiMagno EP, Go VL, Summerskill WH. Relations between pancreatic enzyme outputs and malabsorption in severe pancreatic insufficiency. N Engl J Med 1973;288(16):813–5.

79. Konstan MW, Stern RC, Trout JR, et al. Ultrase MT12 and Ultrase MT20 in the treatment of exocrine pancreatic insufficiency in cystic fibrosis: safety and efficacy. Aliment Pharmacol Ther 2004;20(11–12):1365–71.

80. Raimondo M, DiMagno EP. Lipolytic activity of bacterial lipase survives better than that of porcine lipase in human gastric and duodenal content. Gastroenterology 1994;107(1):231–5.

81. Isaksson G, Lilja P, Lundquist I, et al. Influence of dietary fiber on exocrine pancreatic function in the rat. Digestion 1983;27(2):57–62.

82. Cui Y, Andersen DK. Pancreatogenic Diabetes: Special Considerations for Management. Pancreatology 2011;11(3):279–94.

83. American Diabetes Association: Standards of medical care in diabetes – 2011. Diab Care 2011;34(suppl 1):S11–61.

The Minimally Invasive Approach to Surgical Management of Pancreatic Diseases

Lea Matsuoka, MD, Dilip Parekh, MD*

KEYWORDS

- Laparoscopy • Pancreas • Pancreatic cancer
- Pancreatic necrosis • Pancreatectomy

Laparoscopic surgery offers several significant advantages over open surgery, including more rapid recovery, lower wound complication rates, shorter hospital stay with its associated cost savings, and avoidance of large, chevron-type incisions typically required for open pancreatic surgery with their significant long-term morbidity. The acceptance and widespread utilization of laparoscopic techniques in pancreatic surgery, however, has had a slow evolution for several reasons, including substantial technical challenges, the risk of serious complications because of the proximity of the pancreas to major vascular structures, and the need for skills in both advanced laparoscopic surgery and expertise in open pancreatic surgery. Since the first reported case of laparoscopic distal pancreatectomy,[1] case studies and series have been accumulating in the literature describing the laparoscopic treatment of pancreatic diseases such as pancreatic necrosis, chronic pancreatitis, and benign and malignant pancreatic tumors. **Fig. 1** shows the different surgical procedures on the pancreas. In this review, the focus is on the results of the laparoscopic procedures that have gained more widespread acceptance, such as left-sided pancreatic resections, enucleation of pancreatic tumors, pancreatic debridement, and pancreaticoduodenectomy for pancreatic head lesions.

SURGICAL TECHNIQUES FOR LAPAROSCOPIC SURGERY ON THE PANCREAS

Different techniques have evolved for the minimal-access surgical approach to pancreatic surgery. In the pure laparoscopic approach, the surgical procedure is performed utilizing standard laparoscopic equipment and techniques. The advantage

The authors have nothing to disclose.
Department of Surgery, University of Southern California, 1510 San Pablo Street, Suite 400, Los Angeles, CA 90033, USA
* Corresponding author.
E-mail address: dparekh@surgery.usc.edu

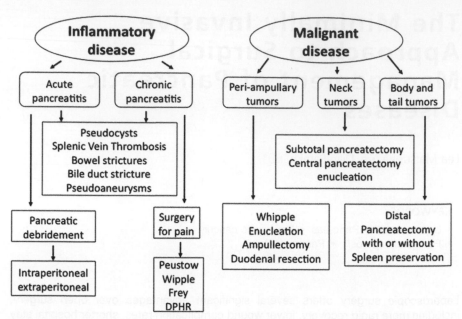

Fig. 1. Surgical procedures for benign, malignant, and inflammatory disorders of the pancreas.

of this approach is that patients have only tiny incisions associated with the insertion of laparoscopic ports. The disadvantages of this approach include the absence of tactile sensation, the inability to retract tissues, and the increased difficulty in obtaining hemostasis if bleeding is encountered during surgery. A hand-assisted laparoscopic approach has evolved in which a specialized device, a handport, is utilized during laparoscopic surgery (**Fig. 2**). The handport allows for the maintenance of pneumoperitoneum and provides all the advantages of laparoscopic surgery, with the added benefit of having a hand in the abdomen. The disadvantage of this approach is that a surgical incision of about 2 to 4 inches is required to accommodate the surgeon's hand. In the hybrid approach, the procedure is performed laparoscopically for mobilization and resection of the tumor; then, a small open incision is created, through which the procedure is completed. For example, this small open incision may be utilized for intestinal anastomosis during pancreaticoduodenectomy. It is unclear as to whether the hybrid approach provides any advantage over open surgery. Pure laparoscopic techniques and hand-assisted techniques are widely utilized for pancreatic surgery. Additionally, few reports have been published on the use of the DaVinci robot system for pancreatic surgery.[2] At present, there is no evidence that the robotic approach provides any additional benefit over that of standard laparoscopic approaches.

MINIMALLY INVASIVE APPROACH TO THE TREATMENT OF PANCREATIC NECROSIS

Pancreatic necrosis, a complication of acute pancreatitis, is defined as a focal or diffuse area of nonviable pancreatic and peripancreatic tissue, and it can be associated with organ failure, hemorrhage, or infection. Sterile pancreatic necrosis is

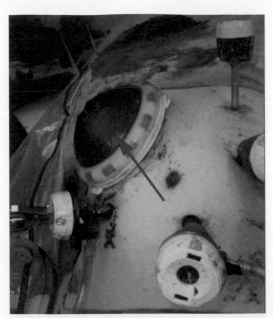

Fig. 2. Hand-assisted laparoscopic surgery is a useful technique for complex procedures on the pancreas. Port placement and a hand access device (Gelport) are illustrated (*arrow*).

associated with a mortality rate of up to 12%. Infected pancreatic necrosis develops in up to 40% to 70% of cases and increases the mortality rate to as high as 30%.[3] The traditional treatment for infected pancreatic necrosis has been open surgical debridement. The median mortality rate, however, of open surgical intervention is 25%, and ranges from 6% to 56%.[4] A major development in the treatment of pancreatic necrosis has been the observation that areas of pancreatic necrosis that initially present as phlegmon or as diffuse necrosis undergo organization and localization—a process of forming a walled-off pancreatic necrosis (WON). This process usually takes at least 3 to 4 weeks after the initial insult to develop.[4] Mortality rates drop sharply if operative intervention for pancreatic necrosis is delayed until WON has formed, because it facilitates complete necrosectomy (**Figs. 3** and **4**). Present surgical practice strongly recommends against any intervention until there is evidence of WON on imaging studies. Minimally invasive techniques described to address pancreatic necrosis all require the presence of WON.

In treating a patient with necrotizing pancreatitis, it is important to distinguish a fluid collection from persistent pancreatic necrosis. Percutaneous drainage is useful for fluid collection owing to infected pseudocysts, but does not treat pancreatic necrosis in an area of WON or unorganized, diffuse, retroperitoneal pancreatic necrosis. Failure to recognize persistent pancreatic necrosis in WON can lead to significant delays in care and substantial morbidity. Magnetic resonance imaging, which is useful for detecting solid components of a collection, may prompt the treating physician to consider pancreatic debridement rather a simple percutaneous drainage of the WON or fluid collection, if there is debris within the collection (see **Fig. 3**).

The literature for minimally invasive techniques for pancreatic necrosis is limited to case studies and series. Percutaneous, endoscopic, retroperitoneal, and laparoscopic approaches have all been described. Percutaneous drainage is an important

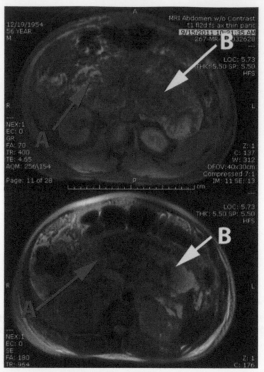

Fig. 3. Transaxial T1-weighted (*top*) and T2-weighted (*bottom*) images from a noncontrast magnetic resonance image. No normal pancreas is seen. Areas of high T2 signal intensity suggest drainable fluid (*bottom arrow; B*); however, the diffusely increased T1 signal intensity confirms that this material represents complex, proteinaceous fluid and/or fat necrosis (*top arrow; A and B*). No drainable collections are present. This patient would be unsuitable for endoscopic approach or VARD because of a centrally located periduodenal area of WON (*arrow; B*); however, laparoscopic pancreatic debridement with complete drainage of all visualized areas of necrosis was feasible in this patient.

adjunct in the treatment of pancreatic necrosis because it assists in delaying operative intervention until WON has formed. It is also useful for taking care of residual collections formed after surgical debridement. Percutaneous drainage has also become an important component of the step-up approach for the treatment of sterile or infected WON. Horvath and colleagues[5] reported on the efficacy of percutaneous drainage as part of the step-up approach in a multicenter, prospective, single arm, phase 2 study of video-assisted retroperitoneal debridement (VARD). Twenty-seven percent of patients in the study were treated primarily with percutaneous drainage and the authors found that a 75% reduction of the collection at 10 to 14 days after drainage was a predictor of successful percutaneous drainage alone. The Dutch group reported their results of a randomized, control study comparing the step-up approach to open necrosectomy for necrotizing pancreatitis.[6] In this study of randomly assigned 88 patients, 35% of 44 patients randomized to the step-up approach responded to percutaneous drainage alone. These studies have suggested that patients requiring intervention for necrotizing pancreatitis should first have a percutaneous drain placed in the necrosis cavity. Patients who fail to respond within

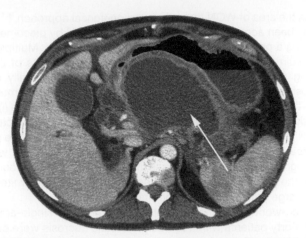

Fig. 4. Abdominal CT demonstrating a lesser sac WON that was treated by a laparoscopic transgastric drainage approach.

a short period of 1 to 2 weeks should then be crossed over to a surgical or an endoscopic intervention.

The use of percutaneous catheters as the definitive treatment of necrotizing pancreatitis has been reported in several small series of 20 to 30 patients, with success rates ranging from 30% to 100% of patients.[3,6–8] Many patients treated with percutaneous catheters were hemodynamically stable and relatively healthy, thus making results difficult to extrapolate to patients with necrotizing pancreatitis, who are much more ill. Treatment using percutaneous catheters is very labor intensive, and requires multiple imaging studies with catheter placements, exchanges and debridement sessions.[8,9] Gastrointestinal fistulas have been a significant complication of this method.[8,9] Therefore, we do not recommend percutaneous drainage as the primary treatment for pancreatic necrosis.

Endoscopic debridement techniques that create an opening between the posterior gastric wall and the WON cavity have been described.[3,9,10] In the majority of studies, an endoscopic ultrasound-guided approach is used. The endoscopic approach requires that the WON be optimally located and adherent to the stomach or duodenum. Patients with extension of necrosis into the paracolic gutters, and perinephric, retroduodenal, and other areas difficult to access through the endoscopic approach, or with large amounts of necrosis, are not suitable for endoscopic pancreatic debridement. A short metal stent is sometimes placed to maintain access to the WON cavity because multiple endoscopic procedures are usually required and the cavity is debrided using retrieval baskets and forceps. A successful debridement rate of 81% to 91% has been reported after median of 3 to 6 procedures per patient.[3,9,10] Complications, which occurred in 15% to 26% of patients, included perforation, peritonitis, bleeding, and air embolism, requiring further treatment with angiographic or operative intervention.[3,9,10] Endoscopic therapy requires highly specialized expertise found in a tertiary medical center. Additionally, multiple procedures performed nearly every other day may be required, which may be problematic in critically ill patients.

Minimally invasive surgical approaches that have been described include VARD and a laparoscopic intra-abdominal approach. In VARD, an endoscope or nephroscope is inserted after progressively dilating a drain tract or small incision so that a port can access the area of WON through a retroperitoneal approach.[3,11,12] Once the WON cavity has been accessed, debridement is performed by piecemeal removal of the necrosis using a grasper inserted through the nephroscope. Multiple procedures are typically required for an adequate debridement. The benefits of this approach include avoiding opening the abdominal cavity, thereby potentially reducing the incidence of postdebridement sepsis with its associated systemic immune inflammatory syndrome–like response. The disadvantages of this approach are (i) the need for multiple procedures, (ii) the inability to address other intra-abdominal pathology such as gallstones, (iii) the inability to drain collections in areas, such as the periduodenal areas, transverse mesocolon, lesser sac, or root of the mesentery, which are not accessible through the retroperitoneum, and (iv) the possibility of inadequate debridement, because the small channel of the nephroscope provides limited access for debridement of large amounts of necrotic material.

Horvath and co-workers[5] recently reported on a phase 2 single-arm multicenter study of VARD. Forty patients with infected pancreatic necrosis were evaluated with the step-up approach; of these, 31 patients required surgery. VARD was initially possible in 25 (81%) of surgical patients; however, 10 of these 25 patients (40%) ultimately required open surgery because of the technical inability to drain centrally located collections that were not accessible by VARD. Therefore, only 48% of the eligible 31 surgical patients were treated primarily by VARD, and in 51% of the surgical patients, open surgery was required to treat collections that were not accessible to VARD. Van Santvoort and associates[6] reported on the results of a randomized, controlled trial comparing open necrosectomy with a step-up approach. Eighty-eight patients were randomized into either an open necrosectomy arm or a step-up arm. In the step-up arm 43 patients were initially treated with percutaneous drainage. Fifteen (35%) patients required percutaneous drainage only for the resolution of their necrosis. In the step-up arm, 26 patients were candidates for surgery owing to failure of percutaneous drainage alone. Twenty-four patients underwent VARD; in 14 of these patients (58%), further surgical procedures were necessary to address residual areas of necrosis or complications associated with VARD. Therefore, only 38% of patients requiring surgery in the step-up arm in this study were treated primarily by VARD. Patients who underwent the step-up approach with VARD had a lower rate of major complications or death and reduced utilization of health care resources compared with patients who underwent open necrosectomy.[6] It is unclear whether these benefits can be attributed to VARD, because this study is fundamentally flawed. The step-up approach was utilized only in the VARD group (in 35% of patients in the step-up group, surgery was avoided with percutaneous drainage), whereas all patients in the open surgery arm underwent surgery. One plausible explanation for the poorer outcome for those in the open necrosectomy group is that those patients were not afforded the benefit of percutaneous drainage that those in the step-up arm received, allowing them to avoid surgery. It is possible that, if percutaneous drainage had been added as a treatment for the open necrosectomy group, a smaller number of patients may have required open necrosectomy with potentially better results. These multicenter studies demonstrate the limitations of VARD; only 40% to 50% of eligible patients were treated primarily by this approach because of the inaccessibility of centrally located areas of necrosis and the limited access for debridement of large amounts of necrotic material.

Gagner[13] reported the first cases describing a laparoscopic approach to the treatment of necrotizing pancreatitis. Since that time, only a few case reports and small case series of patients undergoing laparoscopic pancreatic debridement have

Table 1
Studies on laparoscopic treatment of pancreatic necrosis

Author/Year	Patients (n)	Approach	Mortality	LOS (d)	Complications
Parekh/2010	49	Transgastric, retrocolic, lesser sac, retroduodenal	6%	NR	35% Major complications
Bucher/2008	8	Via drain tract	0	NR	13% Pancreatic fistula
Parekh/2006	18	Infracolic, lesser sac	11%	16	58% Pancreatic fistula
Zhou/2003	13	Lesser sac, utz-guided	0	NR	8% Pancreatic pseudocyst
Ammori/2002	1	Transgastric	0	14	None
Zhu/2001	10	Lesser sac	10%	10–30	None
Hamad/2000	1	Lesser sac	0	7	100% Pancreatic fistula
Alverdy/2000	2	Via drain tract	0	NR	100% Pancreatic fistula
Cuschieri/2000	2	Infracolic	0	21–30	None
Gagner/1996	7	Transgastric, retrocolic retrogastric	0	51	None

Abbreviations: LOS, length of stay; NR, not reported.

been reported[14–21] (**Table 1**). We have reported the largest experience of laparoscopic pancreatic necrosectomy, which initially included a series of 19 patients who underwent hand-assisted laparoscopic debridement of pancreatic necrosis as the initial treatment of necrotizing pancreatitis.[21] One patient was converted to an open procedure secondary to an intraoperative enteric injury. Of the 18 patients who successfully underwent the initial laparoscopic pancreatic debridement, 4 patients required further surgical explorations: 2 of these were operated on during the early part of our experience and their subsequent procedures were performed by open surgery and the other 2 were reexplored laparoscopically. Thus, a total of 20 laparoscopic procedures were completed in 18 patients and 16 patients were treated by the laparoscopic route alone. There were 2 deaths in this series for a mortality rate of 11%. Mean length of stay was 16 days and external pancreatic fistulae developed in 11 (61%) patients.

We have recently reported our updated experience on 56 consecutive patients treated surgically for pancreatic debridement from 2001 to 2010.[22] Seven patients underwent open surgery and 49 patients underwent laparoscopic pancreatic debridement. The reasons for open surgery in the 7 patients were colon perforation (n = 2) and severe abdominal distension or adherence of bowel to the anterior abdominal wall that would have prevented an adequate pneumoperitoneum (n = 4); 1 patient, who was moribund, would not have tolerated a laparoscopic procedure. Of the 49 patients who were approached primarily with a hand-assisted laparoscopic procedure, the procedure was completed laparoscopically in 47 patients. Two patients were converted to open surgery (one because of an enteric injury and the other because of the patient's severe portal hypertension, which made the laparoscopic procedure unsafe), for a conversion rate of 4%. The surgery duration was an average of 132 minutes, blood loss was 295 mL, and median blood transfusion was zero units. Twenty-two additional procedures were performed laparoscopically on this group of patients, including 15 cholecystectomies. Fifty-five percent of patients had an infected necrosis confirmed on intraoperative cultures. Twenty reoperations were

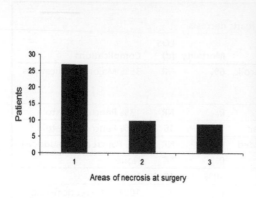

LOCATION	#
Lesser Sac	46
Left perinephric/ paracolic gutter	13
Right paranephric space	2
Subhepatic	2
Root of the mesentary	8
Retroduodenal	6
Total	77
Average/patient	1.6

Fig. 5. Number of areas of WON per patient (*left panel*) and distribution of areas of necrosis (*right panel*) at surgery during laparoscopic pancreatic debridement.

performed in 21% of the patients for recurrent collections; 10 of these procedures were performed laparoscopically and 10 were open. The overall incidence of serious postoperative complications was 35% with the majority of the complications being non–life-threatening (Clavien grade 3 in 27%, grade 4 in 4.2%, and grade 5 in 4.2%). The mortality rate was 6%.

Endoscopic therapy and minimally invasive retroperitoneal approaches for pancreatic debridement require that the WON be located in an accessible location: The lesser sac adherent to the stomach for endoscopic approaches and the retroperitoneum for VARD. Both of these approaches are unsuitable when areas of necrosis are present in multiple compartments of the abdomen (see **Fig. 3**). **Fig. 5** shows the 77 areas of necrosis found in the 47 patients in our study that underwent laparoscopic pancreatic debridement. There were 1.6 areas of necrosis per patient and all compartments of the abdomen were affected. Forty percent of patients had more than 1 area of necrosis in the abdomen. The wide distribution of the collections in different compartments of the abdomen suggests that many of these patients would have been unsuitable for minimally invasive endoscopic or VARD approaches. Utilizing the transabdominal laparoscopic approach, all identified areas of necrosis on the preoperative computed tomography (CT) were debrided at the initial procedure; we did not convert any patient to open surgery because of an inaccessible location or incomplete debridement of the pancreatic necrosis.

The transgastric approach for necrosectomy—opening the necrotic cavity into the stomach through the posterior gastric wall, which is similar to the endoscopic approach—avoids the creation of an external pancreatic fistula, providing a major advantage to these patients. We have thus far approached 2 patients laparoscopically with this technique of transgastric necrosectomy, with no morbidity or mortality (see **Fig. 4**). The laparoscopic transgastric approach provides an additional technique for debriding in selected patients with pancreatic necrosis.

Since 2001, we have laparoscopically debrided 67 patients with pancreatic necrosis successfully, with a mortality of 6% and a conversion rate of 3%. Our experience suggests that laparoscopic pancreatic debridement is an effective and safe procedure that allows for removal of both solid and liquid components of pancreatic necrosis in all intra-abdominal compartments with very low mortality and morbidity compared with open surgery. In patients with WON, a single procedure is usually required and conversion to open surgery is uncommon. It is a less traumatic way of achieving complete debridement of necrotic tissue in critically ill patients and may lead to a decreased systemic immune inflammatory syndrome–like response in the postoperative period, fewer complications, and a shorter hospital stay compared with open surgery.[21] Other intra-abdominal pathology, such as gallstones, can be addressed simultaneously with the laparoscopic approach. Furthermore, our experience demonstrates that laparoscopic transgastric pancreatic necrosectomy may be preferred in selected clinically stable patients with a single area of lesser sac WON.

Laparoscopic pancreatic necrosectomy is a feasible option for the vast majority of patients requiring debridement for pancreatic necrosis. In our experience, the contraindications for the laparoscopic approach are few and are limited to (i) critically ill or moribund patients who will not tolerate pneumoperitoneum, (ii) patients with a markedly distended abdomen with adherence of bowel to the anterior abdominal wall making laparoscopic access to the abdominal cavity difficult, and (iii) patients who have other severe complications such as colonic necrosis, pseudoaneurysms, or severe left-sided portal hypertension from splenic vein or portal vein thrombosis.

Optimal treatment of necrotizing pancreatitis requires a multidisciplinary approach. Treatment procedures should be tailored to the patient based on the severity of the systemic illness, presence of infected necrosis, imaging localization of the WON areas, and the center's expertise in minimally invasive techniques. Recent data suggest that the step-up approach may reduce morbidity and mortality compared with open necrosectomy. We agree with the recommendation that all patients requiring intervention for a sterile or infected necrosis should be treated with a percutaneous drain placed into the dominant collection. If there is a failure to respond rapidly, as demonstrated by improvement in the clinical condition and reduction of the cavity by about two thirds over a period of 1 to 2 weeks, then the patient should be crossed over to an endoscopic or surgical intervention.

Cumulative published data on minimally invasive approaches to pancreatic debridement suggest that it is a safe and effective option for all patients ranging from those who have an infected pseudocyst to those with large areas of walled off necrosis. Although VARD has been advocated as the preferred minimally invasive approach, recent studies show that only 40% to 50% of patients are suitable candidates for VARD as the primary approach.[5,6] There are 2 major limitations of this approach: (i) Difficulty in accessing all the areas of necrosis in the abdomen and (ii) very limited access available through a nephroscope channel to remove large amounts of necrotic material. Our results suggest that the transabdominal laparoscopic approach may be preferred, because all the potential areas of necrosis in the abdominal cavity can be accessed through this approach. Open surgery for pancreatic debridement should be limited to the occasional patient who is unsuitable for minimally invasive approaches.

The specific minimally invasive approach selected depends on the expertise of the physician performing the procedure. Endoscopic and VARD approaches may be suitable for patients who have a small amount of necrosis and in whom the WON cavity is appropriately located, making the procedure technically feasible (**Table 2**). Patients who have lesser sac collections that are adherent to the stomach may be treated through a transgastric approach by either an endoscopic or laparoscopic procedure (see **Fig. 4**). The laparoscopic procedure may be preferred if the physician has limited endoscopic experience and in patients who have large amounts of solid necrosis. Patients who are septic or critically ill and have a large or multiple areas of necrosis in different compartments of the abdomen on imaging should be considered primarily for the laparoscopic approach. The laparoscopic approach is presently

Table 2
Relationship between WON, degree of necrosis in WON cavity, and length of hospital stay

	n	LOS (d)
Walled off largely liquid collection	4	5 ± 2.7
Walled off solid necrosis	29	17.03 ± 2.36
Partially walled off or diffuse solid necrosis	6	78.8 ± 15.83

Abbreviation: LOS, length of stay.
$P \le .001$.

underutilized; our experience suggests that it warrants a wider role in the treatment of necrotizing pancreatitis, because it is a technically feasible option in the vast majority of patients who require pancreatic debridement.

THE ROLE OF LAPAROSCOPY IN THE TREATMENT OF CHRONIC PANCREATITIS

Chronic pain and pseudocyst formation are common indications for operative treatment of chronic pancreatitis. Laparoscopic techniques have been described in the treatment of these conditions.

Pain Relief

Unremitting debilitating pain is the most common indication for surgery in chronic pancreatitis. Traditionally, Peustow-type longitudinal pancreaticojejunostomy (LPJ) was the preferred procedure in a patient with a dilated pancreatic duct. Techniques for laparoscopic LPJ are well-established; however, LPJ is associated with long-term pain relief in about 70% of patients.[23,24] The Frey and Beger procedures are modern surgical therapies for pain in chronic pancreatitis that address inflammation in the pancreatic head, and relief from pain occurs in about 80% of patients after these procedures.[25]

Laparoscopic LPJ is the most common procedure reported for chronic pancreatitis. The pancreatic duct is identified by aspiration or ultrasonography during the laparoscopic procedure and electrocautery is used to longitudinally open the duct. The duct is inspected and any impacted stones are removed. The procedure is then completed with a Roux-en-Y, side-to-side pancreaticojejunostomy. The largest series of LPJ in the literature describes 17 patients who underwent laparoscopic LPJ.[26] The most common symptoms were abdominal pain and weight loss. There was a 23.5% conversion rate to open surgery secondary to bleeding or inability to isolate the pancreatic duct. Morbidity was 11.8% and there was no mortality. Length of hospital stay was 5.2 days. A recent review of the literature examined a total of 37 reported patients who underwent laparoscopic LPJ.[27] There was an overall 13.5% conversion rate, 0% mortality rate, and 13.5% morbidity rate. Mean hospital length of stay was 5.5 days. This compares with morbidity rates that range from 22% to 25% and lengths of stay from 8 to 14 days for open LPJ. Laparoscopic LPJ requires experience in laparoscopic techniques and may result in lower morbidity rates and shorter length of stay when compared with open LPJ.[27]

We have reported the first laparoscopic Frey (**Fig. 6**) and Beger procedures (**Fig. 7**).[28,29] The first laparoscopic Frey procedure was performed in a patient with familial chronic pancreatitis who had a previous failed open LPJ. Resection of the head of the pancreas was performed with a hand-assisted technique and the LPJ was

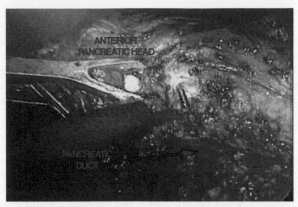

Fig. 6. Intraoperative image of a laparoscopic Frey procedure. Resection of the anterior head of the pancreas, including all the tissue anterior to the pancreatic duct.

performed with the DaVinci robot system. The patient is currently 4 years post laparoscopic surgery with substantial relief of pain. We have performed 7 laparoscopic, duodenum-preserving, Beger-type pancreatic head resections for chronic pancreatitis or for intraductal papillary mucinous neoplasms (IPMN) involving the head of the pancreas with 37% morbidity and no mortality. The procedure is technically challenging and requires further experience to define its role in treatment of chronic pancreatitis.

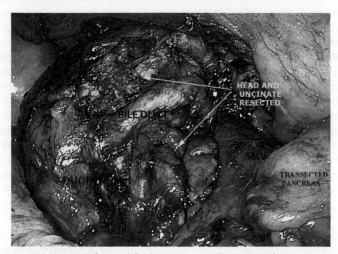

Fig. 7. Intraoperative image of a modified Beger procedure: Complete resection of the head and uncinate process of the pancreas with preservation of the duodenum and the bile duct. The transected left pancreas is shown on this image, reconstruction is usually with a Roux-en-Y pancreaticojejunostomy to the transected left sided pancreas. The modified Beger procedure with a total pancreatic head resection and preservation of the duodenum is an option for patients with small benign neuroendocrine and cystic lesions of the head of the pancreas.

Patients with chronic pancreatitis often have poorly understood hyperalgesia that may be opioid induced or from a central mechanism, and large open incisions are frequently morbid in this group, combined with long periods of disability from the surgery.[30] Laparoscopic procedures for surgical treatment of pain in chronic pancreatitis are technically, feasible as shown in case reports or small case series. More experience is necessary before these procedures can be routinely recommended. Laparoscopic surgery may provide a further surgical option in the treatment of patients with chronic pancreatitis and warrant further study.

Pseudocysts

Pancreatic pseudocysts arise after disruption of the pancreatic duct, leading to extravasation of pancreatic juice into surrounding tissues. These fluid-filled cavities develop a fibrous wall and can lead to obstruction, bleeding, or infection. Pseudocysts occur in 5% to 16% of patients with acute pancreatitis and in 20% to 40% of patients with chronic pancreatitis.[31] The historical standard of care has been open surgical intervention.

Laparoscopic pancreatic cystgastrostomy is performed through an anterior gastrostomy. Communication is then established with the pseudocyst through the posterior gastric wall and an endoscopic stapler is used to create a wide side-by-side cystgastrostomy. Laparoscopic pancreatic cystjejunostomy is performed most often for pseudocysts visualized through the transverse mesocolon. The pseudocyst is opened through the transverse mesocolon and a stapled or hand-sewn cystjejunostomy is performed.

Reports on the laparoscopic treatment of pancreatic pseudocysts describe minimal complications and recurrences, and short hospital lengths of stay.[32–35] Park and co-workers[33] described 28 patients who underwent laparoscopic cystgastrostomy or cystjejunostomy for pancreatic pseudocysts.[33] There was 1 conversion to open procedure secondary to extensive gastric varices. The mean operating time was 2.8 hours and mean postoperative length of stay 4.4 days. Palanivelu and associates[35] described 90 patients who underwent laparoscopic cystgastrostomy and 8 patients who underwent cystjejunostomy. The patients receiving cystgastrostomy had a mean operating time of 86 minutes. Two patients suffered postoperative bleeding and 1 patient had a recurrent pseudocyst. The cystjejunostomy patients had a mean operating time of 126 minutes and 1 patient was reported to have a postoperative infection. There were no conversions and no mortalities reported.

The treatment of pancreatic pseudocysts has evolved significantly over the past 2 decades. For many pseudocysts, endoscopic therapy is probably the procedure of choice. If a patient requires surgery, then the laparoscopic approach may be preferred, because laparoscopic treatment of pancreatic pseudocysts is not restricted by location or size of the pseudocyst and large openings can be created to prevent closure of the cyst anastomosis and recurrence of the pseudocyst.

THE LAPAROSCOPIC APPROACH TO THE TREATMENT OF PANCREATIC TUMORS

The laparoscopic approach for resection of pancreatic tumors is rapidly gaining acceptance in the surgical community. Laparoscopic enucleation has been reported mostly in the treatment of small neuroendocrine tumors (NET) and cystic neoplasms of the head of the pancreas. Laparoscopic left-sided pancreatectomy or distal pancreatectomy (LDP) involves resection of the pancreas to the left of the portal vein for tumors of the pancreatic body and tail. This procedure can be performed with or without splenectomy (LDP with splenic preservation). Spleen-preserving laparoscopic pancreaticoduodenectomy (LPD) is important in children and young adults. LDP has been widely reported in the literature and is probably the procedure of choice today for patients with left-sided tumors. LPD, on the other hand, is more technically challenging, is sparsely reported in the literature, and is performed only in a few specialized centers.

Operative Strategies for Resection of Benign and Malignant Pancreatic Neoplasms

Surgical considerations differ depending on whether the patient has a benign or a malignant tumor in the pancreas (see **Fig. 1**). For malignant disease, radical resection of the pancreas, and surrounding soft tissue and regional lymph node dissection are important for complete extirpation of the tumor. For benign pancreatic tumors, the overarching goal should be pancreas preservation and removal of the tumor with a minimal amount of normal pancreatic tissue.

If the patient has a suspected malignant tumor in the body or tail of the pancreas, the operative procedure of choice is a radical distal or a subtotal pancreatectomy and splenectomy, including the surrounding soft tissue envelope to ensure a negative surgical margin (this may include resection of Gerota's fascia, adrenal gland, transverse mesocolon, partial colectomy, and partial gastrectomy). For suspected malignant tumors in the head of the pancreas, pancreaticoduodenectomy is a standard recommended surgical procedure.

In patients with suspected benign tumors of the pancreas, a major surgical goal is conservation of pancreatic tissue. For pancreatic body and tail lesions, a spleen-preserving distal pancreatectomy should be considered. For lesions in the neck of the pancreas, a central pancreatectomy with a Roux-en-Y pancreaticojejunostomy should be considered; this procedure preserves the body and tail of the pancreas. For pancreatic head lesions, enucleation of the pancreatic tumor or a duodenum-preserving pancreatic head resection should be considered as alternative procedures to a classic pancreaticoduodenectomy (see **Fig. 1**). Laparoscopic techniques of all the surgical procedures listed have been described.

Laparoscopic Left-Sided Pancreatectomy

Since the first report of laparoscopic distal pancreatectomy in 1996, outcomes of LDP have been compared with outcomes after open distal pancreatectomy (ODP) in multiple studies.[36-43] The demographics and outcomes reported from studies that have included more than 30 patients are shown in **Tables 3** and **4**. We have recently reported the largest single surgeon experience of 120 laparoscopic left-sided pancreatectomies, of which 42 (35%) patients had splenic preservation and 78 (65%) patients had a concomitant splenectomy.[44] One hundred three procedures (86%) were performed for benign disease and 17 (14%) were performed for malignant lesions. There was no mortality in the 120 patients and 5 (4%) required conversion to open surgery. Of the 5 patients converted to open surgery, invasion of the superior mesenteric or portal vein by the tumor accounted for the conversion in 3 patients, and technical reasons or failure to progress led to the conversion in the other 2. Our overall rate of significant complications was 25% (Clavien grade 2–4). Significant pancreatic fistulae developed in 12% of patients and nonpancreatic fistulae developed in 13%. The median length of stay was 3 days, blood loss was 256 mL, and median transfusion requirements were 0 units. These results compare extremely favorably with published results from open surgery where overall morbidity rates have ranged from 22% to 44%, mortality rates from 1% to 11%, and length of stay from 6 to 10 days.[36-43] These data show that laparoscopic left-sided pancreatectomy with or without splenic preservation is an extremely safe operation when compared with open surgery.

Table 3
Laparoscopic versus open distal pancreatectomy studies: demographics and pathology

Author	No of Patients		Age (y)		BMI		% Benign		Tumor size (cm)	
	LDP	ODP	LDP	ODP	LDP	ODP	LDP	ODP	LDP	ODP
DiNorcia et al	71	168	58.2	60.2	NR	NR	87.3	61.5	2.5	3.6
Vijan et al	100	100	59	58.6	27.4	27.9	77	77	3.3	4
Aly et al	40	35	47	52	21	21	100	100	3	4
Jayaraman et al	107	236	60	64	27	27	83	53	3	3
Eom et al	31	62	46.7	47.5	22.2	23	90.3	93.7	3.9	6.2
Kim et al	93	35	52	52.9	23.4	23.9	100	100	3	3
Kooby et al	142	200	59	58.4	28	26.9	62	58	3.2	3.3
Finan et al	44	104	60.5	55.5	28.3	29.9	75	57.5	3.3	7.7
Parekh et al	120	N/A	58.9	N/A	27.7	N/A	84	N/A	2.97	N/A

Abbreviations: BMI, body mass index; NR, not reported.

Other authors have reported similar results. Kooby and colleagues[39] reported on a multicenter comparison of data from 8 centers between 2002 and 2006. In a matched comparison, 142 LDP patients were compared with 200 ODP patients. The conversion rate was a 13%. Operating times (230 vs 216 min) and rates of pancreatic leak (26% vs 32%) were equivalent between the 2 groups, but patients undergoing LDP had less blood loss (357 vs 588 mL), fewer overall complications (40% vs 57%), and shorter hospital lengths of stay (5.9 vs 9.0 days). The authors felt that the strength of their study was the fact that cases came from both low- and high-volume centers, diminishing any bias secondary to expertise. The conclusions of the study were that LDP is a safe procedure that results in less blood loss, lower morbidity, and shorter

Table 4
Laparoscopic versus open distal pancreatectomy studies: outcomes

Author	Conversion Rate (%)		Operating Time (min)		EBL (mL)		Morbidity (%)		Mortality (%)		LOS (d)	
	LDP	ODP	LDP	ODP	LDP	ODP	LDP	ODP	LDP	ODP	LDP	ODP
DiNorcia et al	25.3	N/A	191	195	150	900	28.2	43.8	0	1	5	6
Vijan et al	4	N/A	214	208	171	519	34	29	3	1	6.1	8.6
Aly et al	10	N/A	342	250	363	600	20	31	0	0	22	27
Jayaraman et al	30	N/A	193	164	150	350	27	40	1	0	5	7
Eom et al	NR	N/A	218	195	NR	NR	36	24	0	0	11.5	13.5
Kim et al	NR	N/A	195	190	110	110	24.7	29	0	0	10	16
Kooby et al	13	N/A	230	216	357	588	40	57	0	1	5.9	9
Finan et al	12	N/A	156	200	158	720	NR	NR	0	5	5.9	8.6
Parekh et al	120	N/A	175	N/A	256	N/A	25	N/A	0	N/A	3	N/A

Abbreviations: EBL, estimated blood loss; LOS, length of stay; NR, not reported; N/A, not applicable.

hospital stay when compared with ODP. Similarly, Jayaraman and co-workers[38] of Memorial Sloan Kettering Cancer Center compared 107 LDP patients with a matched cohort of 236 ODP patients. This study reported a 30% rate of conversion to open procedure and also found that LDP patients had less blood loss, shorter lengths of hospital stay, fewer overall complications, and equivalent rates of pancreatic leak. Operating times, however, were longer in patients undergoing LDP compared with those undergoing ODP (194 vs 163 min). Nigri and colleagues[45] reported on a meta-analysis of 10 studies published between 2006 and 2009, comparing 340 LDP and 380 ODP patients. There were no differences between the groups with regard to operative times or mortality; however, the LDP group had significantly less blood loss, shorter hospital lengths of stay, fewer overall complications, and fewer pancreatic fistulae.

There has been some controversy over the role of LDP for malignant disease. In published studies, the majority of patients undergoing LDP have had benign disease. Our experience is similar; only 14% of our patients had malignant disease. In studies describing outcomes for LDP, the percentage of patients with malignancy ranged from 0% to 47%.[33,36–43,46–49] Jayaraman and co-workers[38] found that LDP patients who underwent conversion to open procedure were more likely to have a malignant diagnosis, and this subset had more blood loss and higher complication rates. The authors thus advised against laparoscopic resection in patients with malignant disease. This experience has not been supported by other studies. For example, in our patient population, in matched groups of patients with no vascular involvement, the conversion rate, complication rate, blood loss, and lengths of stay were similar between patients with benign and malignant disease (unpublished data). The conversion rate in the Jayaraman study was 30%, which is substantially higher compared with recent reports, suggesting there may be a learning curve bias in the study.

The adequacy of laparoscopic resection of malignant pancreatic tumors satisfying accepted oncologic principles has been a subject of some debate in the literature. Kooby and associates[50] performed a multi-institutional study specifically examining the role of LDP in patients with pancreatic adenocarcinoma. A 3:1 matched analysis resulted in 23 patients who underwent LDP for adenocarcinoma and 70 patients who underwent ODP for adenocarcinoma. When the groups were compared, there was no difference in positive margin rates, tumor size, or number of nodes. The overall survival in LDP patients (16 months) and ODP patients (16 months) was not different. The study supported the use of LDP for patients with distal pancreatic cancer. In our study, an average of 22 nodes per patient were retrieved in the group undergoing LDP with splenectomy.[44] Four percent of all patients had positive margins and 12% of patients with a final diagnosis of pancreatic cancer had a positive radial margin. In 25 (32%) patients, additional resections were performed en bloc with LPD with splenectomy, including Gerota's fascia, adrenalectomy, transverse mesocolon, partial gastrectomy, and transverse colectomy (**Fig. 8**). This extent of soft tissue resection, margin status, and nodal excision is at least as good as the experience reported in large series of patients undergoing open left-sided pancreatectomy and splenectomy.[36–43] Although further studies are necessary, early experience suggest that the extent of soft tissue resection, nodal excision, margin status, and long-term outcome seem to be similar between patients undergoing LPD compared with those undergoing open left-sided pancreatectomy for pancreatic cancer.

LPD

The first LPD procedure was reported by Gagner and Pomp in 1994.[51] Gagner and Pomp subsequently published a case series in 1997 of 10 patients who underwent

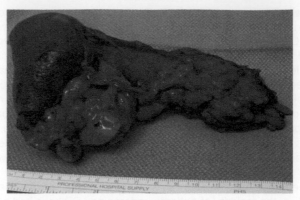

Fig. 8. Gross specimen image of a laparoscopic left-sided pancreatectomy showing the extent of soft tissue resected during this procedure. In this patient, a portion of Gerota's fascia was resected to maintain a soft tissue envelope around the resected tumor.

LPD.[52] Eight of these patients had periampullary adenocarcinoma and 2 had chronic pancreatitis. The conversion rate was 40%, average length of surgery was 8.5 hours, and average length of hospital stay was 22.3 days. Complications included delayed gastric emptying, splenic bleeding treated by splenectomy, and pancreatic leak. Based on these results, the authors concluded there was no benefit from LPD.

Since the pioneering work of Gagner and Pomp reported in 1997, advances in laparoscopic technology have led to dramatically improved results from experienced specialty centers.[52–56] We performed our first LPD in 2001 and since then we have performed over 40 laparoscopic pancreaticoduodenectomies without any mortality. In our experience, once the learning curve has been passed, the open and laparoscopic Whipple operations can be performed with similar operating room times. The largest published series from India by Palanivelu and colleagues[55] described 75 patients who underwent LPD. The majority of cases were performed for malignancy and there were no conversions to an open procedure. The mortality rate was 1.3%, incidence of postoperative pancreatic fistula was 7%, mean operative time was 357 minutes, and mean length of stay was 8.2 days. Margins were histologically positive in 2.5% of patients and the mean number of lymph nodes retrieved was 14. Dulucq and co-workers[54] from France describe 25 patients who underwent LPD. Three required conversion to open procedure, there was a 32% morbidity rate, and the mean length of stay was 16.2 days. All soft tissue pathologic margins were negative and the mean number of lymph nodes retrieved was 18. Kendrick and colleagues[57] have reported the largest study from North America. Sixty-two patients with a mean age of 66 years underwent total LPD. Median operative time was 368 minutes and median blood loss was 240 ml. Diagnosis was pancreatic adenocarcinoma (n = 31), IPMN (n = 12), periampullary adenocarcinoma (n = 8), NET (n = 4), chronic pancreatitis (n = 3), cholangiocarcinoma (n = 1), metastatic renal cell carcinoma (n = 1), cystadenoma (n = 1), and duodenal adenoma (n = 1). The median tumor size was 3 cm and the median number of lymph nodes harvested was 15. Perioperative morbidity occurred in 42% patients and included pancreatic fistula (18%), delayed gastric emptying (15%), bleeding (8%), and deep vein thrombosis (3%). There was 2% postoperative mortality and the median length of hospital stay was 7 days. A 2011 review by Gumbs and associates[58] of cases published in the literature included

285 cases of LPD procedures performed since 1994. The most common malignancy treated was pancreatic adenocarcinoma, accounting for 32% of all cases. Eighty-seven percent were performed entirely laparoscopically, and 13% were performed with a hand-assisted approach to facilitate the reconstruction step of the procedure. The rate of conversion to an open procedure was 9%. Estimated blood loss had a weighted average (WA) of 189 mL. Average length of stay had a WA of 12 days, and average follow-up had a WA of 14 months. The overall complication rate was 48%, and the overall mortality rate was 2%. Average lymph nodes retrieved ranged from 7 to 36, with a WA of 15, and positive margins of resection were reported in 0.4% of patients with malignant disease. These early results from small case series of LPD suggest LPD can be performed safely as the perioperative results, number of lymph nodes retrieved, and the extent of reported soft tissue resections are similar to those reported for open pancreaticoduodenectomies.[59,60]

In our experience, patients who have a pancreatic neoplasm confined to the head of the pancreas, distal cholangiocarcinoma, or ampullary tumors would be candidates for LPD. If the fat plane between the superior mesenteric vein and tumor is obliterated on a 4-phase CT scan, suggesting that the tumor may be adherent to the superior mesenteric vein, or if there is partial encasement of the superior mesenteric vein or artery, then this would constitute a contraindication to LPD because the patient will probably require an en-bloc portal vein resection for tumor clearance and negative surgical margins. Similarly, patients who fall into the category of borderline resectable pancreatic cancer should not be approached laparoscopically. LPD is technically a very difficult operation and at present should be limited to high-volume centers that specialize in laparoscopic pancreatic surgery. The limited worldwide experience does not suggest widespread application of this procedure until its safety record is better established.

Laparoscopic Enucleation of Tumors of the Head of the Pancreas

Laparoscopic enucleation of tumors in the head of the pancreas provides a surgical alternative to pancreaticoduodenectomy for benign tumors of the head of the pancreas. Enucleation has been the preferred option for benign NET of the head of the pancreas, such as insulinomas (**Fig. 9**). Enucleation is also an option for benign cystic neoplasms of the head of the pancreas, such as serous and mucinous cyst adenomas and side branch IPMN (**Fig. 10**).

Insulinomas account for 10% to 20% of pancreatic NET. The majority of these tumors are single and benign. Surgical resection can lead to cure, and enucleation is an option for tumors in the head of the pancreas. In the largest study published to date, Zhao and co-workers[61] described outcomes for 292 patients who underwent surgical management of insulinoma. Forty-six cases were approached laparoscopically, and 19 of these patients were converted to open surgery for a conversion rate of 46.3%. Twenty-seven patients were completed laparoscopically: 18 underwent enucleation and 9 underwent distal pancreatectomy. These 27 patients were compared with 255 patients undergoing open tumor enucleation or distal pancreatectomy. There was no difference between the open and laparoscopic group with respect to blood loss, operating time, and postoperative complications. Fernandez-Cruz and colleagues[49] performed 20 laparoscopic enucleations for small NET, including 14 insulinomas, 5 nonfunctioning tumors, and 1 gastrinoma.[49] The mean operating time was 120 minutes, there were no mortalities, and the pancreatic fistula rate was slightly higher compared with open procedures at 35%, with 15% of these fistulae being clinically relevant grade B fistulas. Length of stay was reported at 5.5 days. A 2009 review by Briggs and colleagues[62] of all cases published in the literature

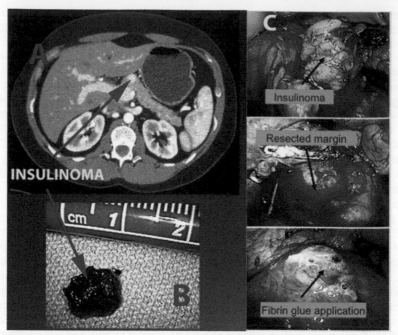

Fig. 9. Laparoscopic enucleation of an insulinoma in the neck of the pancreas. (*A*) Hypervascular lesion in the neck of the pancreas on a CT scan. (*B*) Resected specimen. (*C*) Intraoperative images: Circumferential excision of insulinoma. The resected area is covered with fibrin glue.

since 1996 included 108 patients who underwent a laparoscopic enucleation of the pancreatic tumor in the head of the pancreas. The weighted mean duration of surgery was 132 minutes, conversion rate 23.3%, hospital stay 7.8 days, overall mobility 48%, and the rate of postoperative pancreatic fistula of any type 29.3%. There were no mortalities reported in this series of patients. Crippa and colleagues[63] reported on the largest series of open enucleation of tumors in the body and head of the pancreas. Fifty-seven patients underwent open enucleation of pancreatic neoplasms. The mean duration of surgery was 162 minutes, morbidity was 43%, incidence of pancreatic fistula was 38% (8% of patients underwent reoperation for pancreatic fistulae), and length of stay was 14 days; there was no mortality in this series. Although comparative large studies of open and laparoscopic pancreatic enucleation are lacking in the literature, the outcomes of laparoscopic enucleation series are similar to those reported for open pancreatic enucleation.

In our experience, benign lesions in the head of the pancreas are the primary indication for enucleation, which avoids pancreaticoduodenectomy. Laparoscopic enucleation is not technically difficult and is feasible for both NET and cystic neoplasms. It is important to maintain the dissection close to the tumor to prevent injury to the underlying pancreatic duct. In patients with side branch IPMN, we have found that the lesion can be completely enucleated and the side branch giving rise to the IPMN can be identified and followed close to its origin (see **Fig. 9**). It seems laparoscopic enucleation is a safe and beneficial procedure and should be considered in the management of small NET, especially insulinomas, and cystic tumors of the pancreas.

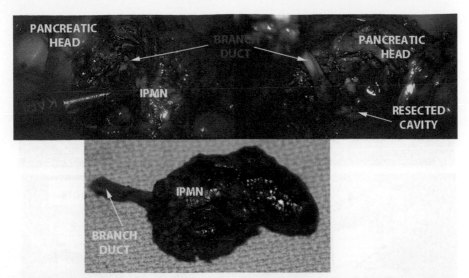

Fig. 10. Laparoscopic enucleation of a cystic lesion from a side-branch IPMN in the head of the pancreas. Upper panels show intraoperative images after complete enucleation of the cystic lesion, the offending side-branch duct is clearly demonstrated and is followed into the substance of the pancreas and resected. (*Bottom*) Gross image of the excised specimen.

Total Pancreatectomy

Total pancreatectomy is often considered in patients with diffuse multifocal disease, such as main duct IPMN or multifocal NET, and as a prophylactic procedure in patients with familial pancreatic cancer. Although total pancreatectomy with islet cell transplant has been advocated as primary treatment for pain in chronic pancreatitis, it has not received widespread acceptance. Widespread application of total pancreatectomy in the past was limited because of significant perioperative morbidity and mortality and severe long-term morbidity and mortality from malabsorption, steatorrhea, profound nutritional deficiencies, and brittle diabetes mellitus associated with frequent severe hypoglycemic attacks owing to concomitant loss of glucagon secretion. Improved results in last 2 decades from better operative techniques and perioperative care, growth of high-volume centers, and new treatments for diabetes mellitus and malabsorption have led to renewed interest in this procedure, particularly for benign disease. Recent studies have demonstrated that morbidity and mortality rates and the quality of life achieved after total pancreatectomy is similar that after more limited pancreatic resections.[64,65]

There are very few anecdotal case reports of laparoscopic total pancreatectomy in the literature.[66,67] We have performed laparoscopic total pancreatectomy in 7 patients (2 with multiple endocrine tumors and 5 with multiple cystic neoplasms or diffuse main duct IPMN; **Fig. 11**; unpublished data). The median operative time was 431 minutes and blood loss was 300 mL. The mean length of stay was 10 days, hospital mortality was 0%, and morbidity was 29%. These results are at least as good as that published for open surgery, suggesting that laparoscopic total pancreatectomy may be a feasible option in selected patients with diffuse pancreatic neoplasms.[68,69]

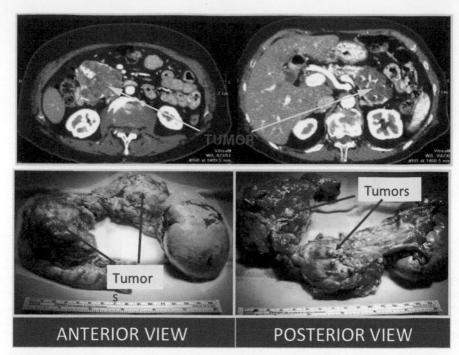

Fig. 11. Laparoscopic total pancreatectomy for a multifocal cystic lesion of the head, body, and tail of the pancreas. (*Upper panels*) Preoperative CT images of the tumor. (*Lower panel*) Gross images demonstrating the extent of tissue resection during the laparoscopic total pancreatectomy procedure.

Central Pancreatectomy

Central pancreatectomy provides a surgical alternative to pancreaticoduodenectomy or extended subtotal pancreatectomy for benign tumors located in the neck of the pancreas. The advantage of this procedure is the preservation of pancreatic tissue, thereby minimizing the possibility of diabetes or pancreatic malabsorption. Central pancreatectomy is a preferred option for benign NET, cystic neoplasms such as serous and mucinous cyst adenomas, and side branch IPMN of the neck of the pancreas.

The reported experience of laparoscopic central pancreatectomy is limited. Sa Cunha and colleagues[70] reported on a small series of 6 patients who underwent laparoscopic central pancreatectomy. Laparoscopic central pancreatectomy was successful in all patients. In 1 case, a laparotomy was performed to retrieve the specimen. The median operative time was 225 minutes. None of the patients required blood transfusion in the perioperative period, and there was no mortality. Symptomatic pancreatic fistula occurred in 2 patients (33%). Oral feeding was resumed after a median of 11 days. The median postoperative hospital stay was 18 days. At a median follow-up of 15 months, all patients were alive without exocrine or endocrine insufficiency.

We have performed three central pancreatectomies with reconstruction of the transected left pancreas with Roux-en-Y pancreaticojejunostomies. Our limited experience supports Sa Cunha and co-workers,[68] who report that laparoscopic

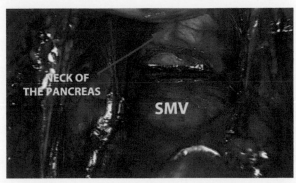

Fig. 12 Intraoperative image during a laparoscopic central pancreatectomy demonstrating the separation of the neck of the pancreas from the underlying superior mesenteric vein. The view provided by the laparoscope allows excellent visualization of the superior mesenteric vein and the dissection is done under complete vision as the neck of the pancreas is progressively separated from the superior mesenteric vein.

central pancreatectomy is a feasible procedure. The critical step in performing this operation either by open or by laparoscopic techniques is dissection to separate the pancreatic neck from the superior mesenteric vein. Having performed these procedures both by open surgery and laparoscopically, we have found that the dissection to separate the pancreatic neck from the superior mesenteric vein is easier when using the laparoscopic technique owing to the magnification of the anatomy (**Fig. 12**). Although laparoscopic central pancreatectomy seems to be a feasible procedure, we cannot recommend it because of the limited information available on the safety of this procedure. At present, it should probably be performed only in high-volume centers with highly specialized expertise in laparoscopic pancreatic surgery.

SUMMARY

Laparoscopic pancreas surgery has undergone rapid development over the past decade. Although acceptability among traditional surgeons has been low, emerging specialty centers are reporting excellent outcomes for advanced and complex operations, such as pancreaticoduodenectomy. A note of caution is necessary: These outstanding results are from skilled surgeons, many of whom are pioneers in the field, who have overcome the learning curve over many years of innovation. As the procedures gain wider practice, outcomes need to be carefully watched because many of these procedures are extremely demanding technically. Although many have suggested that controlled, randomized studies comparing laparoscopic pancreatic resections with open resections are necessary to establish the efficacy of laparoscopic procedure, the cumulative data on the safety and efficacy of the laparoscopic procedure argues against such an approach. The logistic difficulties of conducting such studies will be considerable given patient preferences, the need for multicenter studies, and the rapid adoption of the laparoscopic procedure among experienced pancreatic surgeons. A more reasonable approach to truly evaluate the safety of these procedures is the establishment of a national registry that can measure progress of the field and record outcomes in the wider, nonspecialty community. Hepatobiliary training programs should also establish a minimal standard of training for many of the advanced procedures, such as the pancreaticoduodenectomy, so that the benefit of laparoscopic surgery can be made available outside of just a few specialty centers.

REFERENCES

1. Cuschieri A. Laparoscopic surgery of the pancreas. J R Coll Surg Edinb 1994;39: 178–84.
2. Zeh HJ 3rd, Bartlett DL, Moser AJ. Robotic-assisted major pancreatic resection. Adv Surg 2011;45:323–40.
3. Navaneethan U, Vege SS, Chari ST, et al. Minimally invasive techniques in pancreatic necrosis. Pancreas 2009;38:867–75.
4. Besselink MG, Verwer TJ, Schoenmaeckers EJ, et al. Timing of surgical intervention in necrotizing pancreatitis. Arch Surg 2007;142:1194–201.
5. Horvath K, Freeny P, Escallon J, et al. Safety and efficacy of video-assisted retroper-itoneal debridement for infected pancreatic collections: a multicenter, prospective, single-arm phase 2 study. Arch Surg 2010;145:817–25.
6. van Santvoort HC, Besselink MG, Bakker OJ, et al. A step-up approach or open necrosectomy for necrotizing pancreatitis. N Engl J Med 2010;362:1491–502.
7. Echenique AM, Sleeman D, Yrizarry J, et al. Percutaneous catheter-directed debride-ment of infected pancreatic necrosis: results in 20 patients. J Vasc Interv Radiol 1998;9:565–71.
8. Freeny PC, Hauptmann E, Althaus SJ, et al. Percutaneous CT-guided catheter drainage of infected acute necrotizing pancreatitis: techniques and results. AJR Am J Roentgenol 1998;170:969–75.
9. Papachristou GI, Takahashi N, Chahal P, et al. Peroral endoscopic drainage/debride-ment of walled-off pancreatic necrosis. Ann Surg 2007;245:943–51.
10. Voermans RP, Veldkamp MC, Rauws EA, et al. Endoscopic transmural debridement of symptomatic organized pancreatic necrosis (with videos). Gastrointest Endosc 2007;66:909–16.
11. Connor S, Ghaneh P, Raraty M, et al. Minimally invasive retroperitoneal pancreatic necrosectomy. Dig Surg 2003;20:270–7.
12. Gambiez LP, Denimal FA, Porte HL, et al. Retroperitoneal approach and endoscopic management of peripancreatic necrosis collections. Arch Surg 1998;133:66–72.
13. Gagner M. Laparoscopic treatment of acute necrotizing pancreatitis. Semin Laparosc Surg 1996;3:21–8.
14. Hamad GG, Broderick TJ. Laparoscopic pancreatic necrosectomy. J Laparoendosc Adv Surg Tech A 2000;10:115–8.
15. Ammori BJ. Laparoscopic transgastric pancreatic necrosectomy for infected pancre-atic necrosis. Surg Endosc 2002;16:1362.
16. Alverdy J, Vargish T, Desai T, et al. Laparoscopic intracavitary debridement of peripancreatic necrosis: preliminary report and description of the technique. Surgery 2000;127:112–4.
17. Cuschieri A. Laparoscopic hand-assisted surgery for hepatic and pancreatic disease. Surg Endosc 2000;14:991–6.
18. Zhou ZG, Zheng YC, Shu Y, et al. Laparoscopic management of severe acute pancreatitis. Pancreas 2003;27:e46–50.
19. Zhu JF, Fan XH, Zhang XH. Laparoscopic treatment of severe acute pancreatitis. Surg Endosc 2001;15:146–8.
20. Bucher P, Pugin F, Morel P. Minimally invasive necrosectomy for infected necrotizing pancreatitis. Pancreas 2008;36:113–9.
21. Parekh D. Laparoscopic-assisted pancreatic necrosectomy: A new surgical option for treatment of severe necrotizing pancreatitis. Arch Surg 2006;141:895–902.

22. Kulkarni S, Selby R, Boswell W, et al. Laparoscopic-assisted transabdominal pancreatic debridement: a safe and effective treatment option for necrotizing pancreatitis [abstract]. Gastroenterology 2010;140:S383.
23. Sielezneff I, Malouf A, Salle E, et al. Long term results of lateral pancreaticojejunostomy for chronic alcoholic pancreatitis. Eur J Surg 2000;166:58–64.
24. Kalady MF, Broome AH, Meyers WC, et al. Immediate and long-term outcomes after lateral pancreaticojejunostomy for chronic pancreatitis. Am Surg 2001;67:478–83.
25. Beger HG, Schlosser W, Friess HM, et al. Duodenum-preserving head resection in chronic pancreatitis changes the natural course of the disease: a single-center 26-year experience. Ann Surg 1999;230:512–9.
26. Tantia O, Jindal MK, Khanna S, et al. Laparoscopic lateral pancreaticojejunostomy: our experience of 17 cases. Surg Endosc 2004;18:1054–7.
27. Khaled YS, Ammori MB, Ammori BJ. Laparoscopic lateral pancreaticojejunostomy for chronic pancreatitis: a case report and review of the literature. Surg Laparosc Endosc Percutan Tech 2011;21:e36–40.
28. Kulkarni S, Parekh D, Selby R, et al. Laparoscopic-assisted Frey procedure: a new option for treatment of pain in chronic pancreatitis [abstract]. Gastroenterology 2010;140:S993.
29. Parekh D, Berrera K. Hand-assisted laparoscopic duodenum-preserving pancreatic head resection and total pancreatectomy. In: Asbun HJ, editor. ACS multimedia atlas of surgery pancreas surgery. Chicago: American College of Surgeons; 2010. p. 77–102.
30. Buscher HC, Wilder-Smith OH, van Goor H. Chronic pancreatitis patients show hyperalgesia of central origin: a pilot study. Eur J Pain 2006;10:363–70.
31. Aghdassi A, Mayerle J, Kraft M, et al. Diagnosis and treatment of pancreatic pseudocysts in chronic pancreatitis. Pancreas 2008;36:105–12.
32. Hauters P, Weerts J, Navez B, et al. Laparoscopic treatment of pancreatic pseudocysts. Surg Endosc 2004;18:1645–8.
33. Park AE, Heniford BT. Therapeutic laparoscopy of the pancreas. Ann Surg 2002;236:149–58.
34. Fernandez-Cruz L, Saenz A, Astudillo E, et al. Laparoscopic pancreatic surgery in patients with chronic pancreatitis. Surg Endosc 2002;16:996–1003.
35. Palanivelu C, Senthilkumar K, Madhankumar MV, et al. Management of pancreatic pseudocyst in the era of laparoscopic surgery: experience from a tertiary centre. Surg Endosc 2007;21:2262–7.
36. DiNorcia J, Schrope BA, Lee MK, et al. Laparoscopic distal pancreatectomy offers shorter hospital stays with fewer complications. J Gastrointest Surg 2010;14:1804–12.
37. Vijan SS, Ahmed KA, Harmsen WS, et al. Laparoscopic vs open distal pancreatectomy: a single-institution comparative study. Arch Surg 2010;145:616–21.
38. Jayaraman S, Gonen M, Brennan MF, et al. Laparoscopic distal pancreatectomy: evolution of a technique at a single institution. J Am Coll Surg 2010;211:503–9.
39. Kooby DA, Gillespie T, Bentrem D, et al. Left-sided pancreatectomy: a multicenter comparison of laparoscopic and open approaches. Ann Surg 2008;248:438–46.
40. Finan KR, Cannon EE, Kim EJ, et al. Laparoscopic and open distal pancreatectomy: a comparison of outcomes. Am Surg 2009;75:671–9.
41. Kim SC, Park KT, Hwang JW, et al. Comparative analysis of clinical outcomes for laparoscopic distal pancreatic resection and open distal pancreatic resection at a single institution. Surg Endosc 2008;22:2261–8.
42. Eom BW, Jang JY, Lee SE, et al. Clinical outcomes compared between laparoscopic and open distal pancreatectomy. Surg Endosc 2008;22:1334–8.

43. Aly MY, Tsutsumi K, Nakamura M, et al. Comparative study of laparoscopic and open distal pancreatectomy. J Laparoendosc Adv Surg Tech A 2010;20:435–40.
44. Barrera K, Parekh D, Boswell W, et al. Laparoscopic-assisted spleen preserving left-sided pancreatectomy (DP-SP): a safe effective option for benign tumors of the pancreas [abstract]. Gastroenterology 2010;140:S1056.
45. Nigri GR, Rosman AS, Petrucciani N, et al. Metaanalysis of trials comparing minimally invasive and open distal pancreatectomies. Surg Endosc 2011;25:1642–51.
46. Taylor C, O'Rourke N, Nathanson L, et al. Laparoscopic distal pancreatectomy: the Brisbane experience of forty-six cases. HPB (Oxford) 2008;10:38–42.
47. Laxa BU, Carbonell AM 2nd, Cobb WS, et al. Laparoscopic and hand-assisted distal pancreatectomy. Am Surg 2008;74:481–6.
48. Dulucq JL, Wintringer P, Stabilini C, et al. Are major laparoscopic pancreatic resections worthwhile? A prospective study of 32 patients in a single institution. Surg Endosc 2005;19:1028–34.
49. Fernandez-Cruz L, Cosa R, Blanco L, et al. Curative laparoscopic resection for pancreatic neoplasms: a critical analysis from a single institution. J Gastrointest Surg 2007;11:1607–21.
50. Kooby DA, Hawkins WG, Schmidt CM, et al. A multicenter analysis of distal pancreatectomy for adenocarcinoma: is laparoscopic resection appropriate? J Am Coll Surg 2010;210:779–85.
51. Gagner M, Pomp A. Laparoscopic pylorus-preserving pancreatoduodenectomy. Surg Endosc 1994;8:408–10.
52. Gagner M, Pomp A. Laparoscopic pancreatic resection: is it worthwhile? J Gastrointest Surg 1997;1:20–5.
53. Pugliese R, Scandroglio I, Sansonna F, et al. Laparoscopic pancreaticoduodenectomy: a retrospective review of 19 cases. Surg Laparosc Endosc Percutan Tech 2008;18:13–8.
54. Dulucq JL, Wintringer P, Mahajna A. Laparoscopic pancreaticoduodenectomy for benign and malignant diseases. Surg Endosc 2006;20:1045–50.
55. Palanivelu C, Jani K, Senthilnathan P, et al. Laparoscopic pancreaticoduodenectomy: technique and outcomes. J Am Coll Surg 2007;205:222–30.
56. Sohn TA, Yeo CJ, Cameron JL, et al. Resected adenocarcinoma of the pancreas-616 patients: results, outcomes, and prognostic indicators. J Gastrointest Surg 2000;4: 567–79.
57. Kendrick ML, Cusati D. Total laparoscopic pancreaticoduodenectomy: feasibility and outcome in an early experience. Arch Surg 2010;145:19–23.
58. Gumbs AA, Rodriguez Rivera AM, Milone L, et al. Laparoscopic pancreatoduodenectomy: a review of 285 published cases. Ann Surg Oncol 2011;18:1335–41.
59. Winter JM, Cameron JL, Campbell KA, et al. 1423 pancreaticoduodenectomies for pancreatic cancer: a single-institution experience. J Gastrointest Surg 2006;10: 1199–210.
60. McPhee JT, Hill JS, Whalen GF, et al. Perioperative mortality for pancreatectomy: a national perspective. Ann Surg 2007;246:246–53.
61. Zhao YP, Zhan HX, Zhang TP, et al. Surgical management of patients with insulinomas: Result of 292 cases in a single institution. J Surg Oncol 2011;103:169–74.
62. Briggs CD, Mann CD, Irving GR, et al. Systematic review of minimally invasive pancreatic resection. J Gastrointest Surg 2009;13:1129–37.
63. Crippa S, Bassi C, Salvia R, et al. Enucleation of pancreatic neoplasms. Br J Surg 2007;94:1254–9.
64. Muller MW, Friess H, Kleeff J, et al. Is there still a role for total pancreatectomy? Ann Surg 2007;246:966–74.

65. Billings BJ, Christein JD, Harmsen WS, et al. Quality-of-life after total pancreatectomy: is it really that bad on long-term follow-up? J Gastrointest Surg 2005;9:1059–66.

66. Kim DH, Kang CM, Lee WJ. Laparoscopic-assisted spleen-preserving and pylorus-preserving total pancreatectomy for main duct type intraductal papillary mucinous tumors of the pancreas: a case report. Surg Laparosc Endosc Percutan Tech 2011;21:e179–82.

67. Kitasato A, Tajima Y, Kuroki T, et al. Hand-assisted laparoscopic total pancreatectomy for a main duct intraductal papillary mucinous neoplasm of the pancreas. Surg Today 2011;41:306–10.

68. Crippa S, Tamburrino D, Partelli S, et al. Total pancreatectomy: indications, different timing, and perioperative and long-term outcomes. Surgery 2011;149:79–86.

69. Janot MS, Belyaev O, Kersting S, et al. Indications and early outcomes for total pancreatectomy at a high-volume pancreas center. HPB Surg 2010;2010. pii: 686702.

70. Sa Cunha A, Rault A, Beau C, et al. Laparoscopic central pancreatectomy: single institution experience of 6 patients. Surgery 2007;142:405–9.

Pancreatic Cystic Neoplasms: Diagnosis and Management

Won Jae Yoon, MD[a], William R. Brugge, MD[b],*

KEYWORDS

- Pancreatic cystic neoplasm
- Intraductal papillary mucinous neoplasm
- Mucinous cystic neoplasm • Serous cystic neoplasm
- Solid-pseudopapillary neoplasm

Pancreatic cystic lesions are being detected with increasing frequency, at least partly because of the increased use of cross-sectional imaging for the evaluation of abdominal complaints or screening for other conditions.[1] Image-based studies report prevalences of pancreatic cystic lesions ranging from 1.2% to 19.6%.[2–4] In a study of 1064 pancreatic cystic neoplasm (PCN) patients pathologically confirmed over a 12.5-year period, 108 (10.5%) of the patients had pancreatic lesions that were detected while undergoing workup for other diseases.[5]

PCNs are reported to account for up to 60% of all pancreatic cystic lesions, followed by injury-related and inflammation-related cysts (30%).[6] PCNs include intraductal papillary mucinous neoplasm (IPMN), mucinous cystic neoplasm (MCN), serous cystic neoplasm (SCN), solid-pseudopapillary neoplasm (SPN), cystic neuroendocrine neoplasm, ductal adenocarcinoma with cystic degeneration, and acinar-cell cystic neoplasm.[7] The proportion of PCNs varies with population. In the Western Hemisphere, SCNs account for 32% to 39%, MCNs for 10% to 45%, IPMNs for 21% to 33%, and SPNs for less than 10% of all PCNs.[7] A nationwide survey from Korea reports the proportions of PCN which are composed of IPMNs (41.0%), MCNs (25.2%), SPNs (18.3%), SCNs (15.2%), and others (0.3%).[5]

THE MAJOR PANCREATIC CYSTIC NEOPLASMS

The 4 major types of PCNs are IPMN, MCN, SCN, and SPN. Distinguishing among the 4 most common types of cysts is important, since the management varies with each type of cyst.

The authors have nothing to disclose.
[a] Gastrointestinal Unit, Massachusetts General Hospital, 55 Fruit Street, Boston, MA 02114, USA
[b] Harvard Medical School, Gastrointestinal Unit, Massachusetts General Hospital, Boston, MA 02114, USA
* Corresponding author.
E-mail address: wbrugge@partners.org

Gastroenterol Clin N Am 41 (2012) 103–118
doi:10.1016/j.gtc.2011.12.016
0889-8553/12/$ – see front matter © 2012 Published by Elsevier Inc.

Intraductal Papillary Mucinous Neoplasms

IPMNs are defined as intraductal grossly visible (typically ≥1.0 cm) epithelial neoplasms of mucin-producing cells, arising in the main pancreatic duct or its branches.[8] The first report was 4 cases with the triad of mucus secretion, main pancreatic duct dilatation, and a swollen duodenal papilla.[9] Since then, the number of IPMN cases reported has been increasing significantly. This may be due to a true increase in the incidence, improvement in the understanding of IPMN, and/or increased use of cross-sectional imaging in clinical practice.[1,7]

IPMNs are usually diagnosed in the elderly, often diagnosed in the seventh decade of life.[5,10–13] There is a slight male preponderance.[5,10,11,13] Although the true incidence of IPMN is unknown, IPMNs are reported to be the most common PCN. IPMN accounts for approximately 1% to 3% of pancreatic exocrine neoplasms and 20% to 50% of all PCNs.[5,7,8,14, 15] Most patients diagnosed with IPMN are asymptomatic and are usually incidentally diagnosed. Symptomatic patients present with abdominal pain, pancreatitis, weight loss, diabetes mellitus, and jaundice.[5,10–13]

The World Health Organization (WHO) classification of tumors of the pancreas, including IPMN, was modified in 2010. In the 2000 WHO classification, IPMNs were separated according to the degree of dysplasia into intraductal papillary mucinous adenoma; intraductal papillary mucinous neoplasm with moderate dysplasia; intraductal papillary mucinous carcinoma, noninvasive; and intraductal papillary mucinous carcinoma, invasive.[16] In the 2010 WHO classification, IPMNs were classified into IPMN with low- or intermediate-grade dysplasia (which includes the former intraductal papillary mucinous adenoma and intraductal papillary mucinous neoplasm with moderate dysplasia), IPMN with high-grade dysplasia (which is equivalent to the intraductal papillary mucinous carcinoma, noninvasive), and IPMN with an associated invasive carcinoma (changed from intraductal papillary mucinous carcinoma, invasive).[8]

Macroscopically, depending on the pancreatic ductal system involved, IPMNs are classified as either main-duct IPMN (MD-IPMN), branch-duct (BD-IPMN), or combined-type IPMN.[17] The clinicopathologic behavior of combined-type IPMN is similar to that of MD-IPMN.[13] Intraductal proliferation of columnar mucin-producing cells is the main histologic characteristics of IPMN. The neoplastic epithelium may show diverse architecture and cytology. Four subtypes of IPMNs have been characterized: gastric, intestinal, pancreatobiliary, and oncocytic.[18] In a recent report, the 4 subtypes of IPMNs were associated with significant differences in survival. Patients with gastric-type IPMN had the best prognosis, whereas those with pancreatobiliary type had the worst prognosis.[19]

Most IPMNs are diagnosed incidentally. Even symptomatic patients present with nonspecific symptoms such as abdominal pain, malaise, nausea/vomiting, and weight loss. In patients with an associated invasive carcinoma, symptoms and signs of pancreatic ductal adenocarcinoma such as weight loss, diabetes mellitus, and/or painless jaundice may be observed.[11,20,21]

Routine blood tests, such as complete blood count, liver function test, amylase, and lipase, are usually within normal limits or show nonspecific changes.[22] Serum CA 19-9 and carcinoembryonic antigen (CEA) are generally not of diagnostic value. However, there is a report that serum CA 19-9 was elevated in 74% of patients with invasive IPMN and in 14% of patients with noninvasive IPMN. Furthermore, it is reported that 80% of patients with invasive IPMN had elevated serum levels of CA 19-9 and/or CEA, compared with 18% of patients with noninvasive IPMN.[23]

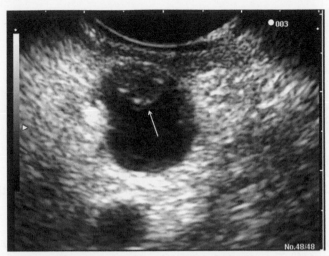

Fig. 1. EUS finding of a BD-IPMN with a mural nodule (*arrow*).

Endoscopic retrograde cholangiopancreatography (ERCP) was the standard diagnostic tool for IPMN in the past. In MD-IPMN, the hallmark finding is a diffusely dilated main pancreatic duct with filling defects correlating to mucinous filling or papillary tumors.[24]

For BD-IPMN, the affected branch ducts are cystically dilated and communicate with the main pancreatic duct.[24] In some occasions, the cystic side branch ducts do not fill with contrast due to mucus plugging.[25] In some cases, duodenoscopy during ERCP reveals a patulous duodenal papilla and mucin extrusion through the orifice.[9,26]

The use of ERCP for the diagnosis of IPMN is limited by its invasiveness and risk of complications. In some cases, visualization of the entire pancreatic duct system is not possible because of copious amount of mucin.[27] However, ERCP offers the advantages of cytologic sampling and intervention. In addition, it may serve as a platform for developing endoscopic technologies.[28]

Endoscopic ultrasonography (EUS) is being increasingly used to differentiate the types of IPMNs (**Fig. 1**). EUS demonstrates a detailed morphologic analysis of pancreatic cystic lesions, guides fine-needle aspiration (FNA), and provides fluid for subsequent cyst fluid analysis such as cytology, CEA, and DNA analysis.[29–31] Furthermore, EUS may play a role in the treatment of IPMN, such as the intracystic injection of ethanol or ethanol/paclitaxel for cyst ablation.[32–34] EUS findings associated with malignancy in IPMN patients include marked dilatation of the main pancreatic duct (≥10 mm) in MD-IPMN and large tumors (>40 mm) with irregular septa in BD-IPMN; mural nodule greater than 10 mm in height was associated with malignancy in both MD-IPMN and BD-IPMN.[35] The drawbacks of EUS include operator dependence[35,36] and the inability to differentiate between malignancy and areas of focal inflammation that infiltrate pancreatic parenchyma and mimic malignancy.[37] Cyst fluid analysis often demonstrates a high concentration of CEA, reflecting the presence of a mucinous epithelium. A cut-off CEA level of 192 ng/mL has the sensitivity of 73%, specificity of 84%, and accuracy of 79% for differentiating mucinous from nonmucinous pancreatic cystic lesions.[29] However, cyst fluid CEA differentiates neither malignant mucinous cysts from benign mucinous cysts[38] nor malignant IPMNs from benign IPMNs.[39] Cyst fluid cytology is rarely sufficiently

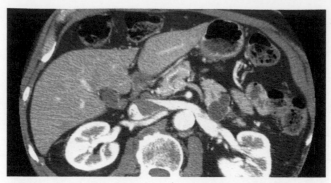

Fig. 2. CT finding of a BD-IPMN at the tail of the pancreas. Note the fine septations.

diagnostic to distinguish IPMN from MCN; the result is a generic cytology report of a "mucinous cyst."[40] The reported sensitivity, specificity, positive predictive value, negative predictive value, and accuracy of EUS-FNA for malignant IPMN were 75%, 91%, 79%, 89%, and 86%.[39]

Computed tomography (CT) and magnetic resonance imaging (MRI)/magnetic resonance cholangiopancreatography (MRCP) are used to describe the anatomic location of the IPMNs, the relationship between the lesion with surrounding organs and vessels, and the presence of distant metastasis (**Fig. 2**). MD-IPMNs show diffuse or focal involvement of the main pancreatic duct.[24] BD-IPMNs appear as either a cyst or a cluster of cysts, usually located in the head, particularly in the uncinate process.[41] BD-IPMNs may be multifocal. In a report of 145 resected cases of BD-IPMN, multifocality was observed in 14.5% of patients.[42] In another report of 190 patients with radiologically and/or histologically diagnosed BD-IPMN, 27.4% of the patients had multifocal disease.[27] MRCP has been reported to be superior to CT in detecting ductal communication in BD-IPMN.[43] However, with advances in multidetector CT, imaging details of CT including visualization of ductal communication have improved similar to those of MRI/MRCP.[41]

Surgical resection is often used to manage advanced IPMNs. For BD-IPMN, resection is advocated if one or more of the following criteria are met: (1) greater than 30 mm in size; (2) mural nodule(s); (3) dilated main pancreatic duct; (4) malignant pancreatic juice cytology; and (5) symptoms associated with pancreatic cysts.[44] For resected IPMNs, the prognosis is mainly determined by the presence of an associated invasive carcinoma.[8] For patients with resected noninvasive IPMN, the 5-year survival rate is 90% to 95%.[45,46] In contrast, for patients with IPMNs with an associated invasive carcinoma, the 5-year survival rates are reported to be between 36% and 60%.[11,20,47–49]

Mucinous Cystic Neoplasms

The 2010 WHO classification of tumors defines MCN as a cyst-forming epithelial neoplasm that is usually without communication with the pancreatic duct and composed of columnar, mucin-producing epithelium with an underlying ovarian-type stroma.[50] Similar to IPMNs, MCNs are classified according to the grade of dysplasia (ie, MCN with low- or intermediate-grade dysplasia, MCN with high-grade dysplasia, and MCN with an associated invasive carcinoma).[50]

MCNs almost exclusively occur in women, with a peak incidence in the fifth decade.[7,51] The body and the tail of the pancreas are predominantly affected.[5,51] Up to one-third of MCNs are reported to harbor an invasive carcinoma.[50] Risk factors for the presence of malignancy include large tumor size, associated mass or mural nodules, and advanced age.[51,52]

Around 30% of the patients may be without symptoms or signs. Symptomatic patients may complain of abdominal pain, palpable mass, weight loss, anorexia, fatigue, or jaundice.[5,51] Some patients may present with pancreatitis.[51] The results of routine laboratory testing are usually nonspecific. Patients with bile duct obstruction display a cholestatic liver function abnormality.

Macroscopically, MCNs present as single spherical masses. The lesions may be unilocular or multilocular. The cysts contain thick mucin or a mixture of mucin and hemorrhagic-necrotic material.[50] There is no communication between the tumor and the pancreatic duct, unless there is fistula formation.[50] The frequency of the lesion communicating with the pancreatic duct system may be high. In a recent Japanese multi-institutional report, 18.1% (25 of 138 patients) of MCNs demonstrated communication with the pancreatic duct.[53]

Histologically, MCNs comprise 2 distinctive components: an epithelial lining and an ovarian-type stroma.[50] Tall mucinous columnar cells line the epithelium. The ovarian-type stroma, which consists of densely packed spindle-shaped cells with round or oval nuclei, is a distinctive finding in MCN. The ovarian-type stroma is considered a requisite for the diagnosis of MCN.[44]

On CT, MCNs appear as large cysts with thin septae; the septae are best shown after the administration of intravenous contrast. Calcifications may be seen, which are lamellated and located on the periphery of the lesion, in contrast to the central, stellate calcifications of the SCN.[54] On MRI, the cysts have high signal intensity (bright) on T2-weighted images. On T1-weighted images with intravenous gadolinium administration, the wall and the septae are more conspicuously demonstrated.[55]

EUS findings of MCN are thin-walled, septated fluid-filled cavities with diameter greater than 1 to 2 cm. Duct communication is rarely seen.[56] Increased size, cyst-wall irregularity and thickening, intracystic solid regions, or an adjacent solid mass are findings suggestive of malignancy.[56] Cyst CEA levels are high as a result of secretion by the mucinous epithelium.[29,38] As mentioned, it is difficult to distinguish MCN from IPMN on the basis of cyst fluid cytology.[40] Since MCNs rarely communicate with the pancreatic duct, ERCP is not routinely performed in the evaluation of MCNs.[57]

Current consensus guideline advocates that all MCNs should be resected, unless there are contraindications for operation.[44] Surgical resection is curative in nearly all patients with noninvasive MCN.[51,58] For MCNs with an associated invasive carcinoma, prognosis depends on the extent of the invasive component, tumor stage, and resectability.[50] The 2-year survival rate and 5-year survival rate of patients with resected MCN with an associated invasive carcinoma are about 67% and 50%, respectively.[50,59]

Serous Cystic Neoplasms

SCNs are cystic neoplasms composed of cuboidal, glycogen-rich epithelial cells. The lesions are filled with serous fluid.[60] According to the degree of dysplasia, they are classified as either serous cystadenoma or serous cystadenocarcinoma.

SCNs occur more frequently in women.[5,7] Patients are usually diagnosed with SCN in their late 50s or early 60s. They occur more frequently in the body or the tail of the pancreas. Most patients are without symptoms or signs on diagnosis. Symptomatic patients may present with abdominal pain, palpable mass, anorexia, jaundice, fatigue/malaise, or weight loss.[5,61] Nearly 90% of von Hippel–Lindau (VHL) syndrome patients are reported to develop SCNs.[60] SCNs are rarely malignant; only about 25 malignant cases have been reported to this date.[60]

SCNs are usually single, round lesions, with diameters that can be greater than 20 cm. On cross-section, the cysts are composed of numerous microcysts filled with serous fluid. SCNs do not communicate with the pancreatic duct. A dense fibronodular scar is often located in the center of the lesion. A single layer of cuboidal epithelial cells lines the cysts. The central scar is composed of acellular hyalinized tissue and a few clusters of tiny cysts.[60]

Four variants of serous cystadenoma are known. The serous epithelial components of these variants are identical to those of serous cystadenoma. They are macrocystic serous cystadenoma, solid serous adenoma, VHL-associated SCN, and mixed serous neuroendocrine neoplasm.[60] Macrocystic serous cystadenomas include previous serous oligocystic and ill-demarcated serous adenoma. Solid serous adenomas are well-circumscribed neoplasms that have a solid gross appearance; they share the cytologic and immunohistologic features of classic SCN. VHL-associated SCN describes multiple serous cystadenomas and macrocystic variants that occur in VHL syndrome patients. In patients with VHL, SCNs typically involve the pancreas diffusely or in a patchy fashion. The mixed serous neuroendocrine neoplasm is the rare entity of serous cystadenomas associated with pancreatic neuroendocrine neoplasms. This is highly suggestive of VHL syndrome.[60]

On CT, SCNs may have the classic microcystic appearance or the less common oligocystic appearance (**Fig. 3**). Microcystic-type lesions comprise multiple small cysts. A central fibrous scar with calcification, which occurs up to 30% in SCNs, is considered pathognomonic.[62] The dense tissue is arranged in a stellate form. In some cases, the small cysts and dense fibrous component may make the lesions appear solid on CT.[63]

The oligocystic pattern is often difficult to differentiate from MCN on CT. Oligocystic SCNs should be suspected when a unilocular cystic lesion with lobulated contour without wall enhancement is located in the pancreatic head.[64] On T1-weighted fat-suppressed MRI, the fluid component shows lower signal intensity compared to the fibrous matrix. On T2-weighted images, the fluid becomes bright.[54]

On EUS, the typical SCN has multiple small, anechoic cystic areas and thin septations. Because of the vascular nature of the SCN, aspirants from EUS-FNA may be bloody or contain hemosiderin-laden macrophages.[65] Aspirated cyst fluid is low in CEA concentration.[29,66] The yield of cytology with EUS-FNA is poor.[67,68]

The prognosis for patients with SCN is excellent.[60] Even in the rare cases of serous cystadenocarcinoma, there are reports of a long-term survival after resection.[69,70] Currently, proposed indications for surgical resection are presence of symptoms, size of greater than 4 cm, and uncertainty about the nature of the cystic neoplasm.[62] Although increased size does not predict malignancy, large SCNs are reported to grow at a faster rate and are more likely to cause symptoms.[61]

Solid-pseudopapillary Neoplasms

SPNs are low-grade malignant neoplasms composed of monomorphic epithelial cells that form solid and pseudopapillary structures. SPNs frequently undergo hemorrhagic-cystic degeneration.[71]

SPNs occur predominantly in young women. The mean age at diagnosis is in the patient's 20s[72] or 30s.[5,73] Symptomatic patients may present with pain, mass, anorexia, nausea/vomiting, jaundice, or weight loss.[5,72] SPNs are reported to occur evenly throughout the pancreas.[71]

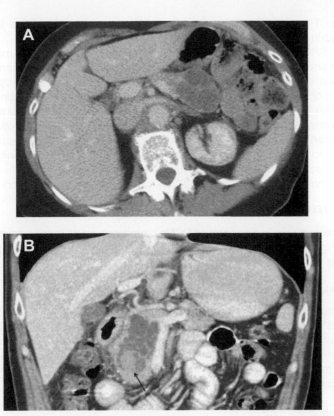

Fig. 3. CT findings of SCN. (*A*) Axial image. Note the septa coming from the central scar. (*B*) Sagittal image. Note the focal high-intensity lesion within a cyst representing hemorrhage (*arrow*).

Macroscopically, SPNs are large, round, single masses (average size, 8–10 cm). They are well demarcated and often fluctuant. The cut section discloses lobulated solid areas and zones with a mixture of hemorrhage, necrosis, and cystic degeneration. Microscopically, they are a combination of solid pseudopapillary component and hemorrhagic-necrotic pseudocystic components. The solid portion is formed with poorly cohesive monomorphic cells and myxoid stromal bands containing thin-walled blood vessels. When the poorly cohesive neoplastic cells fall out, the remaining neoplastic cells and the stroma form the pseudopapillae. The neoplastic cells have eosinophilic or clear vacuolated cytoplasms. Mucin is absent, and glycogen is not conspicuous. SPNs without histologic criteria of malignant behavior, such as perineural invasion, angioinvasion, or infiltration of the surrounding parenchyma, may metastasize. Therefore, all SPNs are classified as low-grade malignant neoplasms.[71]

On CT, SPNs appear as well-circumscribed, encapsulated masses with varying areas of soft tissue and necrotic foci. The capsule is usually thick and enhancing. Peripheral calcification has been reported up to 30% of patients.[74] No septations are visualized.[75] On MRI, the neoplasm is shown as a well-defined lesion with a mix of high and low signal intensity on T1- and T2-weighted images, which reflects the complex nature of the mass. Areas filled with blood products demonstrate high signal intensity on T1-weighted images and low or inhomogeneous signal intensity on T2-weighted images.[76,77]

On EUS, SPNs are usually well-defined, hypoechoic masses. They may be solid, mixed solid and cystic, or cystic. Internal calcifications can be seen in some patients. The reported diagnostic accuracy of EUS-FNA for SPN based on cytology and immunohistochemistry is 65%.[78] Aspirated cyst fluid may display necrotic debris. The cyst fluid CEA is low, reflecting the presence of nonmucinous epithelium.[7]

The mainstay of treatment is surgery. After complete surgical resection, 85% to 95% of patients are cured.[71] Even in cases with local invasion, recurrences, or metastases, long-term survival have been documented.[72,79,80] No definite biological or morphologic predictors of outcome have been documented. Suggested indicators of poor outcome include old age and SPNs with an aneuploidy DNA content.[71]

RECENT DEVELOPMENTS

Recent developments in diagnosis of PCNs have been made in the analysis of cystic fluid and high-resolution imaging. For the treatment of PCNs, EUS-guided cyst ablation has shown promising results.

Cyst Fluid Analysis

DNA analysis of pancreatic cyst fluid demonstrated that KRAS mutation is highly specific (96%) for mucinous cysts. Elevated amounts of cyst fluid DNA, high-amplitude mutations, and specific mutation sequences were indicators of malignancy. High-amplitude KRAS mutation followed by allelic loss was the most specific marker for malignancy.[31] Cyst fluid interleukin-1β concentration has been shown to be higher in malignant IPMN than benign IPMN.[81]

High-resolution Imaging

Ex vivo optical coherence tomography (OCT) of freshly resected pancreatectomy specimens demonstrated that mucinous cysts could be differentiated from nonmucinous cysts with high sensitivity (>95%), specificity (>95%), and almost perfect interobserver agreement.[82] OCT is an interferometric technique that typically uses near-infrared light. It allows noninvasive micron-scale cross-sectional imaging of biological tissues by measuring their optical reflections.[83]

Confocal laser endomicroscopy (CLE) is a novel imaging technology that uses low-power laser to obtain in vivo histology of the gastrointestinal mucosa.[84] Needle-based CLE (nCLE) enables the performance of CLE in intra-abdominal organs under EUS guidance or via natural-orifice transluminal endoscopic surgery procedures.[85] Konda and colleagues reported the feasibility of nCLE during EUS-FNA of pancreatic lesions in 18 patients with pancreatic lesions (16 cysts and 2 masses).[86] The nCLE miniprobe was introduced into the lesion through a 19-gauge FNA needle. Technical feasibility was achieved in 17 cases. Image quality was good to very good in 10 cases. Two serious adverse events of pancreatitis requiring hospitalization were reported.

Pancreatic Cyst Ablation

The introduction of curvilinear EUS and EUS-FNA made EUS-guided injection therapy possible.[87] EUS-guided pancreatic cyst ablation is achieved by the injection of a cytotoxic agent after puncture of the pancreatic cyst under EUS guidance. Injection of a cytotoxic agent may result in ablation of the cyst epithelium.[88]

The first cytotoxic agent used was ethanol. In the initial study, various concentrations of ethanol (5%–80%) were injected into the pancreatic cysts of 25 patients.

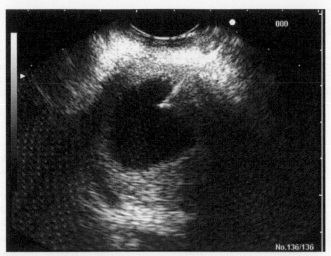

Fig. 4. EUS-FNA of a pseudocyst in a 43-year-old woman with alcoholic chronic pancreatitis. Cyst fluid amylase was 19,612 U/L, and CEA was 176.5 ng/mL. Cyst cytology was negative for malignant cells, and no definitive epithelial cells were identified.

There were no reported complications. Eight patients had complete resolution of pancreatic cysts. Histologic evidence of epithelial ablation was seen in 5 patients who underwent resection.[89] A prospective randomized multicenter trial comparing lavage of pancreatic cysts with 80% ethanol to lavage with saline was conducted in 2 centers. Ethanol lavage resulted in a greater mean percentage of cyst surface area decrease than saline. The overall pancreatic cyst resolution defined by CT was 33.3%. Histology of 4 resected specimens demonstrated 0% epithelial ablation in 1 saline lavage case and 50% to 100% epithelial ablation in 3 ethanol lavage cases. Complication rates were similar in both groups, with one major complication of acute pancreatitis requiring hospitalization in the ethanol group.[32] Long-term follow-up results of patients from this study were reported in 2010. In 9 patients, follow-up CTs performed after a median follow-up period of 26 months after initial documentation of cyst resolution demonstrated no evidence of cyst recurrence.[33]

EUS-guided ethanol lavage with paclitaxel injection (EUS-ELPI) for pancreatic cysts was recently introduced in Korea. This technique involves the aspiration of cyst fluid under EUS guidance, lavaging the cyst with 99% ethanol, re-aspiration of ethanol, and injecting paclitaxel (concentration of 3 mg/mL) into the cyst. The volume of the injected paclitaxel is the same as the volume of the aspirated cyst fluid.[90] A study involving 52 patients who underwent EUS-ELPI for pancreatic cysts was reported in 2011. Forty-three patients were followed for longer than 12 months, and 4 patients underwent surgery for persistent cysts; 5 patients were excluded from analysis. A complete response was observed in 29 patients, partial response in 6, and persistent cyst in 12. For 4 patients who underwent resection, histopathology revealed variable epithelial ablation extent of 0%, 25%, 40%, and 100%. Small cyst volume was the only independent factor associated with complete cyst resolution. Complications reported were fever without bacteremia (n = 1), abdominal discomfort of 2-weeks' duration (n = 1), pancreatitis (n = 1), pericystic spillage (n = 1), and splenic vein obliteration with collateral formation (n = 1).[34]

Table 1
Diagnostic summary

	IPMN	MCN	SCN	SPN
Cross-sectional imaging (CT and/or MRI)	Finely septated cystic lesions that may be multifocal	Solitary round septated lesions located in the body or tail	Solitary complex cystic lesion with central scar	Complex solitary cystic mass
Cyst fluid cytology	Mucinous epithelium with a range of neoplasia	Mucinous epithelium with a range of neoplasia	Bloody acellular nondiagnostic fluid with hemosiderin-laden macrophages	Highly cellular specimen with monotonous sheets of densely packed cells
Cyst fluid CEA	High	High	Low or absent	Low or absent
Malignant potential	High	High	Low or absent	Moderate

The early results of EUS-guided pancreatic cyst ablation are promising. However, more data on long-term follow-up and efficacy are needed to define precise indications.

APPROACH TO INCIDENTAL PANCREATIC CYSTIC LESIONS

There are many suggested algorithms on the management of pancreatic cystic lesions. Much emphasis is placed on the size and the morphology of the pancreatic cystic lesions.

Once confronted with a pancreatic cystic lesion, the first step is to differentiate PCNs from pseudocysts. The diagnosis of pseudocysts is primarily based on a patient history compatible with pancreatitis, with additional information from biochemical and imaging features (**Fig. 4**).[91] However, patients with PCNs may present with pancreatitis; patients with pseudocysts may have no apparent history suggestive of pancreatitis.[91]

Once pseudocysts have been excluded, the type of PCN should be determined. The primary focus should be on differentiating between mucinous (IPMN and MCN) and serous (SCN) cysts. Once a mucinous cyst has been diagnosed, patients with MD-IPMN, combined-type IPMN, and MCN should undergo a surgical consultation. Patients with BD-IPMN should be managed using the algorithm of the consensus guideline.[44] SCNs should be observed, unless they are symptomatic or large (>4 cm).

There are no strict published guidelines on the indication for EUS-FNA of pancreatic cystic lesions. In general, there is little need for EUS-FNA of cystic lesions with a clear diagnosis by cross-sectional imaging unless the results will impact patient management. IPMN lesions measuring more than 2 cm should be aspirated if the findings of a benign cytology will indicate the need for continued surveillance. If there is diagnostic uncertainty, the cyst fluid should be analyzed for CEA and KRAS. Each analysis can be performed with less than 0.3 mL of fluid. If the primary question is whether the cyst is malignant or benign, the fluid should be sent for cytology. Cyst fluid for DNA mutations may supplement the results of cytology, particularly when a small volume of cyst fluid is available.

The indication for surgical resection should reflect the risks of surgery based on the location of the cyst, the comorbid conditions of the patient, and the patient's need for diagnostic certainty. In general, low-risk lesions (small BD-IPMNs) located in the head of the pancreas should not be resected. Moderate-risk lesions (>2 cm or containing atypical cytology) located in the tail of the pancreas should be considered for surgical resection. All patients with a high-risk lesion (>3 cm in diameter, presence of a mural nodule, or containing malignant cytology) should be evaluated with a surgical consultation.

SUMMARY

PCNs are composed of a wide range of lesions from benign cysts to malignancies (**Table 1**). Although a cross-sectional imaging provides a sensitive screening test, EUS with FNA and cyst fluid analysis greatly increase the diagnostic certainty. Cyst fluid CEA offers the greatest accuracy in the differentiation between mucinous and nonmucinous PCNs. In the future, endoscopic ablation therapy might offer an alternative to the traditional surgical approach.

REFERENCES

1. Scheiman JM. Cystic lesion of the pancreas. Gastroenterology 2005;128:463–9.
2. Spinelli KS, Fromwiller TE, Daniel RA, et al. Cystic pancreatic neoplasms: observe or operate. Ann Surg 2004;239:651–7 [discussion: 657–9].
3. Laffan TA, Horton KM, Klein AP, et al. Prevalence of unsuspected pancreatic cysts on MDCT. AJR Am J Roentgenol 2008;191:802–7.
4. Zhang XM, Mitchell DG, Dohke M, et al. Pancreatic cysts: depiction on single-shot fast spin-echo MR images. Radiology 2002;223:547–53.
5. Yoon WJ, Lee JK, Lee KH, et al. Cystic neoplasms of the exocrine pancreas: an update of a nationwide survey in Korea. Pancreas 2008;37:254–8.
6. Basturk O, Coban I, Adsay NV. Pancreatic cysts: pathologic classification, differential diagnosis, and clinical implications. Arch Pathol Lab Med 2009;133:423–38.
7. Brugge WR, Lauwers GY, Sahani D, et al. Cystic neoplasms of the pancreas. N Engl J Med 2004;351:1218–26.
8. Adsay NV, Fukushima N, Furukawa T, et al. Intraductal neoplasms of the pancreas. In: Bosman FT, Carneiro F, Hruban RH, et al, editors. World Health Organization classification of tumours of the digestive system. 4th edition. Lyon (France): IARC; 2010. p. 304–13.
9. Ohhashi K, Murakami Y, Maruyama M. Four cases of mucin-producing cancer of the pancreas on specific findings of the papilla of Vater. Prog Dig Endosc 1982;20:348–51.
10. Suzuki Y, Atomi Y, Sugiyama M, et al. Cystic neoplasm of the pancreas: a Japanese multiinstitutional study of intraductal papillary mucinous tumor and mucinous cystic tumor. Pancreas 2004;28:241–6.
11. Sohn IA, Yeo CJ, Cameron JL, et al. Intraductal papillary mucinous neoplasms of the pancreas: an updated experience. Ann Surg 2004;239:788–97; discussion 797–9.
12. Schmidt CM, White PB, Waters JA, et al. Intraductal papillary mucinous neoplasms: predictors of malignant and invasive pathology. Ann Surg 2007;246:644–51[discussion: 651–4].
13. Crippa S, Fernandez-Del Castillo C, Salvia R, et al. Mucin-producing neoplasms of the pancreas: an analysis of distinguishing clinical and epidemiologic characteristics. Clin Gastroenterol Hepatol 2010;8:213–9.
14. Kosmahl M, Pauser U, Peters K, et al. Cystic neoplasms of the pancreas and tumor-like lesions with cystic features: a review of 418 cases and a classification proposal. Virchows Arch 2004;445:168–78.

15. Allen PJ, D'Angelica M, Gonen M, et al. A selective approach to the resection of cystic lesions of the pancreas: results from 539 consecutive patients. Ann Surg 2006;244: 572–82.

16. Longnecker DS, Adler G, Hruban RH, et al. Intraductal papillary-mucinous neoplasms of the pancreas. In: Hamilton SR, Aaltonen LA, editors. World Health Organization classification of tumours. Pathology and genetics of tumours of digestive system. 3rd edition. Lyon (France): IARC Press; 2000. p. 237–40.

17. Hruban RH, Takaori K, Klimstra DS, et al. An illustrated consensus on the classification of pancreatic intraepithelial neoplasia and intraductal papillary mucinous neoplasms. Am J Surg Pathol 2004;28:977–87.

18. Furukawa T, Kloppel G, Volkan Adsay N, et al. Classification of types of intraductal papillary-mucinous neoplasm of the pancreas: a consensus study. Virchows Arch 2005;447:794–9.

19. Furukawa T, Hatori T, Fujita I, et al. Prognostic relevance of morphological types of intraductal papillary mucinous neoplasms of the pancreas. Gut 2011;60:509–16.

20. Salvia R, Fernandez-del Castillo C, Bassi C, et al. Main-duct intraductal papillary mucinous neoplasms of the pancreas: clinical predictors of malignancy and long-term survival following resection. Ann Surg 2004;239:678–85 [discussion: 685–7].

21. D'Angelica M, Brennan MF, Suriawinata AA, et al. Intraductal papillary mucinous neoplasms of the pancreas: an analysis of clinicopathologic features and outcome. Ann Surg 2004;239:400–8.

22. Sakorafas GH, Smyrniotis V, Reid-Lombardo KM, et al. Primary pancreatic cystic neoplasms revisited. Part III. Intraductal papillary mucinous neoplasms. Surg Oncol 2011;20:e109–18.

23. Fritz S, Hackert T, Hinz U, et al. Role of serum carbohydrate antigen 19-9 and carcinoembryonic antigen in distinguishing between benign and invasive intraductal papillary mucinous neoplasm of the pancreas. Br J Surg 2011;98:104–10.

24. Lim JH, Lee G, Oh YL. Radiologic spectrum of intraductal papillary mucinous tumor of the pancreas. Radiographics 2001;21:323–37 [discussion: 337–40].

25. Salvia R, Crippa S, Falconi M, et al. Branch-duct intraductal papillary mucinous neoplasms of the pancreas: to operate or not to operate? Gut 2007;56:1086–90.

26. Yamaguchi K, Tanaka M. Mucin-hypersecreting tumor of the pancreas with mucin extrusion through an enlarged papilla. Am J Gastroenterol 1991;86:835–9.

27. Woo SM, Ryu JK, Lee SH, et al. Branch duct intraductal papillary mucinous neoplasms in a retrospective series of 190 patients. Br J Surg 2009;96:405–11.

28. Turner BG, Brugge WR. Diagnostic and therapeutic endoscopic approaches to intraductal papillary mucinous neoplasm. World J Gastrointest Surg 2010;2:337–41.

29. Brugge WR, Lewandrowski K, Lee-Lewandrowski E, et al. Diagnosis of pancreatic cystic neoplasms: a report of the cooperative pancreatic cyst study. Gastroenterology 2004;126:1330–6.

30. Pitman MB, Michaels PJ, Deshpande V, et al. Cytological and cyst fluid analysis of small (< or =3 cm) branch duct intraductal papillary mucinous neoplasms adds value to patient management decisions. Pancreatology 2008;8:277–84.

31. Khalid A, Zahid M, Finkelstein SD, et al. Pancreatic cyst fluid DNA analysis in evaluating pancreatic cysts: a report of the PANDA study. Gastrointest Endosc 2009;69:1095–102.

32. DeWitt J, McGreevy K, Schmidt CM, et al. EUS-guided ethanol versus saline solution lavage for pancreatic cysts: a randomized, double-blind study. Gastrointest Endosc 2009;70:710–23.

33. DeWitt J, DiMaio CJ, Brugge WR. Long-term follow-up of pancreatic cysts that resolve radiologically after EUS-guided ethanol ablation. Gastrointest Endosc 2010; 72:862–6.
34. Oh HC, Seo DW, Song TJ, et al. Endoscopic ultrasonography-guided ethanol lavage with paclitaxel injection treats patients with pancreatic cysts. Gastroenterology 2011; 140:172–9.
35. Kubo H, Chijiiwa Y, Akahoshi K, et al. Intraductal papillary-mucinous tumors of the pancreas: differential diagnosis between benign and malignant tumors by endoscopic ultrasonography. Am J Gastroenterol 2001;96:1429–34.
36. Ahmad NA, Kochman ML, Lewis JD, et al. Can EUS alone differentiate between malignant and benign cystic lesions of the pancreas? Am J Gastroenterol 2001;96: 3295–300.
37. Brandwein SL, Farrell JJ, Centeno BA, et al. Detection and tumor staging of malignancy in cystic, intraductal, and solid tumors of the pancreas by EUS. Gastrointest Endosc 2001;53:722–7.
38. Cizginer S, Turner B, Bilge AR, et al. Cyst fluid carcinoembryonic antigen is an accurate diagnostic marker of pancreatic mucinous cysts. Pancreas 2011;40: 1024–8.
39. Pais SA, Attasaranya S, Leblanc JK, et al. Role of endoscopic ultrasound in the diagnosis of intraductal papillary mucinous neoplasms: correlation with surgical histopathology. Clin Gastroenterol Hepatol 2007;5:489–95.
40. Pitman MB, Lewandrowski K, Shen J, et al. Pancreatic cysts: preoperative diagnosis and clinical management. Cancer Cytopathol 2010;118:1–13.
41. Sahani DV, Kadavigere R, Blake M, et al. Intraductal papillary mucinous neoplasm of pancreas: multi-detector row CT with 2D curved reformations—correlation with MRCP. Radiology 2006;238:560–9.
42. Rodriguez JR, Salvia R, Crippa S, et al. Branch-duct intraductal papillary mucinous neoplasms: observations in 145 patients who underwent resection. Gastroenterology 2007;133:72–9 [quiz: 309–10].
43. Waters JA, Schmidt CM, Pinchot JW, et al. CT vs MRCP: optimal classification of IPMN type and extent. J Gastrointest Surg 2008;12:101–9.
44. Tanaka M, Chari S, Adsay V, et al. International consensus guidelines for management of intraductal papillary mucinous neoplasms and mucinous cystic neoplasms of the pancreas. Pancreatology 2006;6:17–32.
45. Traverso LW, Peralta EA, Ryan JA Jr, et al. Intraductal neoplasms of the pancreas. Am J Surg 1998;175:426–32.
46. White R, D'Angelica M, Katabi N, et al. Fate of the remnant pancreas after resection of noninvasive intraductal papillary mucinous neoplasm. J Am Coll Surg 2007;204: 987–93 [discussion: 993–5].
47. Chari ST, Yadav D, Smyrk TC, et al. Study of recurrence after surgical resection of intraductal papillary mucinous neoplasm of the pancreas. Gastroenterology 2002; 123:1500–7.
48. Schnelldorfer T, Sarr MG, Nagorney DM, et al. Experience with 208 resections for intraductal papillary mucinous neoplasm of the pancreas. Arch Surg 2008;143:639– 46; discussion 646.
49. Shimada K, Sakamoto Y, Sano T, et al. Invasive carcinoma originating in an intraductal papillary mucinous neoplasm of the pancreas: a clinicopathologic comparison with a common type of invasive ductal carcinoma. Pancreas 2006; 32:281–7.

50. Zamboni G, Fukushima N, Hruban RH, et al. Mucinous cystic neoplasms of the pancreas. In: Bosman FT, Carneiro F, Hruban RH, et al, editors. World Health Organization classification of tumours of the digestive system. 4th edition. Lyon (France): IARC; 2010. p. 300–3.

51. Crippa S, Salvia R, Warshaw AL, et al. Mucinous cystic neoplasm of the pancreas is not an aggressive entity: lessons from 163 resected patients. Ann Surg 2008;247: 571–9.

52. Goh BK, Tan YM, Chung YF, et al. A review of mucinous cystic neoplasms of the pancreas defined by ovarian-type stroma: clinicopathological features of 344 patients. World J Surg 2006;30:2236–45.

53. Yamao K, Yanagisawa A, Takahashi K, et al. Clinicopathological features and prognosis of mucinous cystic neoplasm with ovarian-type stroma: a multi-institutional study of the Japan pancreas society. Pancreas 2011;40:67–71.

54. Megibow AJ. Pancreatic neoplams. In: Gore RM, Levine MS, editors. Textbook of gastrointestinal radiology. 3rd edition. Philadelphia: Elsevier Saunders; 2008. p.1915–31.

55. Buetow PC, Rao P, Thompson LD. From the archives of the AFIP. Mucinous cystic neoplasms of the pancreas: radiologic-pathologic correlation. Radiographics 1998; 18:433–49.

56. Levy MJ. Pancreatic cysts. Gastrointest Endosc 2009;69:S110–6.

57. Sakorafas GH, Smyrniotis V, Reid-Lombardo KM, et al. Primary pancreatic cystic neoplasms revisited: part II. Mucinous cystic neoplasms. Surg Oncol 2011;20:e93–101.

58. Sarr MG, Carpenter HA, Prabhakar LP, et al. Clinical and pathologic correlation of 84 mucinous cystic neoplasms of the pancreas: can one reliably differentiate benign from malignant (or premalignant) neoplasms? Ann Surg 2000;231:205–12.

59. Hruban RH, Pitman MB, Klimstra D. Tumors of the pancreas. Atlas of tumor pathology, 4th series, fascicle 6. Washington, DC: Armed Forces Institute of Pathology; 2007.

60. Terris B, Fukushima N, Hruban RH. Serous neoplasms of the pancreas. In: Bosman FT, Carneiro F, Hruban RH, et al, editors. World Health Organization classification of tumours of the digestive system. 4th edition. Lyon (France): IARC; 2010. p. 296–9.

61. Tseng JF, Warshaw AL, Sahani DV, et al. Serous cystadenoma of the pancreas: tumor growth rates and recommendations for treatment. Ann Surg 2005;242:413–9 [discussion: 419–21].

62. Sakorafas GH, Smyrniotis V, Reid-Lombardo KM, et al. Primary pancreatic cystic neoplasms revisited. Part I: serous cystic neoplasms. Surg Oncol 2011;20:e84–92.

63. Procacci C, Graziani R, Bicego E, et al. Serous cystadenoma of the pancreas: report of 30 cases with emphasis on the imaging findings. J Comput Assist Tomogr 1997;21:373–82.

64. Cohen-Scali F, Vilgrain V, Brancatelli G, et al. Discrimination of unilocular macrocystic serous cystadenoma from pancreatic pseudocyst and mucinous cystadenoma with CT: initial observations. Radiology 2003;228:727–33.

65. Penman ID, Lennon AM. EUS in the evaluation of pancreatic cysts. Endosonography. 2nd edition. In: Hawes RH, Fockens P, Varadarajulu S, editors. Philadelphia: Elsevier Saunders; 2011. p. 166–77.

66. Lewandrowski KB, Southern JF, Pins MR, et al. Cyst fluid analysis in the differential diagnosis of pancreatic cysts. A comparison of pseudocysts, serous cystadenomas, mucinous cystic neoplasms, and mucinous cystadenocarcinoma. Ann Surg 1993; 217:41–7.

67. Huang P, Staerkel G, Sneige N, et al. Fine-needle aspiration of pancreatic serous cystadenoma: cytologic features and diagnostic pitfalls. Cancer 2006;108:239–49.

68. Belsley NA, Pitman MB, Lauwers GY, et al. Serous cystadenoma of the pancreas: limitations and pitfalls of endoscopic ultrasound-guided fine-needle aspiration biopsy. Cancer 2008;114:102–10.
69. Eriguchi N, Aoyagi S, Nakayama T, et al. Serous cystadenocarcinoma of the pancreas with liver metastases. J Hepatobiliary Pancreat Surg 1998;5:467–70.
70. King JC, Ng TT, White SC, et al. Pancreatic serous cystadenocarcinoma: a case report and review of the literature. J Gastrointest Surg 2009;13:1864–8.
71. Kloppel G, Hruban RH, Klimstra D, et al. Solid-pseudopapillary neoplasm of the pancreas. In: Bosman FT, Carneiro F, Hruban RH, et al, editors. World Health Organization classification of tumours of the digestive system. 4th edition. Lyon (France): IARC; 2010. p. 327–30.
72. Papavramidis T, Papavramidis S. Solid pseudopapillary tumors of the pancreas: review of 718 patients reported in English literature. J Am Coll Surg 2005;200:965–72.
73. Tipton SG, Smyrk TC, Sarr MG, et al. Malignant potential of solid pseudopapillary neoplasm of the pancreas. Br J Surg 2006;93:733–7.
74. Buetow PC, Buck JL, Pantongrag-Brown L, et al. Solid and papillary epithelial neoplasm of the pancreas: imaging-pathologic correlation on 56 cases. Radiology 1996;199:707–11.
75. Choi BI, Kim KW, Han MC, et al. Solid and papillary epithelial neoplasms of the pancreas: CT findings. Radiology 1988;166:413–6.
76. Coleman KM, Doherty MC, Bigler SA. Solid-pseudopapillary tumor of the pancreas. Radiographics 2003;23:1644–8.
77. Choi JY, Kim MJ, Kim JH, et al. Solid pseudopapillary tumor of the pancreas: typical and atypical manifestations. AJR Am J Roentgenol 2006;187:W178–86.
78. Jani N, Dewitt J, Eloubeidi M, et al. Endoscopic ultrasound-guided fine-needle aspiration for diagnosis of solid pseudopapillary tumors of the pancreas: a multicenter experience. Endoscopy 2008;40:200–3.
79. Lee SE, Jang JY, Hwang DW, et al. Clinical features and outcome of solid pseudopapillary neoplasm: differences between adults and children. Arch Surg 2008;143:1218–21.
80. Kim CW, Han DJ, Kim J, et al. Solid pseudopapillary tumor of the pancreas: can malignancy be predicted? Surgery 2011;149:625–34.
81. Maker AV, Katabi N, Qin LX, et al. Cyst fluid interleukin-1beta (IL1beta) levels predict the risk of carcinoma in intraductal papillary mucinous neoplasms of the pancreas. Clin Cancer Res 2011;17:1502–8.
82. Iftimia N, Cizginer S, Deshpande V, et al. Differentiation of pancreatic cysts with optical coherence tomography (OCT) imaging: an ex vivo pilot study. Biomed Opt Express 2011;2:2372–82.
83. Huang D, Swanson EA, Lin CP, et al. Optical coherence tomography. Science 1991;254:1178–81.
84. Dunbar K, Canto M. Confocal endomicroscopy. Curr Opin Gastroenterol 2008;24:631–7.
85. Becker V, Wallace MB, Fockens P, et al. Needle-based confocal endomicroscopy for in vivo histology of intra-abdominal organs: first results in a porcine model (with videos). Gastrointest Endosc 2010;71:1260–6.
86. Konda VJ, Aslanian HR, Wallace MB, et al. First assessment of needle-based confocal laser endomicroscopy during EUS-FNA procedures of the pancreas (with videos). Gastrointest Endosc 2011;74:1049–60.
87. Ashida R, Chang KJ. Interventional EUS for the treatment of pancreatic cancer. J Hepatobiliary Pancreat Surg 2009;16:592–7.

88. Brugge WR. EUS-guided ablation therapy and celiac plexus interventions. In: Hawes RH, Fockens P, Varadarajulu S, editors. Endosonography: 2nd edition. Philadelphia: Elsevier Saunders; 2011. p. 275–82.

89. Gan SI, Thompson CC, Lauwers GY, et al. Ethanol lavage of pancreatic cystic lesions: initial pilot study. Gastrointest Endosc 2005;61:746–52.

90. Oh HC, Seo DW, Lee TY, et al. New treatment for cystic tumors of the pancreas: EUS-guided ethanol lavage with paclitaxel injection. Gastrointest Endosc 2008;67: 636–42.

91. Goh BK, Tan YM, Thng CH, et al. How useful are clinical, biochemical, and cross-sectional imaging features in predicting potentially malignant or malignant cystic lesions of the pancreas? Results from a single institution experience with 220 surgically treated patients. J Am Coll Surg 2008;206:17–27.

Management of Pancreatic Neuroendocrine Tumors

Daniel M. Halperin, MD[a], Matthew H. Kulke, MD[b,c,]*

KEYWORDS

- Neuroendocrine tumor • Pancreatic neuroendocrine tumor
- Islet cell tumor • Diagnosis • Prognosis • Management

Pancreatic neuroendocrine tumors (PNETs) account for less than 5% of all pancreatic cancers and have an estimated overall incidence of 5 cases per 1 million population annually.[1,2] In recent years the diagnosed incidence of neuroendocrine tumors has been increasing, probably due at least in part to improved detection and diagnosis.[3] PNETs are best known for their association with characteristic syndromes of hormone hypersecretion. Such symptoms can often be effectively controlled with medical therapy, and when tumors are localized they can be successfully resected. However, the majority of PNETs are clinically silent, presenting at a more advanced clinical stage. Treatment options for patients with advanced PNET have previously been limited. Recently, new biologically targeted therapies have been approved for these tumors and offer improved treatment opportunities for patients with this disease.

CAUSES AND GENETICS

PNETs, also termed *islet cell tumors*, were originally thought to arise from the hormone-producing islet cells of the pancreas. Recent studies have suggested that PNETs may, in fact, arise from ductal progenitor cells, which are putative embryonic and adult pancreatic stem cells.[4] A minority of PNETs are associated with inherited genetic syndromes, including multiple endocrine neoplasia type I (MEN1), von Hippel-Lindau disease, von Recklinghausen disease/neurofibromatosis, and the tuberous sclerosis complex. PNETs are present in the majority of MEN1 patients but are less commonly associated with the other inherited genetic syndromes.[5]

Financial disclosures: DMH has no financial disclosures to report. MHK has served as a consultant to Novartis, Pfizer, Ipsen, and Molecular Insight.

[a] Department of Medicine, Brigham and Women's Hospital, 75 Francis Street, Boston, MA 02115, USA

[b] Department of Medical Oncology, Dana-Farber Cancer Institute, 44 Binney Street, Boston, MA 02115, USA

[c] Harvard Medical School, Boston, MA, USA

* Corresponding author. Department of Medical Oncology, Dana-Farber Cancer Institute, 44 Binney Street, Boston, MA 02115.

E-mail address: Matthew_Kulke@dfci.harvard.edu

CLINICAL PRESENTATION AND DIAGNOSIS

Approximately 70% of PNETs are not associated with symptoms of hormone hypersecretion and instead present with vague abdominal complaints related to mass effect. Much attention has been focused on the potential use of secreted biomarkers for the detection and diagnosis of such tumors. Chromogranin A is a ubiquitous component of dense-core granules in all neuroendocrine cells and is cosecreted with neurohumoral products.[6] Although chromogranin A may be a useful adjunct to other diagnostic modalities, most studies suggest it is not sufficiently sensitive or specific to serve as an independent biomarker. In one study, elevated chromogranin A had a sensitivity of 67.9% and specificity of 85.7% in patients with neuroendocrine tumors.[7] In those patients who do present with symptoms of hormone hypersecretion, symptoms depend in large part on the specific hormone secreted. Characteristic syndromes are summarized in **Table 1** and are described further in the following sections.

Insulinoma

Insulinomas were first described by Whipple and Frantz[8] in 1935 as causing a syndrome of hypoglycemia and neuroglycopenic or sympathetic symptoms that resolve with feeding. When this triad is identified, serum assessment of insulin, proinsulin, C peptide, and glucose are generally used to confirm an endogenous hyperinsulinemic state.[9–11] Absence of ketosis or sulfonylurea metabolites in the blood or urine is another criterion used for diagnosis of insulinoma. For many patients, frequent small meals can normalize the blood glucose sufficiently to

Table 1
Pancreatic neuroendocrine tumors: clinical presentation and medical management of symptoms of hormone secretion

Tumor	Symptoms or Signs	Medical Management
Insulinoma	Hypoglycemia resulting in intermittent confusion, sweating, weakness, nausea. Loss of consciousness may occur in severe cases.	Frequent small meals, diazoxide, dextrose infusions, everolimus
Glucagonoma	Rash (necrotizing migratory erythema), cachexia, diabetes, deep venous thrombosis.	Somatostatin analogs
VIPoma, Verner-Morrison Syndrome, WDHA Syndrome	Profound secretory diarrhea, electrolyte disturbances.	Somatostatin analogs
Gastrinoma, Zollinger-Ellison Syndrome	Acid hypersecretion resulting in refractory peptic ulcer disease, abdominal pain, and diarrhea.	Proton pump inhibitors, somatostatin analogs
Nonfunctioning	May be first diagnosed because of mass effect.	Therapy for tumor control in patients with unresectable disease

Abbreviation: WDHA, watery diarrhea, hypokalemia, acidosis.

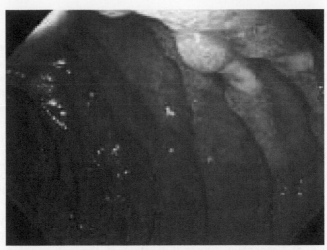

Fig. 1. Multiple duodenal ulcers observed in a patient with gastrinoma.

relieve symptoms. For others, continuous infusions of dextrose can be used. Diazoxide, a nondiuretic antihypertensive seldom used for that indication, has also been used to normalize blood glucose levels.[12,13] More recent reports have suggested that treatment with the mammalian target of rapamycin (mTOR) inhibitor everolimus is highly effective in normalizing glucose levels in patients with symptomatic insulinoma.[14] However, over 90% of these tumors are small, solitary, and successfully treated with surgical resection.[9]

Gastrinoma

Gastrinomas result in a syndrome of hypergastrinemia and refractory peptic ulcer disease originally described by Zollinger and Ellison.[15] Patients typically present with gastroesophageal reflux, abdominal pain, diarrhea, and multiple duodenal ulcers (**Fig. 1**). The diagnosis can be confirmed with elevated fasting gastrin levels, which can be stimulated to supraphysiologic levels in a secretin stimulation test.[16] Importantly, hypercalcemia due to primary hyperparathyroidism in MEN1 patients may independently increase gastrin secretion and stomach acidification in the absence of true gastrinoma.[17] Symptoms of gastrinoma can be controlled with proton pump inhibitors,[18,19] which block the effect of the gastrin without reducing its serum concentration or altering the tumor biology.[20] Treatment with somatostatin analogs is also commonly used to suppress gastrin secretion and in some cases to control tumor growth.

Gastrinomas may present not only in the pancreas but also in extrapancreatic locations within the "gastrinoma triangle." Localizing gastrinomas can be challenging and not uncommonly requires careful imaging with magnetic resonance imaging, somatostatin receptor scintigraphy, or endoscopic ultrasound. Although advances in somatostatin receptor scintigraphy have improved preoperative localization of PNETs, 30% of tumors are still undetected, including over 60% of tumors smaller than 1 cm.[21] Empiric surgery with duodenotomy has therefore been considered in selected hypergastrinemic patients suspected of having gastrinoma.[22]

Glucagonoma

Glucagonomas are associated with the development of migratory necrolytic erythema (dermatitis), diabetes, and an increased risk of deep venous thrombosis.[23] Demonstration of elevated plasma glucagon levels confirms the presence of glucagonoma syndrome. Glucagonomas frequently present as large tumors and at a more advanced stage than other secretory neuroendocrine tumors. Surgical resection is performed when feasible; otherwise, treatment with somatostatin analogs is used to control symptoms.

Vasoactive Intestinal Peptide Tumors (VIPomas)

Patients with tumors that secrete vasoactive intestinal peptide (VIPomas) present with a syndrome of massive (frequently greater than 3 liters daily) secretory diarrhea associated with hypokalemia in the absence of gastric ulceration. This syndrome, caused by excess secretion of vasoactive intestinal peptide, was originally described by Verner and Morrison[24] and has also been described as pancreatic cholera. Elevated levels of vasoactive intestinal peptide in the setting of a pancreatic neuroendocrine tumor are diagnostic of this syndrome. The secretory symptoms associated with VIPoma are highly responsive to somatostatin analogs.

Other PNETs

PNETs have also been reported to secrete somatostatin, adrenocorticotrophic hormone producing Cushing syndrome,[25–27] growth hormone-releasing factor producing acromegaly,[28,29] and various other hormones including erythropoietin and luteinizing hormone.

IMAGING MODALITIES

Detection of both primary lesions and metastases has been significantly improved with the development of increasingly sensitive imaging techniques. Because of its speed and availability, computed tomography (CT) is typically the initial imaging technique used to localize the primary tumor when a hormonal syndrome is identified. Nonfunctioning tumors are most commonly identified incidentally on CT while evaluating mass-related symptoms. Given the vascularity of these lesions, intravenous contrast and multiphasic imaging (including arterial and portal venous phases) is usually recommended. Dynamic magnetic resonance imaging with gadolinium is an alternative imaging modality with a modest increase in sensitivity compared with CT.[30] Use of somatostatin receptor scintigraphy with an indium-111–labeled somatostatin analog ([^{111}In-DTPA^0]octreotide) provides a further imaging modality with relatively high sensitivity[30] and specificity[31] for pancreatic neuroendocrine tumors (Fig. 2).

Traditional imaging techniques are nevertheless often insufficient for localization of all PNETs, especially those smaller than 1 cm in diameter. Endoscopic ultrasound may be more sensitive for detection, particularly for these smaller lesions, and it also provides the potential opportunity to perform a diagnostic biopsy.[32–35] Recent studies have reported that the use of echogenic contrast can improve sensitivity and specificity for both exocrine carcinoma and neuroendocrine tumors in lesions smaller than 2 cm. When used in conjunction with fine-needle aspiration, this technique's sensitivity for malignancy is 100%, improved from 92% when contrast was not used.[33]

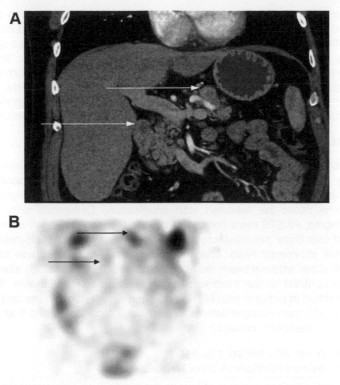

Fig. 2. Characteristics of PNET: CT (*A*) and somatostatin receptor scintigraphy (*B*) in a single patient. Arrows indicate the primary pancreatic tumor and a regional lymph node metastasis.

STAGING, GRADE, AND PROGNOSIS

Several organizations, including the European Neuroendocrine Tumor Society (ENETS)[36,37] and the American Joint Committee on Cancer (AJCC) have proposed staging systems for pancreatic neuroendocrine tumors using the commonly accepted TNM (tumor status-nodal status-metastatic status) notation.[38] These two systems differ slightly; for example, the ENETS system incorporates tumor diameter in its assessment of T stage, whereas the AJCC system incorporates factors determining tumor resectability. Both systems have been clinically validated and are nearly identical in their definitions of stage IV disease.

Stage has a major impact on prognosis. Patients with early-stage, surgically resectable disease generally have high cure rates. The modified ENETS-TNM system predicts a 5-year survival of 100% for stage I disease (tumors <4 cm, restricted to the pancreas), 93% for stage II disease (tumors >4 cm but still restricted to the pancreas), 65% for stage III disease (tumors invading adjacent structures or with positive lymph nodes), and 35% for stage IV (metastatic) disease.[39] Survival estimates for patients with advanced pancreatic neuroendocrine tumors vary. In the Surveillance, Epidemiology, and End Results (SEER) database, for example, the median survival duration for patients with metastatic neuroendocrine tumors was only 24 months. Survival estimates in institutional series are more encouraging, with some estimates for median survival approaching 6 years.

A number of histologic classification systems have been proposed to subclassify neuroendocrine tumors. Despite some differences, all commonly used classification systems reflect the basic observation that neuroendocrine tumors have a spectrum of malignancy ranging from more indolent, well-differentiated tumors to far more aggressive poorly differentiated ones (**Table 2**). As a general rule, tumors with a high grade (grade 3), a mitotic count greater than 20/10 high-powered fields, or a Ki-67 proliferation index of more than 20% represent highly aggressive malignancies with a clinical behavior that differs markedly from more well-differentiated tumors.[3]

MANAGEMENT OF LOCALIZED DISEASE

Surgical resection is the only curative treatment modality for patients with PNET and is generally recommended for patients with localized disease. The specific surgical approach varies depending on tumor size and location. Smaller low-grade tumors may in some cases be resected with enucleation. Compared with pancreatic adenocarcinoma, PNETS more commonly arise in the pancreatic tail where they can be resected with distal pancreatectomy. Whipple resections are performed for larger tumors in the pancreatic head. There is currently no established role for adjuvant therapy with either external beam radiation or systemic chemotherapy after resection of PNET, in contrast to the treatment for pancreatic adenocarcinoma. The role of surgical resection in patients with MEN1 has been debated, given the fact that many of these patients have multiple tumors throughout the pancreas and that symptoms can usually be medically managed.[35]

MANAGEMENT OF ADVANCED DISEASE
Hepatic Resection and Orthotopic Liver Transplantation

In patients with a limited number of liver metastases and a resected primary tumor, hepatic resection may be considered. Uncontrolled trials have reported benefit from cytoreductive surgery for hepatic metastases, with better outcomes associated with complete resections compared with outcomes for incomplete resections.[40] Orthotopic liver transplantation for hepatic oligometastatic disease has also been attempted. Although 5-year survival durations in most series seem to be encouraging, tumor recurrence rates are high, and transplantation remains highly investigational in this setting.

Hepatic Artery Embolization

Hepatic artery embolization is often considered for patients with hepatic predominant disease that is not amenable to surgical resection. Embolization can be performed via the infusion of gel foam powder into the hepatic artery through an angiography catheter (bland embolization) or in conjunction with chemotherapy (eg, doxorubicin, cisplatin, or streptozocin, on drug-eluting beads). A third embolization technique uses radioactive isotopes (eg, yttrium-90 [90-Y]) that are tagged to glass or resin microspheres and delivered selectively to the tumor via the hepatic artery. In the absence of randomized trials, any of the three techniques (bland embolization, chemoembolization, or radioembolization) are considered reasonable approaches for the palliation of neuroendocrine tumor patients, and response rates reported with all three techniques generally exceed 50%.[41–44]

Somatostatin Analogs

Somatostatin analogs are routinely used to control symptoms of hormone hypersecretion in patients with PNETs. Their role in the control of PNET growth, however,

Table 2
Histologic classification of pancreatic neuroendocrine tumors

Differentiation	Grade	Mitotic Count	Ki-67 Index	Traditional	ENETS, WHO
Well-Differentiated	Low grade (G1)	<2 per 10 HPF	≤2%	Islet cell tumor, pancreatic (neuro)endocrine tumor	Neuroendocrine tumor, grade 1
	Intermediate grade (G2)	2–20 per 10 HPF	3–20%	"atypical neuroendocrine tumor"	Neuroendocrine tumor, grade 2
Poorly Differentiated	High-grade (G3)	>20 per 10 HPF	>20%	Small cell carcinoma	Neuroendocrine carcinoma, grade 3, small cell
				Large cell neuroendocrine carcinoma	Neuroendocrine carcinoma, grade 3, large cell

Abbreviations: ENETS, European Neuroendocrine Tumor Society; HPF, high powered fields; WHO, World Health Organization.
Data from Kulke MH, Siu LL, Tepper JE, et al. Future directions in the treatment of neuroendocrine tumors: consensus report of the National Cancer Institute Neuroendocrine Tumor clinical trials planning meeting. J Clin Oncol 2011;29:934–43.

remains uncertain. A randomized trial recently demonstrated that treatment with the somatostatin analog octreotide is associated with improved time to tumor progression in patients with advanced mid-gut neuroendocrine tumors.[45] Ongoing studies are currently evaluating whether somatostatin analogs will be associated with a similar effect in PNETs.[3]

Cytotoxic Chemotherapy

Treatment with cytotoxic chemotherapy has previously been one of the few systemic options available for patients with advanced pancreatic neuroendocrine tumors. The alkylating agent streptozocin was approved for use in patients with advanced PNETs in 1982, after demonstration of antitumor activity in the 1970s.[46] In a subsequent randomized trial, patients with advanced pancreatic neuroendocrine tumors were randomized to receive streptozocin/doxorubicin, streptozocin/5-FU, or chlorozotocin. The overall tumor response rate associated with streptozocin/doxorubicin was reported to be 69%; treatment with streptozocin/doxorubicin in this study was also associated with a modest survival benefit.[47,48] More recent series using standard radiologic response criteria have confirmed that streptozocin-based regimens are active, although they suggest that the tumor response rate associated with streptozocin-based regimens may be somewhat lower. A retrospective analysis of 84 patients demonstrated an objective response rate of 39% and median survival of 37 months for patients with metastatic PNETs treated with the three-drug regimen of 5-fluorouracil, doxorubicin, and streptozocin (FAS).[49]

Recent retrospective studies have suggested that temozolomide-based regimens may be similar in efficacy to streptozocin-based regimens in PNETs.[50–52] Retrospective series have reported highly variable response rates associated with temozolomide-based therapy. In one study evaluating single-agent temozolomide, the overall response rate in PNET was 8%.[50] In a second retrospective series, the overall response rate reported with a combination of temozolomide and capecitabine was 70%.[53] In the largest of the retrospective series, 18 of 53 patients (34%) with PNETs experienced a partial or complete response to temozolomide-based therapy.[54] In prospective studies, temozolomide has been evaluated in combination with thalidomide, bevacizumab, or everolimus, with response rates ranging from 34% to 45%.[55–57] Taken together, these data suggest that temozolomide has similar efficacy to streptozocin-based therapy in advanced PNET.

Patients with poorly differentiated (G3) disease are generally treated using a different chemotherapeutic approach, with platinum-based regimens similar to those used for small cell carcinoma.[58] Some investigators have also added taxanes to these regimens. Although responses with these regimens are observed, the duration of response is generally brief.[59]

mTOR Inhibitors

Initial observations that pancreatic neuroendocrine tumors were at times associated with the tuberous sclerosis complex raised the possibility that inhibition of the mTOR pathway may prove to be an effective treatment approach in this disease. In an initial phase II trial, 60 patients with advanced neuroendocrine tumors, including 30 with PNETs, were treated with octreotide and either 5 mg or 10 mg of everolimus. The overall response rate in PNETs was 27%.[60] A large multicentered phase II study (RADIANT-1) performed in patients with metastatic PNETs who had received prior cytotoxic chemotherapy confirmed antitumor activity associated with everolimus.[61] A third study, RADIANT-3, randomized over 400 patients to receive treatment with either everolimus or placebo. Patients receiving everolimus had a

Table 3
Randomized trials of biologically targeted agents for advanced pancreatic NET

Agent	Patients	Tumor Response Rate (RECIST) (%)	Median PFS (mo)	Reference
Sunitinib	86	9.3	11.4	Raymond et al, 2011[64]
vs				
Placebo	85	0	5.5	
Everolimus	207	5	11	Yao et al, 2011 (RADIANT-3)[62]
vs				
Placebo	203	2	4.6	

Abbreviations: PFS, progression-free survival; RECIST, Response Criteria Evaluation in Solid Tumors.

median progression-free survival rate of 11 months compared with 4.6 months for the placebo group ($P \leq .01$).[62] Patients receiving placebo were crossed over to receive everolimus at the time of tumor progression, and no differences in overall survival were observed between the two arms. The Food and Drug Administration approved everolimus for treatment of advanced PNET, based on the results of this study, in May of 2011.

Vascular Endothelial Growth Factor Receptor Pathway Inhibition

A number of tyrosine kinase inhibitors targeting the vascular endothelial growth factor receptor, as well as other receptor tyrosine kinases, have been evaluated in advanced PNET including pazopanib, sorafenib, and sunitinib. In phase II studies, overall response rates associated with these agents in PNET have ranged from 11% to 19%.[63] Sunitinib was subsequently taken forward in a randomized, placebo-controlled study (**Table 3**). This study, which had originally planned to enroll 340 patients, was closed after the enrollment of 171 patients. At the time of study closure, the median progression-free survival was 11.4 months in the sunitinib group compared with 5.5 months in the placebo group, leading to its Food and Drug Administration approval for advanced PNET.[64]

Peptide Receptor Radionuclide Therapy

Somatostatin receptor–targeted radionuclide therapy has been a theoretically attractive option for patients with advanced neuroendocrine tumors, given the prevalence of somatostatin receptor expression in most neuroendocrine tumor subtypes. In a prospective phase II study of 90 patients with metastatic carcinoid tumor and symptoms refractory to octreotide treated with ^{90}Y-DOTA tyr3-octreotide (90Y-edotreotide), over 50% of patients had improvement in symptom control. Modest tumor responses were noted, including 4% of patients with a partial radiographic response and 70% with stable disease after treatment.[65] ^{177}Lu-DOTA, Tyr3-octreotate has been used in the treatment of over 500 patients with either carcinoid or PNETs. Efficacy results reported for 310 patients suggest an overall tumor response rate of up to 30%.[66] Randomized prospective studies better defining the antitumor activity and long-term toxicity of radiolabeled somatostatin analogs are anticipated.

FUTURE DIRECTIONS

Whereas there have been multiple new developments in the treatment of PNETs, early recognition of symptoms, appropriate diagnosis, and surgical intervention remain the most effective strategies to enhance cure rates. For patients with advanced, inoperable disease, targeted therapies for advanced PNETs represent encouraging new treatment options. A better understanding of the genetic and molecular events driving the growth of PNETs should lead to the identification of molecular subgroups, as well as to the development of predictive markers. The recent identification of characteristic mutations in PNETs involving menin, the mTOR pathway, and chromatin remodeling may provide an initial step in this direction.[5] Additionally, ongoing studies evaluating novel therapies and new therapeutic combinations promise to enhance further outcomes for patients with this unique disease.

REFERENCES

1. Lam KY, Lo CY. Pancreatic endocrine tumour: a 22-year clinico-pathological experience with morphological, immunohistochemical observation and a review of the literature. Eur J Surg Oncol 1997;23:36–42.
2. Yao JC, Eisner MP, Leary C, et al. Population-based study of islet cell carcinoma. Ann Surg Oncol 2007;14:3492–500.
3. Kulke MH, Siu LL, Tepper JE, et al. Future directions in the treatment of neuroendocrine tumors: consensus report of the National Cancer Institute Neuroendocrine Tumor clinical trials planning meeting. J Clin Oncol 2011;29:934–43.
4. Vortmeyer AO, Huang S, Lubensky I, et al. Non-islet origin of pancreatic islet cell tumors. J Clin Endocrinol Metab 2004;89:1934–8.
5. Jensen RT, Berna MJ, Bingham DB, et al. Inherited pancreatic endocrine tumor syndromes: advances in molecular pathogenesis, diagnosis, management, and controversies. Cancer 2008;113:1807–43.
6. Modlin IM, Gustafsson BI, Moss SF, et al. Chromogranin A–biological function and clinical utility in neuro endocrine tumor disease. Ann Surg Oncol 2010;17(9):2427–43.
7. Bajetta E, Ferrari L, Martinetti A, et al. Chromogranin A, neuron specific enolase, carcinoembryonic antigen, and hydroxyindole acetic acid evaluation in patients with neuroendocrine tumors. Cancer 1999;86(5):858–65.
8. Whipple AO, Frantz VK. Adenoma of islet cells with hyperinsulinism: a review. Ann Surg 1935;101:1299–335.
9. Kulke MH, Anthony LB, Bushnell DL, et al. NANETS treatment guidelines: well-differentiated neuroendocrine tumors of the stomach and pancreas. Pancreas 2010; 39:735–52.
10. Hirshberg B, Livi A, Bartlett DL, et al. Forty-eight-hour fast: the diagnostic test for insulinoma. J Clin Endocrinol Metab 2000;85:3222–6.
11. Quinkler M, Strelow F, Pirlich M, et al. Assessment of suspected insulinoma by 48-hour fasting test: a retrospective monocentric study of 23 cases. Horm Metab Res 2007;39:507–10.
12. Gill GV, Rauf O, MacFarlane IA. Diazoxide treatment for insulinoma: a national UK survey. Postgrad Med J 1997;73:640–1.
13. Goode PN, Farndon JR, Anderson J, et al. Diazoxide in the management of patients with insulinoma. World J Surg 1986;10:586–92.
14. Kulke MH, Bergsland EK, Yao JC. Glycemic control in patients with insulinoma treated with everolimus. N Engl J Med 2009;360:195–7.
15. Zollinger RM, Ellison EH. Primary peptic ulcerations of the jejunum associated with islet cell tumors of the pancreas. Ann Surg 1955;142:709–23 [discussion: 724–8].
16. Lamers CG, Van Tongeren JH. Comparative study of the value of the calcium, secretin, and meal stimulated increase in serum gastrin to the diagnosis of the Zollinger-Ellison syndrome. Gut 1977;18:128–35.

17. Norton JA, Venzon DJ, Berna MJ, et al. Prospective study of surgery for primary hyperparathyroidism (HPT) in multiple endocrine neoplasia-type 1 and Zollinger-Ellison syndrome: long-term outcome of a more virulent form of HPT. Ann Surg 2008;247:501–10.

18. Blanchi A, Delchier JC, Soule JC, et al. Control of acute Zollinger-Ellison syndrome with intravenous omeprazole. Lancet 1982;2:1223–4.

19. Lambers CB, Lind T, Moberg S, et al. Omeprazole in Zollinger-Ellison syndrome. Effects of a single dose and of long-term treatment in patients resistant to histamine H2-receptor antagonists. N Engl J Med 1984;310:758–61.

20. Maton PN, Lack EE, Collen MJ, et al. The effect of Zollinger-Ellison syndrome and omeprazole therapy on gastric oxyntic endocrine cells. Gastroenterology 1990;99: 943–50.

21. Alexander HR, Fraker DL, Norton JA, et al. Prospective study of somatostatin receptor scintigraphy and its effect on operative outcome in patients with Zollinger-Ellison syndrome. Ann Surg 1998;228(2):228–38.

22. Norton JA, Alexander HR, Fraker DL, et al. Does the use of routine duodenotomy (DUODX) affect rate of cure, development of liver metastases, or survival in patients with Zollinger-Ellison syndrome? Ann Surg 2004;239(5):617–25 [discussion: 626].

23. Vinik AI, Gonzales MR. New and emerging syndromes due to neuroendocrine tumors. Endocrinol Metab Clin North Am 2011;40:19–63, vii.

24. Verner JV, Morrison AB. Islet cell tumor and a syndrome of refractory watery diarrhea and hypokalemia. Am J Med 1958;25:374–80.

25. Balls KF, Nicholson JT, Goodman HL, et al. Functioning islet-cell carcinoma of the pancreas with Cushing's syndrome. J Clin Endocrinol Metab 1959;19:1134–43.

26. Maton PN, Gardner JD, Jensen RT. Cushing's syndrome in patients with the Zollinger-Ellison syndrome. N Engl J Med 1986;315:1–5.

27. Rosenberg AA. Fulminating adrenocortical hyperfunction associated with islet-cell carcinoma of the pancreas; case report. J Clin Endocrinol Metab 1956;16:1364–73.

28. Gola M, Doga M, Bonadonna S, et al. Neuroendocrine tumors secreting growth hormone-releasing hormone: Pathophysiological and clinical aspects. Pituitary 2006; 9:221–9.

29. Thorner MO, Perryman RL, Cronin MJ, et al. Somatotroph hyperplasia. Successful treatment of acromegaly by removal of a pancreatic islet tumor secreting a growth hormone-releasing factor. J Clin invest 1982;70:965–77.

30. Gibril F, Reynolds JC, Doppman JL, et al. Somatostatin receptor scintigraphy: its sensitivity compared with that of other imaging methods in detecting primary and metastatic gastrinomas. A prospective study. Ann Intern Med 1996;125:26–34.

31. Gibril F, Reynolds JC, Chen CC, et al. Specificity of somatostatin receptor scintigraphy: a prospective study and effects of false-positive localizations on management in patients with gastrinomas. J Nucl Med 1999;40:539–53.

32. Dabizzi E, Panossian A, Raimondo M. Management of pancreatic neuroendocrine tumors. Minerva Gastroenterol Dietol 2010;56(4):467–79.

33. Kitano M, Kudo M, Yamao K, et al. Characterization of small solid tumors in the pancreas: the value of contrast-enhanced harmonic endoscopic ultrasonography. Am J Gastroenterol 2011. [Epub ahead of print].

34. Norton JA, Jensen RT. Resolved and unresolved controversies in the surgical management of patients with Zollinger-Ellison syndrome. Ann Surg 2004;240(5):757–73.

35. Tonelli F, Fratini G, Nesi G, et al. Pancreatectomy in multiple endocrine neoplasia type 1-related gastrinomas and pancreatic endocrine neoplasias. Ann Surg 2006;244(1): 61–70.

36. Liszka Ł, Pajk J, Mrowiec S, et al. Discrepancies between two alternative staging systems (European Neuroendocrine Tumor Society 2006 and American Joint Committee on Cancer/Union for International Cancer Control 2010) of neuroendocrine neoplasms of the pancreas. A study of 50 cases. Pathol Res Pract 2011;207:220–4.

37. Rindi G, Klöppel G, Alhman H, et al. TNM staging of foregut (neuro)endocrine tumors: a consensus proposal including a grading system. Virchows Arch 2006;449:395–401.

38. Edge SB, Byrd DR, Compton CC, et al. AJCC cancer staging manual. 7th edition. New York: Springer; 2010.

39. Scarpa A, Mantovani W, Capelli P, et al. Pancreatic endocrine tumors: improved TNM staging and histopathological grading permit a clinically efficient prognostic stratification of patients. Mod Pathol 2010;23:824–33.

40. Sarmiento JM, Heywood G, Rubin J, et al. Surgical treatment of neuroendocrine metastases to the liver: a plea for resection to increase survival. J Am Coll Surg 2003;197:29–37.

41. Ruszniewski P, Rougier P, Roche A, et al. Hepatic arterial chemoembolization in patients with liver metastases of endocrine tumors. A prospective phase II study in 24 patients. Cancer 1993;71:2624–30.

42. Eriksson BK, Larsson EG, Skogseid BM, et al. Liver embolizations of patients with malignant neuroendocrine gastrointestinal tumors. Cancer 1998;83:2293–301.

43. Gupta S, Johnson MM, Murthy R, et al. Hepatic arterial embolization and chemoembolization for the treatment of patients with metastatic neuroendocrine tumors: variables affecting response rates and survival. Cancer 2005;104:1590–602.

44. Arslan N, Emi M, Alagoz E, et al. Selective intraarterial radionuclide therapy with Yttrium-90 (Y-90) microspheres for hepatic neuroendocrine metastases: initial experience at a single center. Vojnosanit Pregl 2011;68(4):341–8.

45. Rinke A, Müller H-H, Schade-Brittinger C, et al. Placebo-controlled, double-blind, prospective, randomized study on the effect of octreotide LAR in the control of tumor growth in patients with metastatic neuroendocrine midgut tumors: a report from the PROMID Study Group. J Clin Oncol 2009;27:4656–63.

46. Broder LE, Carter SK. Pancreatic islet cell carcinoma. II. Results of therapy with streptozotocin in 52 patients. Ann Intern Med 1973;79:108–18.

47. Moertel CG, Hanley JA, Johnson LA. Streptozocin alone compared with streptozocin plus fluorouracil in the treatment of advanced islet-cell carcinoma. N Engl J Med 1980;303:1189–94.

48. Moertel CG, Lefkopoulo M, Lipsitz S, et al. Streptozocin-doxorubicin, streptozocin-fluorouracil or chlorozotocin in the treatment of advanced islet-cell carcinoma. N Engl J Med 1992;326:519–23.

49. Kouvaraki MA, Ajani JA, Hoff P, et al. Fluorouracil, doxorubicin, and streptozocin in the treatment of patients with locally advanced and metastatic pancreatic endocrine carcinomas. J Clin Oncol 2004;22:4762–71.

50. Ekeblad S, Sundin A, Janson ET, et al. Temozolomide as monotherapy is effective in treatment of advanced malignant neuroendocrine tumors. Clin Cancer Res 2007;13:2986–91.

51. Kulke MH, Bendell J, Kvols L, et al. Evolving diagnostic and treatment strategies for pancreatic neuroendocrine tumors. J Hematol Oncol 2011;4:29.

52. Kulke MH, Hornick JL, Frauenhoffer C, et al. O6-methylguanine DNA methyltransferase deficiency and response to temozolomide-based therapy in patients with neuroendocrine tumors. Clin Cancer Res 2009;15:338–45.

53. Strosberg JR, Fine RL, Choi J, et al. First-line chemotherapy with capecitabine and temozolomide in patients with metastatic pancreatic endocrine carcinomas. Cancer 2011;117(2):268–75.

54. Kulke M, Hornick J, Frauenhoffer C, et al. O6-methylguanine DNA methyltransferase deficiency and response to temozolomide-based therapy in patients with neuroendocrine tumors. Clin Cancer Res 2009;15(1):338–45.

55. Kulke MH, Stuart K, Earle C. A phase II study of temozolomide and bevacizumab in patients with advance neuroendocrine tumors [abstract]. ASCO Annual Meeting Proceedings 2006;24:4044a.

56. Kulke MH, Blaszkowsky L, Zhu A. Phase I/II study of everolimus (RAD001) in combination with temozolomide in patients with advanced pancreatic neuroendocrine tumors [abstract]. Gastrointestinal Cancers Symposium 2010:223a.

57. Kulke MH, Stuart K, Enzinger PC, et al. Phase II study of temozolomide and thalidomide in patients with metastatic neuroendocrine tumors. J Clin Oncol 2006; 24(3):401–6.

58. Moertel CG, Kvols LK, O'Connell MJ, et al. Treatment of neuroendocrine carcinomas with combined etoposide and cisplatin. Evidence of major therapeutic activity in the anaplastic variants of these neoplasms. Cancer 1991;68:227–32.

59. Hainsworth JD, Spigel DR, Litchy S, et al. Phase II trial of paclitaxel, carboplatin, and etoposide in advanced poorly differentiated neuroendocrine carcinoma: a Minnie Pearl Cancer Research Network Study. J Clin Oncol 2006;24(22):3548–54.

60. Yao JC, Phan AT, Chang DZ, et al. Efficacy of RAD001 (everolimus) and octreotide LAR in advanced low- to intermediate-grade neuroendocrine tumors: results of a phase II study. J Clin Oncol 2008;26:4311–8.

61. Yao JC, Lombard-Bohas C, Baudin E, et al. Daily oral everolimus activity in patients with metastatic pancreatic neuroendocrine tumors after failure of cytotoxic chemotherapy: a phase II trial. J Clin Oncol 2010;28:69–76.

62. Yao JC, Shah MH, Ito T, et al. Everolimus for advanced pancreatic neuroendocrine tumors. N Engl J Med 2011;364:514–23.

63. Oberstein PE, Saif MW. Novel agents in the treatment of unresectable neuroendocrine tumors. Highlights from the "ASCO Annual Meeting". 2011 Chicago, IL, USA; June 3–7, 2011. JOP 2011;12(4):358–61.

64. Raymond E, Dahan L, Raoul J-L, et al. Sunitinib malate for the treatment of pancreatic neuroendocrine tumors. N Engl J Med 2011;364:501–13.

65. Bushnell DL Jr, O'Dorisio TM, O'Dorisio MS, et al. 90Y-edotreotide for metastatic carcinoid refractory to octreotide. J Clin Oncol 2010;28(10):1652–9.

66. Kwekkeboom DJ, de Herder WW, Kam BL, et al. Treatment with the radiolabeled somatostatin analog [177 Lu-DOTA 0,Tyr3]octreotate: toxicity, efficacy, and survival. J Clin Oncol 2008;26(13):2124–30.

Pancreas Transplantation

Kiran K. Dhanireddy, MD

KEYWORDS

- Diabetes • Transplantation • Surgical complications
- Retinopathy • Vasculopathy • Nephropathy

In the early part of the 20th century, many research groups were trying to isolate insulin from the other digestive proteins of the pancreas. In 1921, Fredrick Banting and his assistant Charles Best succeeded in purifying insulin and treating diabetes. For the first time, patients with type 1 diabetes could live well into adulthood. In 1966, the world's first simultaneous kidney and pancreas transplant was performed on a 28-year-old woman with diabetes and renal failure at the University of Minnesota by Kelly and Lillehei.[1] In the subsequent 45 years, simultaneous pancreas and kidney transplantation has been adopted as the definitive treatment for type 1 diabetes complicated by end-stage renal disease. Pancreas transplantation is also used to treat type 1 diabetes without renal failure in patients who have life-threatening complications, such as severe hypoglycemic unawareness. Increasingly, pancreas transplantation is being recognized as a beneficial treatment for nonobese patients with type 2 diabetes and its attendant complications.[2–5] Approximately 6% of pancreas transplants are performed for treatment of type 2 diabetes.[6]

Pancreas transplant is typically performed in combination with kidney transplantation (simultaneous pancreas and kidney, or SPK) but can also be performed after kidney transplant (pancreas after kidney, or PAK) or in isolation (pancreas alone, or PA). The goal of pancreas transplantation is exogenous insulin-free euglycemia. Intensive control of blood sugars with insulin administration can delay the onset and slow the progression of diabetic complications but cannot reverse them.[7] On the other hand, pancreas transplantation offers the prospect of excellent glycemic control free of exogenous insulin administration, improvement in quality of life, and reduction in diabetes-associated complications.

PANCREAS ORGAN DONORS

The number of pancreas transplants peaked at 1484 in 2004. Since then the volume of pancreas transplants has been decreasing (**Fig. 1**). The vast majority of pancreas transplants originate from brain-dead donors. Although some centers accept donors after cardiac death, these donors account for less than 5% of total transplants.

The author has nothing to disclose.
Keck School of Medicine, University of Southern California, 1510 San Pablo Street, Suite 200, Los Angeles, CA, USA
E-mail address: Kiran.Dhanireddy@med.USC.edu

Gastroenterol Clin N Am 41 (2012) 133–142
doi:10.1016/j.gtc.2011.12.002
0889-8553/12/$ – see front matter © 2012 Elsevier Inc. All rights reserved.

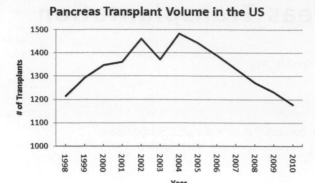

Fig. 1. There has been a steady decline in the total number of pancreas transplants performed in the United States since 2004. (Based on Organ Procurement and Transplantation Network data as of November 1, 2011.)

Additionally, since 2000, approximately 20 live-donor pancreas transplants have been performed (based on Organ Procurement and Transplantation Network data as of November 1, 2011).

The ideal pancreas donor is younger than 30 years old with a body mass index (BMI) under 25. A retrospective analysis of the Scientific Registry of Transplant Recipients was performed to calculate a pancreas donor risk index.[8] Ten donor variables and cold ischemia time were identified as risk factors for grafts loss. The donor factors most strongly associated with poor outcome were increased age, donation after cardiac death, African American race, and higher BMI. There are multiple possible explanations for the decline in overall pancreas transplant numbers, but underutilization of potential donors is a persistent problem.[9–11] Approximately 20% to 25% of potential organ donors are used for pancreas transplant, but a large number of potential donors are refused for reasons that are difficult to ascertain.[10] Use of a group of potential pancreas donors that meet the typical clinical criteria of young age and low BMI could increase pancreas transplant volume by as much as 30%.

SURGICAL PROCEDURE

The pancreas allograft is typically transplanted into the right iliac fossa and receives arterial inflow from the iliac artery. Before implantation, a Y conduit of donor iliac artery is anastomosed to the superior mesenteric and splenic arteries of the graft. The venous and exocrine routes of pancreatic drainage are the two primary technical considerations during a pancreas transplant. The portal vein of the pancreatic allograft can be anastomosed to the portal vein or iliac vein (systemic venous drainage) of the recipient. The exocrine secretions can be drained into the intestine or bladder.

Portal Versus Systemic Venous Drainage

The majority of pancreatic allografts use the iliac vessels for vascular inflow and outflow. Systemic venous drainage may be associated with lower thrombosis rates. On the other hand, portal venous drainage mimics natural physiology by allowing for first-pass degradation of insulin in the liver.

Systemic venous drainage of the pancreatic allograft has been associated with increased peripheral insulin levels and theoretically lower portal insulin levels.[12] Hyperinsulinemia is thought to be an independent risk factor for increased ischemic cardiovascular disease.[13] Pancreatic venous drainage into the liver via the portal vein is thought to decrease circulating insulin levels and potentially offer a metabolic advantage. In fact, portal venous drainage is associated with higher cholesterol levels, and systemic venous drainage is associated with mild hyperinsulinemia and increased insulin resistance.[14] Glucose metabolism does not seem to be affected by the route of venous drainage when comparing patients receiving SPK transplant or kidney transplant alone, thereby controlling for the effects of immunosuppression.[15] Any risk posed by peripheral hyperinsulinemia is more than likely offset by long-term euglycemia. Overall, portal venous drainage does not provide a significant metabolic advantage over systemic venous drainage.

Bladder Versus Enteric Drainage

During surgery the head of the pancreas is placed down into the pelvis, allowing either enteric or bladder exocrine drainage. Enteric drainage allows for delivery of pancreatic secretions into the intestine and was thought to be more physiologically advantageous. Unfortunately, complications with the side-to-side duodenojejunostomy can be life-threatening. Leak from the enteric anastomosis requires surgical exploration and can necessitate allograft pancreatectomy. To mitigate some of the risk associated with enteric drainage, some groups perform Roux-en-Y duodenojejunostomy. Additionally, enteric drainage is associated with an increased rate of graft thrombosis.[16] Undetected early acute rejection in enteric-drained grafts might explain the increased thrombosis rate.[17,18] Severe complications from enteric leaks and sepsis prompted the advent of bladder drainage by Sollinger and colleagues[19] in the 1980s. The primary advantage of bladder drainage is the ease of monitoring the pancreatic graft function. Decreased urinary amylase precedes irreversible hyperglycemia in association with allograft acute cellular rejection.[20] In addition, cystoscopic evaluation of the graft duodenum and graft biopsy is possible. Unfortunately, bladder drainage is associated with multiple genitourinary symptoms such as recurrent urinary tract infection, prostatitis, urethritis, and hematuria.[21] Graft duodenal complications include bleeding and ulceration. Bladder drainage can result in severe metabolic acidosis and dehydration due to urinary bicarbonate loss. Because of these specific complications, conversion to enteric drainage is required in 30% of patients within 5 years and 50% of patients within 15 years.[22] However, a prospective study showed that the route of exocrine drainage does not impact overall patient survival or pancreas graft function.[22,23] Therefore, the majority of SPK transplant patients have enteric exocrine drainage. PA patients have a higher rate of immunologic graft loss and therefore require close surveillance.[6] This group of patients should be considered for bladder drainage to allow for cystoscopy and biopsy.

SURGICAL COMPLICATIONS AFTER PANCREAS TRANSPLANTATION

Pancreas transplantation is complicated by a high rate of early technical failure. In the 1980s, worldwide technical failure rates were approximately 25%. In the subsequent 30 years the rate has fallen to approximately 7% to 9%.[16] Surgical complications require exploration in approximately 30% of patients and almost invariably are associated with graft loss, patient morbidity, and increased cost.[24,25] To a large degree, the high rate of technical failure has inhibited wider adoption of pancreas transplantation as the preferred modality for treating diabetes.

Graft thrombosis is the most frequent serious surgical complication after pancreas transplant. The symptoms of thrombosis include unexplained hyperglycemia, tenderness over the graft, graft enlargement, and in bladder-drained grafts, hematuria and decreased urinary amylase. Donor selection is critical in reducing the risk of thrombosis. The donor factors associated with thrombosis include increased donor age, massive donor volume resuscitation, hemodynamic instability, and cerebrovascular accident as cause of donor death.[26] Poor surgical technique during organ recovery or back table preparation also increases the surgical complication rate. The use of histidine-tryptophan-ketoglutarate preservation solution also seems to increase the rate of surgical complications, particularly if the cold ischemia time exceeds 12 hours.[27] The diagnosis of graft thrombosis is made on ultrasound, computed tomography (CT) angiography, magnetic resonance imaging, or conventional angiography. Once thrombosis is diagnosed, prompt surgical exploration is prudent to prevent leak and sepsis and to reduce the potential for mortality.[24] Nonoperative management of thrombosis is considered in select cases, but careful patient selection is mandatory.[28,29]

Early posttransplant graft pancreatitis can be difficult to definitively diagnose because hyperamylasemia is commonly seen in the early posttransplant period. Risk factors for pancreatitis include advanced donor age, donor obesity, prolonged cold ischemia time, and bladder drainage.[17,24,30] In patients with bladder drainage, reflux pancreatitis can be treated with Foley catheter drainage. Complications of graft pancreatitis are similar to those of native pancreatitis and include peripancreatic abscess, pancreatic necrosis (sterile or infected), pancreatic fistula, and pseudocyst. Late-graft pancreatitis occurs an average of 28 months after transplant.[31] These patients typically present with fever and graft tenderness. Late-graft pancreatitis can be adequately treated with bowel rest, antibiotics, and percutaneous drainage as needed.[31]

Duodenal leaks from bladder-drained pancreas grafts typically occur within the first 3 months, and are easily diagnosed with a cystogram. Prolonged Foley catheter drainage is adequate treatment in up to two-thirds of cases.[32] In complicated cases, surgical exploration and repair or enteric conversion may be required.[33] In contrast, leakage from enteric-drained pancreas grafts frequently results in sepsis and peritonitis secondary to spillage of enteric contents. Early enteric leaks are technical, whereas late leaks are typically due to rejection, infection, or ischemia. Diagnosis of enteric leak is often made on CT scan. Prompt reexploration with conversion to Roux-en-Y drainage or even graft pancreatectomy in severely contaminated cases is required.

Intraabdominal bleeding in the early period after pancreas transplant is typically associated with systemic anticoagulation initiated to prevent graft thrombosis. It is important to rule out venous graft thrombosis of either the pancreas or kidney. Therapy is then directed toward correcting coagulation abnormalities. If a significant perigraft hematoma develops, strong consideration should be given to surgical exploration and evacuation to prevent subsequent infection of the hematoma. Gastrointestinal bleeding within 7 days of enteric-drained pancreas grafts is usually from the anastomotic suture line.[34] This bleeding may require surgical exploration and direct control of bleeding, revision of the duodenojejunal anastomosis, or graft pancreatectomy.[34]

IMPACT OF PANCREAS TRANSPLANTATION ON PATIENT SURVIVAL

There is considerable debate as to whether pancreas transplant translates into an improvement in survival compared with kidney transplant alone (KTA) in diabetic patients with end-stage renal disease. In a large retrospective analysis of the

Scientific Registry of Transplant Recipients, including more than 13,000 patients with type 1 diabetes, the adjusted 10-year survival after SPK transplant was 67%.[35] For patients receiving live-donor KTA the survival was 65%, and for patients receiving deceased-donor KTA the survival was significantly lower at 46%. The survival advantage of SPK transplant was clear in all patient groups compared with deceased-donor KTA, except in recipients older than 50 years. The strong caveat in this study was that the survival advantage for SPK transplant was not seen until 5 years after transplant because of the higher rate of early mortality in patients receiving SPK transplants compared with patients receiving KTA.[35] In patients with preserved renal function, the advantage of pancreas transplant is less clear. A review of data from the United Network for Organ Sharing/Organ Procurement and Transplantation Network suggested that conventional therapy was associated with better survival than PA transplant.[36] Although there are questions about the methodology of this study, at best PA transplant is associated with survival rates similar to convention insulin therapy.[37] Although patients receiving SPK transplant show a clear survival advantage compared with those on the waiting list, the most important prognostic factor for long-term survival in these patients is preservation of pancreatic graft function.[37]

IMPACT OF PANCREAS TRANSPLANTATION ON DIABETES-RELATED COMPLICATIONS

Insulin-dependent diabetes is complicated by long-term microvascular, macrovascular, and neurologic sequelae. Although pancreas transplantation is not necessarily a life-saving procedure, the degree of glycemic control afforded by a functioning pancreas allograft impacts the development and progression of diabetes-related complications.

Cardiovascular Disease

Cardiovascular disease is the leading cause of mortality in patients with diabetes. One potential explanation for improved patient survival after SPK transplant is an improvement in coronary artery disease. In an observational angiographic study comparing 26 patients who had functioning pancreas grafts with 6 patients who had failed pancreas grafts, 38% of patients who had successful grafts showed a reduction in angiographic evidence of coronary atherosclerotic lesions compared with 0% of those who had failed grafts.[38] These improvements are probably directly related to improved glucose control in the patients with functioning grafts. Additionally, rates of cardiovascular mortality, myocardial infarction, and pulmonary edema are improved in patients who had SPK transplants compared with KTA.[39,40] The rate of cardiovascular mortality is 7.6% in SPK transplant patients compared with 20% in KTA patients and 16.1% in patients awaiting transplant.[39]

Ophthalmologic Complications

Diabetes is one of the leading causes of adult-onset blindness and can be associated with multiple ophthalmologic complications such as retinopathy, cataracts, and glaucoma. The most common microvascular complication associated with type 1 diabetes is retinopathy.[7] Approximately 80% of patients with diabetes will have some degree of retinopathy within 15 years of diagnosis.[41] The initial stages of retinal vasculopathy are not associated with vascular proliferation, although proliferative retinopathy develops as the disease progresses.

Patients receiving PA transplant benefit from reduced rates of retinopathy progression compared with patients treated with intensive insulin regimens alone.[42] In patients with nonproliferative retinopathy who underwent PA transplant, 50% of patients showed improvement, and the remainder showed no progression. In patients without transplant, 20% improved, 10% remained unchanged, and 70% worsened. In patients who had laser-treated proliferative retinopathy and who underwent transplant, 86% experienced stabilization of retinal disease and 14% experienced progression. These results compare favorably with patients who did not have a transplant: 43% experienced disease stabilization and 57% experienced disease progression.

Cataracts are the leading cause of blindness worldwide. Diabetes and corticosteroid use are recognized risk factors for cataract development.[43] In a prospective study, SPK transplant patients followed for up to 10 years demonstrated significant increased risk of cataract development.[44] Advanced age and high-dose pulse steroid administration were significant risk factors. Therefore, posttransplant patients require regular screening for visual acuity.

Nephropathy

Diabetic nephropathy is characterized by nodular glomerulosclerosis and proteinuria. Determining the effect of pancreas transplantation on the progression of nephropathy can be challenging because of multiple confounding factors, not least of which is administration of nephrotoxic immunosuppression.[45] Normoglycemia after pancreas transplantation can halt the progression of diabetic nephropathy, but a long period of graft function may be required to reverse diabetic nephropathy.[46–49] In patients receiving PA transplants there was no evidence of amelioration of glomerular lesions 5 years after transplant.[48] Further follow-up of these patients at 10 years showed decrease in the glomerular and tubular basement membrane width. For some patients these measurements fell into the normal range.[49] There was resolution of Kimmelstiel-Wilson nodular lesions and reduction of mesangial expansion. Therefore, a prolonged period of normogylcemia was required before a demonstrable reduction in the glomerular, tubular, and interstitial lesions of diabetic nephropathy. In terms of clinical parameters, PA transplant results in decrease in urinary protein excretion but does not improve serum creatinine or creatinine clearance.[50]

Neuropathy

Polyneuropathy affects approximately 50% of all people with diabetes.[51] Endoneurial microvascular disease of somatic and autonomic nerves results in abnormal nerve conduction.[52] The common symptoms include numbness and tingling of the extremities, gastroparesis, diarrhea, wounds of the lower extremities, and erectile dysfunction. In a 10-year prospective study of 115 pancreas transplant recipients compared with 92 control patients who had insulin-dependent diabetes, motor and sensory nerve conduction indices were improved. Clinical examination and tests of autonomic function improved slightly. In the control population, all measures of neuropathy progressed.[53] Autonomic nervous system dysfunction in persons with diabetes is associated with increased mortality.[54,55] Pancreas transplant may ameliorate some of the mortality risk associated with abnormal cardiorespiratory reflexes due to autonomic neuropathy.[55] Unfortunately, pancreas transplant does not result in resolution of neuropathy; improvement tended to be mild, and typical time to improvement ranged from 1 to 4 years.

Vascular Disease

Patients with Type 1 diabetes are at significant risk for stroke and lower extremity amputation because of cerebrovascular and peripheral vascular disease. The effect of pancreas transplant on the progression of macrovascular disease has been controversial. One measure of overall cerebrovascular and cardiovascular risk is carotid intima media thickness.[56] In one study, patients awaiting pancreas transplant had increased carotid intima media thickness. In patients who had a successful pancreas transplant, carotid intima media thickness was no different than the thickness in matched controls after 4 years.[56] On the contrary, in another study, serial carotid ultrasound suggested progressive worsening of atherosclerotic lesions in patients after SPK transplant.[57] These findings were not associated with an actual increase in the number of strokes. In a small study comparing the prevalence of cerebrovascular, cardiovascular, and peripheral vascular disease in patients who underwent SPK transplant or KTA, no difference was seen until after more than 5 years.[58] As with other complications of diabetes, pancreas transplant may improve macrovascular disease in patients after a prolonged period of normoglycemia and pancreas graft function.

SUMMARY

SPK transplant is the definitive treatment of type 1 diabetes combined with end-stage renal disease. Long-term graft function can lead to improvement in diabetes-related complications and, in patients younger than 50 years, can lead to improved overall survival. PAK transplant and PA transplant do not result in similar improvements in patient survival, but with appropriate patient selection, they can improve quality of life by rendering patients insulin-free. Pancreas transplant is associated with more surgical complications and higher perioperative morbidity and mortality than KTA. Therefore, careful donor and recipient selection along with meticulous surgical technique are mandatory for optimal outcomes.

REFERENCES

1. Kelly WD, Lillehei RC, Merkel FK, et al. Allotransplantation of the pancreas and duodenum along with the kidney in diabetic nephropathy. Surgery 1967;61(6): 827–37.
2. Intensive blood-glucose control with sulphonylureas or insulin compared with conventional treatment and risk of complications in patients with type 2 diabetes (UKPDS 33). Lancet 1998;352(9131):837–53.
3. Light JA, Barhyte DY. Simultaneous pancreas-kidney transplants in type I and type II diabetic patients with end-stage renal disease: similar 10-year outcomes. Transplant Proc 2005;37(2):1283–4.
4. Nath DS, Gruessner AC, Kandaswamy R, et al. Outcomes of pancreas transplants for patients with type 2 diabetes mellitus. Clin Transplant 2005;19(6):792–7.
5. Singh RP, Rogers J, Farney AC, et al. Do pretransplant C-peptide levels influence outcomes in simultaneous kidney-pancreas transplantation? Transplant Proc 2008; 40(2):510–2.
6. Gruessner AC, Sutherland DE, Gruessner RW. Pancreas transplantation in the United States: a review. Curr Opin Organ Transplant 2010;15(1):93–101.
7. The effect of intensive treatment of diabetes on the development and progression of long-term complications in insulin-dependent diabetes mellitus. The Diabetes Control and Complications Trial Research Group. N Engl J Med 1993;329(14):977–86.
8. Axelrod DA, Sung RS, Meyer KH, et al. Systematic evaluation of pancreas allograft quality, outcomes and geographic variation in utilization. Am J Transplant 2010;10(4): 837–45.
9. Stratta RJ, Bennett L. Pancreas underutilization in the United States: analysis of United Network for Organ Sharing data. Transplant Proc 1997;29(8):3309–10.

10. Wiseman AC, Wainright JL, Sleeman E, et al. An analysis of the lack of donor pancreas utilization from younger adult organ donors. Transplantation 2010;90(5):475–80.

11. Krieger NR, Odorico JS, Heisey DM, et al. Underutilization of pancreas donors. Transplantation 27 2003;75(8):1271–6.

12. Diem P, Abid M, Redmon JB, et al. Systemic venous drainage of pancreas allografts as independent cause of hyperinsulinemia in type I diabetic recipients. Diabetes 1990;39(5):534–40.

13. Despres JP, Lamarche B, Mauriege P, et al. Hyperinsulinemia as an independent risk factor for ischemic heart disease. N Engl J Med 1996;334(15):952–7.

14. Petruzzo P, Badet L, Lefrancois N, et al. Metabolic consequences of pancreatic systemic or portal venous drainage in simultaneous pancreas-kidney transplant recipients. Diabet Med 2006;23(6):654–9.

15. Katz H, Homan M, Velosa J, et al. Effects of pancreas transplantation on postprandial glucose metabolism. N Engl J Med 1991;325(18):1278–83.

16. Gruessner AC, Sutherland DE. Pancreas transplant outcomes for United States (US) and non-US cases as reported to the United Network for Organ Sharing (UNOS) and the International Pancreas Transplant Registry (IPTR) as of June 2004. Clin Transplant 2005;19(4):433–55.

17. Drachenberg CB, Papadimitriou JC, Farney A, et al. Pancreas transplantation: the histologic morphology of graft loss and clinical correlations. Transplantation 2001; 71(12):1784–91.

18. White SA, Shaw JA, Sutherland DE. Pancreas transplantation. Lancet 2009; 373(9677):1808–17.

19. Sollinger HW, Cook K, Kamps D, et al. Clinical and experimental experience with pancreaticocystostomy for exocrine pancreatic drainage in pancreas transplantation. Transplant Proc 1984;16(3):749–51.

20. Prieto M, Sutherland DE, Fernandez-Cruz L, et al. Urinary amylase monitoring for early diagnosis of pancreas allograft rejection in dogs. J Surg Res 1986;40(6):597–604.

21. Kleespies A, Mikhailov M, Khalil PN, et al. Enteric conversion after pancreatic transplantation: resolution of symptoms and long-term results. Clin Transplant 2011;25(4): 549–60.

22. Sollinger HW, Odorico JS, Becker YT, et al. One thousand simultaneous pancreas-kidney transplants at a single center with 22-year follow-up. Ann Surg 2009;250(4): 618–30.

23. Stratta RJ, Gaber AO, Shokouh-Amiri MH, et al. A prospective comparison of systemic-bladder versus portal-enteric drainage in vascularized pancreas transplantation. Surgery 2000;127(2):217–26.

24. Cohn JA, Englesbe MJ, Ads YM, et al. Financial implications of pancreas transplant complications: a business case for quality improvement. Am J Transplant 2007;7(6): 1656–60.

25. Troppmann C, Gruessner AC, Dunn DL, et al. Surgical complications requiring early relaparotomy after pancreas transplantation: a multivariate risk factor and economic impact analysis of the cyclosporine era. Ann Surg 1998;227(2):255–68.

26. Troppmann C, Gruessner AC, Benedetti E, et al. Vascular graft thrombosis after pancreatic transplantation: univariate and multivariate operative and nonoperative risk factor analysis. J Am Coll Surg 1996;182(4):285–316.

27. Stewart ZA, Cameron AM, Singer AL, et al. Histidine-tryptophan-ketoglutarate (HTK) is associated with reduced graft survival in pancreas transplantation. Am J Transplant 2009;9(1):217–21.

28. Stockland AH, Willingham DL, Paz-Fumagalli R, et al. Pancreas transplant venous thrombosis: role of endovascular interventions for graft salvage. Cardiovasc Intervent Radiol 2009;32(2):279–83.

29. Gilabert R, Fernandez-Cruz L, Real MI, et al. Treatment and outcome of pancreatic venous graft thrombosis after kidney–pancreas transplantation. Br J Surg Mar 2002; 89(3):355–60.

30. Humar A, Kandaswamy R, Drangstveit MB, et al. Prolonged preservation increases surgical complications after pancreas transplants. Surgery 2000;127(5):545–51.

31. Small RM, Shetzigovski I, Blachar A, et al. Redefining late acute graft pancreatitis: clinical presentation, radiologic findings, principles of management, and prognosis. Ann Surg 2008;247(6):1058–63.

32. Nath DS, Gruessner A, Kandaswamy R, et al. Late anastomotic leaks in pancreas transplant recipients - clinical characteristics and predisposing factors. Clin Transplant 2005;19(2):220–4.

33. West M, Gruessner AC, Metrakos P, et al. Conversion from bladder to enteric drainage after pancreaticoduodenal transplantations. Surgery 1998;124(5):883–93.

34. Orsenigo E, Fiorina P, Dell'Antonio G, et al. Gastrointestinal bleeding from enterically drained transplanted pancreas. Transpl Int 2005;18(3):296–302.

35. Ojo AO, Meier-Kriesche HU, Hanson JA, et al. The impact of simultaneous pancreas-kidney transplantation on long-term patient survival. Transplantation 2001;71(1):82–90.

36. Venstrom JM, McBride MA, Rother KI, et al. Survival after pancreas transplantation in patients with diabetes and preserved kidney function. JAMA 2003;290(21):2817–23.

37. Gruessner RW, Sutherland DE, Gruessner AC. Mortality assessment for pancreas transplants. Am J Transplant 2004;4(12):2018–26.

38. Jukema JW, Smets YF, van der Pijl JW, et al. Impact of simultaneous pancreas and kidney transplantation on progression of coronary atherosclerosis in patients with end-stage renal failure due to type 1 diabetes. Diabetes Care 2002;25(5):906–11.

39. La Rocca E, Fiorina P, di Carlo V, et al. Cardiovascular outcomes after kidney-pancreas and kidney-alone transplantation. Kidney Int 2001;60(5):1964–71.

40. La Rocca E, Fiorina P, Astorri E, et al. Patient survival and cardiovascular events after kidney-pancreas transplantation: comparison with kidney transplantation alone in uremic IDDM patients. Cell Transplant 2000;9(6):929–32.

41. Aiello LP, Gardner TW, King GL, et al. Diabetic retinopathy. Diabetes Care 1998;21(1): 143–56.

42. Giannarelli R, Coppelli A, Sartini MS, et al. Pancreas transplant alone has beneficial effects on retinopathy in type 1 diabetic patients. Diabetologia 2006;49(12):2977–82.

43. Karim AK, Jacob TJ, Thompson GM. The human lens epithelium; morphological and ultrastructural changes associated with steroid therapy. Exp Eye Res 1989;48(2): 215–24.

44. Pai RP, Mitchell P, Chow VC, et al. Posttransplant cataract: lessons from kidney-pancreas transplantation. Transplantation 2000;69(6):1108–14.

45. Nankivell BJ, Borrows RJ, Fung CL, et al. Evolution and pathophysiology of renal-transplant glomerulosclerosis. Transplantation 2004;78(3):461–8.

46. Bohman SO, Tyden G, Wilczek H, et al. Prevention of kidney graft diabetic nephropathy by pancreas transplantation in man. Diabetes 1985;34(3):306–8.

47. Bilous RW, Mauer SM, Sutherland DE, et al. The effects of pancreas transplantation on the glomerular structure of renal allografts in patients with insulin-dependent diabetes. N Engl J Med 1989;321(2):80–5.

48. Fioretto P, Mauer SM, Bilous RW, et al. Effects of pancreas transplantation on glomerular structure in insulin-dependent diabetic patients with their own kidneys. Lancet 1993;342(8881):1193–6.

49. Fioretto P, Steffes MW, Sutherland DE, et al. Reversal of lesions of diabetic nephropathy after pancreas transplantation. N Engl J Med 1998;339(2):69–75.

50. Coppelli A, Giannarelli R, Vistoli F, et al. The beneficial effects of pancreas transplant alone on diabetic nephropathy. Diabetes Care 2005;28(6):1366–70.

51. Tesfaye S, Boulton AJ, Dyck PJ, et al. Diabetic neuropathies: update on definitions, diagnostic criteria, estimation of severity, and treatments. Diabetes Care 2010;33(10):2285–93.

52. Giannini C, Dyck PJ. Ultrastructural morphometric abnormalities of sural nerve endoneurial microvessels in diabetes mellitus. Ann Neurol 1994;36(3):408–15.

53. Navarro X, Sutherland DE, Kennedy WR. Long-term effects of pancreatic transplantation on diabetic neuropathy. Ann Neurol 1997;42(5):727–36.

54. Ewing DJ, Campbell IW, Clarke BF. Mortality in diabetic autonomic neuropathy. Lancet 1976;1(7960):601–3.

55. Navarro X, Kennedy WR, Aeppli D, et al. Neuropathy and mortality in diabetes: influence of pancreas transplantation. Muscle Nerve 1996;19(8):1009–16.

56. Larsen JL, Ratanasuwan T, Burkman T, et al. Carotid intima media thickness decreases after pancreas transplantation. Transplantation 2002;73(6):936–40.

57. Nankivell BJ, Lau SG, Chapman JR, et al. Progression of macrovascular disease after transplantation. Transplantation 2000;69(4):574–81.

58. Biesenbach G, Konigsrainer A, Gross C, et al. Progression of macrovascular diseases is reduced in type 1 diabetic patients after more than 5 years successful combined pancreas-kidney transplantation in comparison to kidney transplantation alone. Transpl Int 2005;18(9):1054–60.

Pancreatic Cancer Screening

Eun Ji Shin, MD, Marcia Irene Canto, MD, MHS*

KEYWORDS

- Pancreatic cancer • Genetic predisposition • Tumor markers
- Screening

PANCREATIC CANCER: WHY CONSIDER SCREENING?

Pancreatic cancer remains one of the most deadly diseases, despite significant advances in medicine over the past decade. Pancreatic adenocarcinoma is the fourth leading cause of cancer deaths in the United States for both males and females, with an estimated 44,030 new cases and 37,660 deaths in 2011.[1] In contrast to the death rates for other leading causes of cancer death (lung, colorectal, breast, and prostate), which have declined since 2003, the death rate from pancreatic adenocarcinoma has increased during the same time period.[1] Unfortunately, the majority of symptomatic patients are incurable. The prognosis for patients with pancreatic adenocarcinoma remains poor: a 5-year relative survival rate of 6% for all stages combined, most likely because of the late stage of disease at the time of diagnosis. Hence, there has been a strong interest in detecting precursor lesions or small asymptomatic cancers that are potentially curable. A widespread screening program does not seem feasible or cost effective given the relatively low incidence of the disease, accounting for 3% of all new cancer cases in the United States, and the lack of accurate, inexpensive, and noninvasive diagnostic tests for early lesions. However, screening may be desirable in the selected population at increased risk for developing pancreatic adenocarcinoma.

GENETIC PREDISPOSITION TO PANCREATIC CANCER

Although the great majority of pancreatic adenocarcinoma cases are thought to be sporadic in nature, up to 10% of cases can be attributed to genetic factors.[2–4] In fact, familial clustering of pancreatic cancer was noted as early as 1967, when Lynch and colleagues reported on an adenocarcinoma-prone family.[5] Familial pancreatic cancer (FPC) is characterized by two or more first-degree relatives (FDRs) with pancreatic adenocarcinoma in the absence of known cancer syndromes or other diseases with known genetic defect. Individuals from a family with a pair of affected FDRs have a higher risk (6.4-fold to 32-fold) of developing pancreatic cancer.[6–9] Thus far, the key causative gene or genes leading to the inherited predisposition in familial pancreatic

---

The authors have nothing to disclose.

Department of Internal Medicine, Division of Gastroenterology and Hepatology, Johns Hopkins University School of Medicine, 1830 East Monument Street, Baltimore, MD 21205, USA

* Corresponding author.

E-mail address: mcanto1@jhmi.edu

Gastroenterol Clin N Am 41 (2012) 143–157

doi:10.1016/j.gtc.2011.12.001

gastro.theclinics.com

cancer have not yet been fully elucidated. Complex segregation analysis suggests that this predisposition may be due to a novel rare major gene with an autosomal dominant inheritance with reduced penetrance.[10–13]

Initial linkage analysis suggested that the mutation of the palladin gene may be involved in the development of pancreatic cancer in a specific kindred.[14] However, the initial excitement has been tempered by the failure of population-based studies in Canada and Europe to demonstrate that mutations in the palladin gene are more common in those with FPC as compared to controls.[15–18] Further, a study evaluating the pattern of palladin protein expression in 177 cases of pancreatic adenocarcinoma determined that although the palladin protein is overexpressed in the stroma, it is not overexpressed in the neoplastic cells in pancreatic cancer.[19]

To date, germline breast cancer 2 (BRCA2) mutation appears to be the most common genetic abnormality in patients from FPC kindreds who develop pancreatic adenocarcinoma, but still have been reported in only 6% to 19% of all FPC kindreds.[20–22] Mutations in the BRCA2 gene can be present even in the absence of breast or ovarian cancer, and in apparently sporadic pancreatic cancer. Recent studies have identified another associated inheritable gene mutation, partner and localizer for breast cancer 2 gene (PALB2), as a pancreatic adenocarcinoma suscep-tibility gene, which may be causative for 3% to 4% of FPC.[7,9] The PALB2 protein directly binds to the breast cancer 1 gene (BRCA1) and acts as a bridge between BRCA1 and BRCA2 to form a complex involved in double-strand break repair.[23] The PALB2 gene is present in 1% to 2% of patients with familial breast cancer. Subsequent testing of patients with a personal history of breast and pancreatic cancer[24] and also of non-BRCA1 and non-BRCA2 breast cancer women with a personal or family history of pancreatic cancer[25] has shown the PALB2 mutation to be a very uncommon mutation. The clinical utility of routine testing of FPC patients for PALB2 has not been proven.

INHERITED CANCER SYNDROMES
Hereditary Pancreatitis

Hereditary pancreatitis is a rare inherited disorder characterized by recurrent attacks of acute pancreatitis in childhood or early adolescence, followed by the development of chronic pancreatitis in late adolescence or early adulthood.[26] It is transmitted as an autosomal dominant disorder with incomplete penetrance.[27] Most are due to germ-line gain-of-function mutations in a cationic trypsinogen gene (PRSS1) on chromo-some 7q35.[28–30] Mutations in PRSS1 cause premature trypsin activation and ineffective autodegradation of active trypsin mutants, leading to autodigestion and acute pancreatitis.[31] Hereditary pancreatitis is associated with one of the highest estimated lifetime risks for developing pancreatic cancer among the inherited pancreatic cancer syndromes, with a lifetime risk approaching 40%.[32,33] Particularly in those individuals with a paternal inheritance pattern, the cumulative risk for developing pancreatic cancer is approximately 75%.[32] Tobacco smoking increases the risk even further in this population, by approximately twofold, and decreases the age at onset of pancreatic cancer by approximately 20 years.[27,34]

Peutz–Jeghers Syndrome

Peutz–Jeghers syndrome is an autosomal dominantly inherited polyposis syndrome with high penetrance. The reported frequency of Peutz–Jeghers syndrome is 1 in 8300 to 280,000 individuals.[35] It is characterized by hamartomatous polyps of the gastrointestinal (GI) tract and mucocutaneous pigmentation. It is caused by an inherited germline mutation of the STK11/LKB1 tumor-suppressor gene.[36] Patients with Peutz–Jeghers syndrome have a significantly increased lifetime risk for multiple GI cancers, including esophageal (0.5%), stomach (29%), small intestinal (13%), and colon (39%).[37] These patients are also at increased risk for non-GI cancers, including breast (54%), lung (15%), ovarian (21%), cervical (10%), uterine (9%), and testicular (9%). The cumulative lifetime risk for developing pancreatic cancer is 36%, with a relative risk (RR) of 132.[37]

Familial Atypical Multiple Mole Melanoma

Familial atypical multiple mole melanoma is an autosomally dominant disease with variable penetrance. It is characterized by familial occurrence of multiple benign melanocytic nevi, dysplastic nevi, and melanoma.[38] It is associated with germline mutations in the *p16/CDKN2A* gene.[39,40] This syndrome is associated with an increased risk of sarcomas and endometrial, breast, and lung cancers.[41,42] There is an approximately 13-fold to 22-fold increased risk of pancreatic cancer in these patients compared to the general population.[42,43]

Lynch Syndrome

Patients with hereditary nonpolyposis colorectal cancer syndrome, also known as Lynch syndrome, have mutations in the mismatch repair genes (*MLH1*, *MSH2*, *MSH6*, and *PMS2*). Lynch syndrome is characterized by early-onset colorectal cancer. Patients with Lynch syndrome are also prone to develop other types of cancers, including endometrial, gastric, renal, ureteral, and small intestinal cancers.[44] Lifetime risk of pancreatic cancer in patients with Lynch syndrome is 3.7% up to the age of 70, which is an 8.6-fold increased risk compared to the general population.[45]

Familial Breast–Ovarian Cancer

Familial breast–ovarian cancer syndrome is an autosomal dominantly inherited syndrome associated with germline mutations in *BRCA1* and *BRCA2* tumor-suppressor genes involved in repair of DNA damage. Carriers of the gene mutations are at a high risk for developing early-onset breast and ovarian cancers, as well as cancers of the gallbladder and bile duct (RR 4.97), prostate (RR 4.65), stomach (RR 2.59), and malignant melanoma (RR 2.58).[46] *BRCA1* mutation is associated with a 2.3-fold to 3.6-fold increased risk for pancreatic cancer,[47,48] and *BRCA2* mutation is associated with a 3-fold to 10-fold increased risk for pancreatic cancer.[46,49,50] In patients with sporadic pancreatic cancer, 7.3% had a germline *BRCA2* mutation.[51] Approximately 1% of the general Ashkenazi Jewish population carries each of the *BRCA1* and *BRCA2* founder mutations.[52, 53] Studies have shown that the *BRCA2* mutation is found in 5.5% to 10% of patients with pancreatic adenocarcinoma who are of Ashkenazi Jewish descent.[52–55]

TARGETS FOR SCREENING AND SURVEILLANCE

The ideal screening strategy for pancreatic cancer would target high-grade benign noninvasive precursor neoplastic lesions (pancreatic intraepithelial neoplasias [PanINs] or intraductal papillary mucinous neoplasms [IPMNs]) before malignant transformation or at an early stage that would allow for curative surgical resection.[56] Although IPMNs can be detected as cystic lesions or a dilated main pancreatic duct or both, PanINs are small branch ducts less than 5 mm in size, often microscopic, and not reliably visualized by clinical imaging tests. Hence, the optimal strategy for detection of early pancreatic neoplasia may need to involve biomarker tests alone or in combination with imaging.

AVAILABLE AND ANTICIPATED TUMOR MARKERS

Currently, there is no biomarker with adequate sensitivity and specificity that can be used for routine clinical screening.[57] Given the typical late stage of disease at the time of diagnosis, there has been much effort invested in identifying accurate tumor markers to aid in earlier diagnosis of pancreatic cancer.

The most widely used serum marker in patients with pancreatic cancer is sialylated Lewis blood group antigen on MUC-1 (Mucin 1, cell surface associated), carbohydrate antigen 19-9 (CA 19-9). It is a cell surface glycoprotein expressed by pancreatic cancer cells, but is also found in normal pancreatic and biliary duct cells and gastric, colonic, endometrial, and salivary epithelia.[58] Consequently, CA 19-9 is not routinely used for diagnosis because of the unacceptably high rate of false-positive results, with specificity ranging from 33% to 100%.[59–61] CA 19-9 is also associated with imperfect sensitivity, ranging from 41% to 86%.[59,61] Approximately 4% to 15% of the general population do not express the Lewis antigen and therefore do not have detectable CA 19-9 levels.[61–65] In patients with resectable pancreatic cancer, only 65% exhibit an elevated level of CA 19-9.[61] The marker is also inadequate to differentiate reliably between pancreatic cancer and chronic pancreatitis, as up to 40% of patient with chronic pancreatitis can exhibit elevated levels of CA 19-9.[61,66] Given its performance characteristics as a biomarker in the general population, serum CA 19-9 is used primarily for monitoring responses to therapy in patients already diagnosed with cancer, rather than for early diagnosis.[61,67–69] A recent feasibility study of 546 individuals with one or more FDRs with pancreatic cancer used serum CA19-9 as a screening test. In the 27 patients with elevated CA 19-9 levels, endoscopic ultrasound (EUS) was performed, and one case of asymptomatic pancreatic ductal adenocarcinoma was detected.[70]

Carcinoembryonic antigen (CEA) was the first biomarker used in diagnostics. Several studies have demonstrated high levels of CEA in the pancreatic juice of patients with pancreatic cancer compared to those with benign pancreatic disease.[71–74] When the CEA cutoff level was set at 50 ng/mL, the positive predictive value, negative predictive value, and accuracy for diagnosing pancreatic cancer were 77%, 95%, and 85%, respectively.[71,75] The main limitation of CEA is its low sensitivity, ranging from 25% to 56%, with relatively high specificity, ranging from 82% to 100% in distinguishing pancreatic cancer from benign pancreatic diseases.[59,76–81]

Much of the initial efforts in identifying novel markers of pancreatic cancer focused on carbohydrate antigens of MUC1 in hopes of improving the performance of CA 19-9. PAM4 is an anti-MUC1 monoclonal antibody that appears to detect MUC1 expressed by pancreatic cancer more specifically than it detects MUC1 antigens derived from other cancers (eg, breast and ovarian).[82] Further, in comparison with CA 19-9, PAM4 demonstrated higher sensitivity and specificity in discriminating patients with pancreatic cancer from those with chronic pancreatitis ($P<.003$).[82] As expected, patients with advanced disease had significantly higher levels that those with early disease. Diagnostic sensitivity of PAM4 for stage 3 and stage 4 disease was 91%; for stage 2, 86%; and for stage 1, 62% (stage 1A, 54%; stage 1B, 75%).[83] Further supporting the potential role of PAM4 in detecting early-stage pancreatic cancer, PAM4 expression was detected in precursor lesions of pancreatic adenocarcinoma, positive in 89% of PanINs and 86% of IMPNs examined, including 94% of the earliest neoplastic lesions, PanIN-1A and 1B.[84]

Recent studies have identified other potential biomarkers for pancreatic cancer, including CA494,[85] carcinoembryonic antigen-related cell adhesion molecule 1 (CEACAM1),[86] parathyroid hormone-related protein (PTHrP),[87] tumor M2-pyruvate kinase (TuM2-PK),[88] anti-mucin antibody CAM 17.1,[78] and serum beta-human chorionic gonadotropin (β-HCG).[89] Although their performance characteristics in initial studies are promising, larger studies are needed to confirm their clinical applicability and they are currently used only in research settings.

Pancreatic juice sample provides a rich medium for genetic and epigenetic marker analysis. Pancreatic juice samples can be obtained at the time of endoscopic ultrasound (secretin-stimulated) or endoscopic retrograde cholangiopancreatography (duodenal aspirate[90] or pure pancreatic juice).[57] Markers that have been studied in pancreatic juice include K-*ras* mutations, *p53* mutations, DNA methylation aberrations, and mitochondrial DNA mutations.[61] Mutant K-*ras* is a marker of particular interest because these mutations are present in 90% of pancreatic adenocarcinomas and it has been measured in pancreatic juice samples. However, its sensitivity and specificity for pancreatic cancer are poor (sensitivity 38%–62%; specificity 88%–90%), most likely because mutant K-*ras* can also be found in chronic pancreatitis and in PanINs without pancreatic cancer.[57,90–96] Mutations at *p53* are found in approximately 70% of invasive pancreatic adenocarcinomas[91] and have been detected in 40% to 50% of pancreatic juice samples and brush cytology specimens of patients with pancreatic cancer.[97] DNA promoter methylation alterations have been investigated in multiple candidate genes, including *p16*,[98,99] *RELN*,[100] *DAB1*,[100] *ppENK*,[101,102] *Cyclin D2*,[103] *SOCS1*,[104] *SPARC*,[105] *TSLC1*,[106] and others.[61,102,107] DNA promoter hypermethylation status was quantified in a panel of candidate genes (*Cyclin D2*, *FOXE1*, *NPTX2*, *ppENK*, *p16*, and *TFP12*) in pure pancreatic juice obtained from patients with pancreatic ductal adenocarcinoma, intraductal papillary mucinous neoplasms, chronic pancreatitis, and controls with no known pancreatic disease, as well as a from a cohort of high-risk individuals from FPC kindreds. This method demonstrated high sensitivity (82%) and specificity (100%) in identifying patients with pancreatic cancer.[108] Mitochondrial DNA mutations are commonly found in multiple cancers.[61,109–113] Using chip technologies, initial studies appear to suggest that mitochondrial mutations can be reliably detected in pancreatic juice samples from patients with pancreatic cancer.[61,111]

APPROACHES TO SCREENING

Currently, there is no sufficiently sensitive, specific, and reliable screening test for the early detection of pancreatic cancer. The great majority of pancreatic cancers, accounting for at least 90% of all patients, are considered sporadic.[2–4] The detection rate is low in average-risk individuals because pancreatic cancer is a rare disease, despite its significant death toll. In screening studies performed in Japan, 5 cancers were found in 2511 individuals.[114] Given the overall low incidence of disease and the current lack of accurate, inexpensive, and noninvasive screening tests, the consensus is that widespread population-based screening for pancreatic cancer in the general population or in those with only one affected FDR is neither feasible nor indicated in most countries.[56] However, selective screening has been performed in high-risk patients from FPC kindreds and in patients with inherited cancer syndromes.[56,115,116]

The various approaches to screening and results of screening tests for asymptomatic pancreatic neoplasms are summarized in **Table 1**. One approach is population-based screening, such as that formed in Japan with abdominal ultrasound (with[114] or without[117] MRI). A second approach uses a serum biomarker such as serum CA19-9 followed by a pancreatic imaging test.[70] A third approach uses only abdominal imaging tests, such as computed tomography (CT), magnetic resonance imaging (MRI), EUS, or endoscopic retrograde cholangiopancreatography (ERCP), in combination or in

Table 1
Approaches to pancreatic screening

	Sequential Serum Biomarker + Imaging	Sequential Abdominal Imaging Tests	Single or Concurrent Imaging Tests
Sporadic population		Transabdominal US followed by noncontrast MRI/MRCP, prospective study in 2511 patients found 5 cancers (4 resectable)[130]	Transabdominal US in 130,951 patients found 3 PDA[117]
High-risk population	Serum CA19-9 followed by EUS if >37 U/mL detected in 546 individuals with ≥1 FDR with pancreatic cancer found pancreatic neoplasms in 5/546 (1 early cancer)	MRI/MRCP or CT followed by EUS in FPC relatives found IPMN and PDA in 8.3%[130] EUS followed by ERCP (when abnormal) detected PanINs[60]	MRI/MRCP only in 79 p16 mutation carriers detected 5 cancers[125] EUS + MRI/MRCP in FPC relatives detected IPMNs or PDA or both[131] EUS + MDCT in FPC relatives detected IPMNs, PNET, and PDA[115,116] EUS only in FPC relatives and mutation carriers detected IPMNs and PDA[126]

Abbreviations: CA 19-9, carbohydrate antigen 19-9; CT, computed tomography; ERCP, endoscopic retrograde cholangiopancreatography; EUS, endoscopic ultrasound; FDR, first-degree relative; FPC, familial pancreatic cancer; IPMNs, intraductal papillary mucinous neoplasms; MDCT, multi-detector computed tomography; MRI/MRCP, nagnetic resonance imaging/magnetic resonance cholangiopancreatography; PanINs, pancreatic intraepithelial neoplasias; PDA, pancreatic ductal adenocarcinoma; PNET, Pancreatic neuroendocrine tumors; US, ultrasound.

sequence (ie, EUS after MRI or magnetic resonance cholangiopancreatography [MRCP], or CT if abnormal).

Multidetector computed tomography (MDCT) is currently the abdominal imaging test of choice for pancreatic disease, particularly for diagnosis of solid tumors and staging of pancreatic cancer.[118,119] Despite its high accuracy for detecting and staging of pancreatic malignancies, the sensitivity of MDCT may be suboptimal, as MDCT misses lesions when used for screening for early pancreatic neoplasia.[115,116,119] The sensitivity of thin-section, triple-phase helical CT to detect lesions smaller than 2 cm is only 70% to 80%.[56,120] Recent studies have shown that MDCT has a negative predictive value of 87% for tumor resectability[121] and an accuracy rate of 85% to 95%.[75,122,123] Further, there is also a concern for radiation exposure if CT is used as part of a long-term screening or surveillance program, particularly in individuals with impaired DNA mismatch repair gene function due to BRCA1, BRCA2, or PALB2 gene mutation. Hence, CT is not the ideal screening or surveillance imaging test for high-risk individuals. Further, MDCP with a pancreatic protocol may not be as sensitive as EUS in at-risk individuals from FPC kindreds[115,116,124] (Canto MI, Hruban RH, Fishman EK, et al. Screening for prevalent early pancreatic neoplasia in high risk individuals: a prospective multicenter blinded study of EUS, CT, and MRI. Submitted for publication).

MRI may be an appropriate choice for noninvasive screening of high-risk patients because it is able to image the entire abdomen and pelvis, unlike EUS, while avoiding radiation exposure, unlike CT. MRCP is able to image pancreatic ductal anatomy noninvasively (unlike ERCP) and small cystic lesions such as IPMNs. Preliminary data from high-risk patients who underwent surgical resection suggest that MRI/MRCP may be superior to CT, particularly for detection of IPMNs (71% vs 14%, $P<.0001$).[56,124] A prospective MRI-based screening study of 79 patients aged 39 to 72 years with a p16 Leiden mutation, which is associated with familial atypical multiple mole melanoma syndrome, has shown that early-stage pancreatic cancers can be detected at baseline and during follow-up.[125] After a median follow-up period of 4 years (range, 0–10 years), pancreatic cancer was diagnosed in seven patients (9%). The mean age at diagnosis was 59 years (range, 49–72 years). Three of the asymptomatic pancreatic cancers were present at the first examination, and four were detected after a negative result in the initial examination. All seven patients with cancer had resectable lesions; five underwent surgery, three had an R0 resection, and two had lymph node metastases. Further, possible precursor lesions (ie, duct ectasias or branch-duct IPMNs, based on MRCP) were found in nine individuals (11%).

EUS has been used to screen high-risk individuals in several screening programs.[60,115,116,126,127] It can provide high-resolution images of the pancreas without the risk of radiation exposure and can image mural nodules (focal thickening of the wall in branch duct IMPNs), which are associated with increased risk of malignancy.[57,119,128] The disadvantages of EUS are that it is operator dependent and is an endoscopic procedure with the inherent risks of procedure and sedation, which may limit its role in a widespread screening and surveillance program. Preliminary analysis of high-risk individuals enrolled in a screening program who underwent surgical resection suggests that EUS can detect almost twice as many neoplastic lesions as CT or MRI/MRCP.[56,124] Published studies using EUS-based screening for high-risk individuals have reported detection of asymptomatic precancerous branch duct IPMNs, large PanINs, incidental pancreatic endocrine tumors, and ductal adenocarcinomas. One Dutch study of BRCA1, BRCA2, or p16 germline mutation carriers, patients with Peutz–Jeghers syndrome, and relatives of patients reported a high one-time yield of EUS-based screening. The authors found a 6.8% prevalence (n = 3 of 44 individuals screened) of asymptomatic pancreatic ductal adenocarcinomas (12, 20, and 50 mm in size).[126] All cancers were completely resected but two already had lymph node metastases at presentation. Further, the diagnostic yield of EUS-based screening for prevalent precursor branch duct IPMNs was 16%.

The clinical utility of ancillary studies such as fine-needle aspiration (FNA) and ERCP is not clear. EUS-guided FNA has been used to investigate pancreatic cystic lesions and can provide a cytologic diagnosis of IPMN in 71% of the cases.[129] The need for routine FNA of pancreatic cysts in a high-risk population has not been proven, given that the majority of cystic lesions detected are typically small branch duct IPMNs that do not require surgical treatment. EUS-guided FNA can also lead to false-positive results if cytologic aspirates show severe dysplasia or findings suspicious for ductal adenocarcinoma, which can lead to potentially unnecessary surgery.[115] ERCP has been used routinely in high-risk patients from FPC kindreds with abnormal EUS, but this resulted in a post-ERCP pancreatitis rate of 7% in one study.[115] Further, ERCP did not reliably demonstrate ductal communication of branch duct IPMNs or lead to additional clinically relevant imaging findings. Hence, most formal screening programs around the world do not recommend routine ERCP for asymptomatic individuals.

SUMMARY

Accumulating data indicate that clinically available abdominal imaging tests such as EUS and MRI/MRCP can detect asymptomatic precursor benign (IPMN, PanIN) and invasive malignant pancreatic neoplasms, such as ductal adenocarcinoma, in individuals with an inherited predisposition. These asymptomatic FPCs detected have been more likely to be resectable, compared to symptomatic tumors. The most challenging part of screening high-risk individuals is the selection of individuals with high-grade precursor neoplasms for preventive treatment (ie, surgical resection before development of invasive cancer). Ongoing and future research should focus on formulating and validating a model for FPC risk and neoplastic progression using patient characteristics, imaging, and biomarkers. The comparative cost and effectiveness of various approaches for screening and surveillance of high-risk individuals also deserves study. For now, screening is best performed in high-risk individuals within the research protocols in academic centers with multidisciplinary teams with expertise in genetics, gastroenterology, radiology, surgery, and pathology.

REFERENCES

1. American Cancer Society. Cancer facts and figures 2011. Available at: http://www.cancer.org/acs/groups/content/epidemiologysurveilance/documents/document/acspc-029771.pdf. Accessed September 1, 2011.
2. Lynch HT, Smyrk T, Kern SE, et al. Familial pancreatic cancer: a review. Semin Oncol 1996;23:251–75.
3. Brand RE, Lynch HT. Hereditary pancreatic adenocarcinoma: a clinical perspective. Med Clin North Am 2000;84:665–75.
4. Klein AP, Hruban RH, Brune KA, et al. Familial pancreatic cancer. Cancer J 2001;7:266–73.
5. Lynch HT, Krush AJ, Larsen AL. Heredity and multiple primary malignant neoplasms: six cancer families. Am J Med Sci 1967;254:322–9.
6. Brune KA, Lau B, Palmisano E, et al. Importance of age of onset in pancreatic cancer kindreds. J Natl Cancer Inst 2010;102:119–26.
7. Jones S, Hruban RH, Kamiyama M, et al. Exomic sequencing identifies PALB2 as a pancreatic cancer susceptibility gene. Science 2009;324:217.

8. Klein AP, Brune KA, Petersen GM, et al. Prospective risk of pancreatic cancer in familial pancreatic cancer kindreds. Cancer Res 2004;64:2634–8.
9. Slater EP, Langer P, Niemczyk E, et al. *PALB2* mutations in European familial pancreatic cancer families. Clin Genet 2010;78:490–4.
10. Klein AP, Beaty TH, Bailey-Wilson JE, et al. Evidence for a major gene influencing risk of pancreatic cancer. Genet Epidemiol 2002;23:133–49.
11. Banke MG, Mulvihill JJ, Aston CE. Inheritance of pancreatic cancer in pancreatic cancer-prone families. Med Clin North Am 2000;84:677–90, x–xi.
12. Rulyak SJ, Lowenfels AB, Maisonneuve P, et al. Risk factors for the development of pancreatic cancer in familial pancreatic cancer kindreds. Gastroenterology 2003; 124:1292–9.
13. Rieder H, Sina-Frey M, Ziegler A, et al. German national case collection of familial pancreatic cancer— clinical-genetic analysis of the first 21 families. Onkologie 2002; 25:262–6.
14. Pogue-Geile KL, Chen R, Bronner MP, et al. Palladin mutation causes familial pancreatic cancer and suggests a new cancer mechanism. PLoS Med 2006;3:e516.
15. Zogopoulos G, Rothenmund H, Eppel A, et al. The P239S palladin variant does not account for a significant fraction of hereditary or early onset pancreas cancer. Hum Genet 2007;121:635–7.
16. Slater E, Amrillaeva V, Fendrich V, et al. Palladin mutation causes familial pancreatic cancer: absence in European families. PLoS Med 2007;4:e164.
17. Klein AP, de Andrade M, Hruban RH, et al. Linkage analysis of chromosome 4 in families with familial pancreatic cancer. Cancer Biol Ther 2007;6:320–3.
18. Earl J, Yan L, Vitone LJ, et al. Evaluation of the 4q32-34 locus in European familial pancreatic cancer. Cancer Epidemiol Biomarkers Prev 2006;15:1948–55.
19. Salaria SN, Illei P, Sharma R, et al. Palladin is overexpressed in the non-neoplastic stroma of infiltrating ductal adenocarcinomas of the pancreas, but is only rarely overexpressed in neoplastic cells. Cancer Biol Ther 2007;6:324–8.
20. Murphy KM, Brune KA, Griffin C, et al. Evaluation of candidate genes *MAP2K4*, *MADH4*, *ACVR1B*, and *BRCA2* in familial pancreatic cancer: deleterious BRCA2 mutations in 17%. Cancer Res 2002;62:3789–93.
21. Hahn SA, Greenhalf B, Ellis I, et al. *BRCA2* germline mutations in familial pancreatic carcinoma. J Natl Cancer Inst 2003;95:214–21.
22. Couch FJ, Johnson MR, Rabe KG, et al. The prevalence of BRCA2 mutations in familial pancreatic cancer. Cancer Epidemiol Biomarkers Prev 2007;16:342–6.
23. Greer JB, Brand RE. New developments in pancreatic cancer. Curr Gastroenterol Rep ;13:131–9.
24. Stadler ZK, Salo-Mullen E, Sabbaghian N, et al. Germline PALB2 mutation analysis in breast-pancreas cancer families. J Med Genet 2011;48:523–5.
25. Hofstatter EW, Domchek SM, Miron A, et al. *PALB2* mutations in familial breast and pancreatic cancer. Fam Cancer 2011;10:225–31.
26. Grover S, Syngal S. Hereditary pancreatic cancer. Gastroenterology 2010;139: 1076–80, 1080 e1–2.
27. Lowenfels AB, Maisonneuve P, Whitcomb DC. Risk factors for cancer in hereditary pancreatitis. International Hereditary Pancreatitis Study Group. Med Clin North Am 2000;84:565–73.
28. Teich N, Nemoda Z, Kohler H, et al. Gene conversion between functional trypsino-gen genes *PRSS1* and *PRSS2* associated with chronic pancreatitis in a six-year-old girl. Hum Mutat 2005;25:343–7.
29. Teich N, Rosendahl J, Toth M, et al. Mutations of human cationic trypsinogen (*PRSS1*) and chronic pancreatitis. Hum Mutat 2006;27:721–30.

30. Sahin-Toth M, Toth M. Gain-of-function mutations associated with hereditary pancreatitis enhance autoactivation of human cationic trypsinogen. Biochem Biophys Res Commun 2000;278:286–9.

31. Whitcomb DC, Ulrich CD 2nd. Hereditary pancreatitis: new insights, new directions. Baillieres Best Pract Res Clin Gastroenterol 1999;13:253–63.

32. Lowenfels AB, Maisonneuve P, DiMagno EP, et al. and International Hereditary Pancreatitis Study Group. Hereditary pancreatitis and the risk of pancreatic cancer. J Natl Cancer Inst 1997;89:442–6.

33. Howes N, Lerch MM, Greenhalf W, et al. Clinical and genetic characteristics of hereditary pancreatitis in Europe. Clin Gastroenterol Hepatol 2004;2:252–61.

34. Lowenfels AB, Maisonneuve P, Whitcomb DC, et al. Cigarette smoking as a risk factor for pancreatic cancer in patients with hereditary pancreatitis. JAMA 2001;286: 169–70.

35. Latchford A, Greenhalf W, Vitone LJ, et al. Peutz-Jeghers syndrome and screening for pancreatic cancer. Br J Surg 2006;93:1446–55.

36. Gruber SB, Entius MM, Petersen GM, et al. Pathogenesis of adenocarcinoma in Peutz-Jeghers syndrome. Cancer Res 1998;58:5267–70.

37. Giardiello FM, Brensinger JD, Tersmette AC, et al. Very high risk of cancer in familial Peutz-Jeghers syndrome. Gastroenterology 2000;119:1447–53.

38. Lynch HT, Fusaro RM, Sandberg AA, et al. Chromosome instability and the FAMMM syndrome. Cancer Genet Cytogenet 1993;71:27–39.

39. Haluska FG, Hodi FS. Molecular genetics of familial cutaneous melanoma. J Clin Oncol 1998;16:670–82.

40. Soufir N, Avril MF, Chompret A, et al. and The French Familial Melanoma Study Group. Prevalence of *p16* and *CDK4* germline mutations in 48 melanoma-prone families in France. Hum Mol Genet 1998;7:209–16.

41. Lynch HT, Brand RE, Hogg D, et al. Phenotypic variation in eight extended *CDKN2A* germline mutation familial atypical multiple mole melanoma-pancreatic carcinoma-prone families: the familial atypical mole melanoma-pancreatic carcinoma syndrome. Cancer 2002;94:84–96.

42. Lynch HT, Fusaro RM, Lynch JF, et al. Pancreatic cancer and the FAMMM syndrome. Fam Cancer 2008;7:103–12.

43. Goldstein AM, Fraser MC, Struewing JP, et al. Increased risk of pancreatic cancer in melanoma-prone kindreds with *p16INK4* mutations. N Engl J Med 1995;333: 970–4.

44. Geary J, Sasieni P, Houlston R, et al. Gene-related cancer spectrum in families with hereditary non-polyposis colorectal cancer (HNPCC). Fam Cancer 2008;7:163–72.

45. Kastrinos F, Mukherjee B, Tayob N, et al. Risk of pancreatic cancer in families with Lynch syndrome. JAMA 2009;302:1790–5.

46. The Breast Cancer Linkage Consortium. Cancer risks in *BRCA2* mutation carriers. J Natl Cancer Inst 1999;91:1310–6.

47. Brose MS, Rebbeck TR, Calzone KA, et al. Cancer risk estimates for *BRCA1* mutation carriers identified in a risk evaluation program. J Natl Cancer Inst 2002;94: 1365–72.

48. Thompson D, Easton DF. Cancer incidence in *BRCA1* mutation carriers. J Natl Cancer Inst 2002;94:1358–65.

49. Lal G, Liu G, Schmocker B, et al. Inherited predisposition to pancreatic adenocarcinoma: role of family history and germ-line *p16*, *BRCA1*, and *BRCA2* mutations. Cancer Res 2000;60:409–16.

50. van Asperen CJ, Brohet RM, Meijers-Heijboer EJ, et al. Cancer risks in *BRCA2* families: estimates for sites other than breast and ovary. J Med Genet 2005;42: 711–9.

51. Goggins M, Schutte M, Lu J, et al. Germline *BRCA2* gene mutations in patients with apparently sporadic pancreatic carcinomas. Cancer Res 1996;56:5360–4.

52. Struewing JP, Abeliovich D, Peretz T, et al. The carrier frequency of the *BRCA1* 185delAG mutation is approximately 1 percent in Ashkenazi Jewish individuals. Nat Genet 1995;11:198–200.

53. Hartge P, Struewing JP, Wacholder S, et al. The prevalence of common *BRCA1* and *BRCA2* mutations among Ashkenazi Jews. Am J Hum Genet 1999;64:963–70.

54. Ozcelik H, Schmocker B, Di Nicola N, et al. Germline *BRCA2* 6174delT mutations in Ashkenazi Jewish pancreatic cancer patients. Nat Genet 1997;16:17–8.

55. Roa BB, Boyd AA, Volcik K, et al. Ashkenazi Jewish population frequencies for common mutations in *BRCA1* and *BRCA2*. Nat Genet 1996;14:185–7.

56. Steinberg WM, Barkin JS, Bradley EL 3rd, et al. Should patients with a strong family history of pancreatic cancer be screened on a periodic basis for cancer of the pancreas? Pancreas 2009;38:e137–50.

57. Canto MI. Strategies for screening for pancreatic adenocarcinoma in high-risk patients. Semin Oncol 2007;34:295–302.

58. Vitone LJ, Greenhalf W, McFaul CD, et al. The inherited genetics of pancreatic cancer and prospects for secondary screening. Best Pract Res Clin Gastroenterol 2006;20:253–83.

59. Bunger S, Laubert T, Roblick UJ, et al. Serum biomarkers for improved diagnostic of pancreatic cancer: a current overview. J Cancer Res Clin Oncol 2011;137:375–89.

60. Brentnall TA, Bronner MP, Byrd DR, et al. Early diagnosis and treatment of pancreatic dysplasia in patients with a family history of pancreatic cancer. Ann Intern Med 1999;131:247–55.

61. Goggins M. Identifying molecular markers for the early detection of pancreatic neoplasia. Semin Oncol 2007;34:303–10.

62. Ritts RE, Pitt HA. CA 19-9 in pancreatic cancer. Surg Oncol Clin N Am 1998;7:93–101.

63. Safi F, Schlosser W, Falkenreck S, et al. CA 19-9 serum course and prognosis of pancreatic cancer. Int J Pancreatol 1996;20:155–61.

64. Tian F, Appert HE, Myles J, et al. Prognostic value of serum CA 19-9 levels in pancreatic adenocarcinoma. Ann Surg 1992;215:350–5.

65. Mann DV, Edwards R, Ho S, et al. Elevated tumour marker CA19-9: clinical interpretation and influence of obstructive jaundice. Eur J Surg Oncol 2000;26: 474–9.

66. Rosty C, Goggins M. Early detection of pancreatic carcinoma. Hematol Oncol Clin North Am 2002;16:37–52.

67. DiMagno EP, Reber HA, Tempero MA, and American Gastroenterological Association. AGA technical review on the epidemiology, diagnosis, and treatment of pancreatic ductal adenocarcinoma. Gastroenterology 1999;117:1464–84.

68. Steinberg W. The clinical utility of the CA 19-9 tumor-associated antigen. Am J Gastroenterol 1990;85:350–5.

69. Lamerz R. Role of tumour markers, cytogenetics. Ann Oncol 1999;10(Suppl 4): 145–9.

70. Zubarik R, Gordon SR, Lidofsky SD, et al. Screening for pancreatic cancer in a high-risk population with serum CA 19-9 and targeted EUS: a feasibility study. Gastrointest Endosc 2011;74:87–95.

71. Futakawa N, Kimura W, Yamagata S, et al. Significance of K-*ras* mutation and CEA level in pancreatic juice in the diagnosis of pancreatic cancer. J Hepatobiliary Pancreat Surg 2000;7:63–71.

72. Basso D, Fabris C, Del Favero G, et al. Serum carcinoembryonic antigen in the differential diagnosis of pancreatic cancer: influence of tumour spread, liver impairment, and age. Dis Markers 1988;6:203–7.

73. Chevinsky AH. CEA in tumors of other than colorectal origin. Semin Surg Oncol 1991;7:162–6.

74. Ona FV, Zamcheck N, Dhar P, et al. Carcinoembryonic antigen (CEA) in the diagnosis of pancreatic cancer. Cancer 1973;31:324–7.

75. Sharma C, Eltawil KM, Renfrew PD, et al. Advances in diagnosis, treatment and palliation of pancreatic carcinoma: 1990–2010. World J Gastroenterol 2011;17: 867–97.

76. Duraker N, Hot S, Polat Y, et al. CEA, CA 19-9, and CA 125 in the differential diagnosis of benign and malignant pancreatic diseases with or without jaundice. J Surg Oncol 2007;95:142–7.

77. Ehmann M, Felix K, Hartmann D, et al. Identification of potential markers for the detection of pancreatic cancer through comparative serum protein expression profiling. Pancreas 2007;34:205–14.

78. Gansauge F, Gansauge S, Parker N, et al. CAM 17.1—a new diagnostic marker in pancreatic cancer. Br J Cancer 1996;74:1997–2002.

79. Groblewska M, Mroczko B, Wereszczynska-Siemiatkowska U, et al. Serum levels of granulocyte colony-stimulating factor (G-CSF) and macrophage colony-stimulating factor (M-CSF) in pancreatic cancer patients. Clin Chem Lab Med 2007;45:30–4.

80. Liao WC, Wu MS, Wang HP, et al. Serum heat shock protein 27 is increased in chronic pancreatitis and pancreatic carcinoma. Pancreas 2009;38:422–6.

81. Mroczko B, Lukaszewicz-Zajac M, Wereszczynska-Siemiatkowska U, et al. Clinical significance of the measurements of serum matrix metalloproteinase-9 and its inhibitor (tissue inhibitor of metalloproteinase-1) in patients with pancreatic cancer: metalloproteinase-9 as an independent prognostic factor. Pancreas 2009;38: 613–8.

82. Gold DV, Modrak DE, Ying Z, et al. New MUC1 serum immunoassay differentiates pancreatic cancer from pancreatitis. J Clin Oncol 2006;24:252–8.

83. Gold DV, Goggins M, Modrak DE, et al. Detection of early-stage pancreatic adenocarcinoma. Cancer Epidemiol Biomarkers Prev 2010;19:2786–94.

84. Gold DV, Karanjawala Z, Modrak DE, et al. PAM4-reactive MUC1 is a biomarker for early pancreatic adenocarcinoma. Clin Cancer Res 2007;13:7380–7.

85. Friess H, Buchler M, Auerbach B, et al. CA 494—a new tumor marker for the diagnosis of pancreatic cancer. Int J Cancer 1993;53:759–63.

86. Simeone DM, Ji B, Banerjee M, et al. CEACAM1, a novel serum biomarker for pancreatic cancer. Pancreas 2007;34:436–43.

87. Bouvet M, Nardin SR, Burton DW, et al. Parathyroid hormone-related protein as a novel tumor marker in pancreatic adenocarcinoma. Pancreas 2002;24:284–90.

88. Kumar Y, Gurusamy K, Pamecha V, et al. Tumor M2-pyruvate kinase as tumor marker in exocrine pancreatic cancer a meta-analysis. Pancreas 2007;35:114–9.

89. Louhimo J, Alfthan H, Stenman UH, et al. Serum HCG beta and CA 72-4 are stronger prognostic factors than CEA, CA 19-9 and CA 242 in pancreatic cancer. Oncology 2004;66:126–31.

90. Watanabe H, Ha A, Hu YX, et al. K-*ras* mutations in duodenal aspirate without secretin stimulation for screening of pancreatic and biliary tract carcinoma. Cancer 1999;86:1441–8.

91. Caldas C, Hahn SA, da Costa LT, et al. Frequent somatic mutations and homozygous deletions of the *p16* (*MTS1*) gene in pancreatic adenocarcinoma. Nat Genet 1994;8:27–32.

92. Trumper L, Menges M, Daus H, et al. Low sensitivity of the ki-ras polymerase chain reaction for diagnosing pancreatic cancer from pancreatic juice and bile: a multicenter prospective trial. J Clin Oncol 2002;20:4331–7.

93. Berger DH, Chang H, Wood M, et al. Mutational activation of K-*ras* in nonneoplastic exocrine pancreatic lesions in relation to cigarette smoking status. Cancer 1999;85: 326–32.

94. Kalthoff H, Schmiegel W, Roeder C, et al. *p53* and K-*RAS* alterations in pancreatic epithelial cell lesions. Oncogene 1993;8:289–98.

95. Schutte M, Hruban RH, Geradts J, et al. Abrogation of the Rb/p16 tumor-suppressive pathway in virtually all pancreatic carcinomas. Cancer Res 1997;57:3126–30.

96. Tada M, Komatsu Y, Kawabe T, et al. Quantitative analysis of K-*ras* gene mutation in pancreatic tissue obtained by endoscopic ultrasonography-guided fine needle aspiration: clinical utility for diagnosis of pancreatic tumor. Am J Gastroenterol 2002; 97:2263–70.

97. Sturm PD, Hruban RH, Ramsoekh TB, et al. The potential diagnostic use of K-*ras* codon 12 and p53 alterations in brush cytology from the pancreatic head region. J Pathol 1998;186:247–53.

98. Sato N, Goggins M. The role of epigenetic alterations in pancreatic cancer. J Hepatobiliary Pancreat Surg 2006;13:286–95.

99. Sato N, Ueki T, Fukushima N, et al. Aberrant methylation of CpG islands in intraductal papillary mucinous neoplasms of the pancreas. Gastroenterology 2002;123:365–72.

100. Sato N, Fukushima N, Chang R, et al. Differential and epigenetic gene expression profiling identifies frequent disruption of the *RELN* pathway in pancreatic cancers. Gastroenterology 2006;130:548–65.

101. Fukushima N, Walter KM, Uek T, et al. Diagnosing pancreatic cancer using methylation specific PCR analysis of pancreatic juice. Cancer Biol Ther 2003;2:78–83.

102. Ueki T, Walter KM, Skinner H, et al. Aberrant CpG island methylation in cancer cell lines arises in the primary cancers from which they were derived. Oncogene 2002;21:2114–7.

103. Matsubayashi H, Sato N, Fukushima N, et al. Methylation of cyclin D2 is observed frequently in pancreatic cancer but is also an age-related phenomenon in gastrointestinal tissues. Clin Cancer Res 2003;9:1446–52.

104. Fukushima N, Sato N, Sahin F, et al. Aberrant methylation of suppressor of cytokine signalling-1 (*SOCS-1*) gene in pancreatic ductal neoplasms. Br J Cancer 2003;89: 338–43.

105. Sato N, Fukushima N, Maehara N, et al. *SPARC*/osteonectin is a frequent target for aberrant methylation in pancreatic adenocarcinoma and a mediator of tumor-stromal interactions. Oncogene 2003;22:5021–30.

106. Jansen M, Fukushima N, Rosty C, et al. Aberrant methylation of the 5' CpG island of TSLC1 is common in pancreatic ductal adenocarcinoma and is first manifest in high-grade PanINs. Cancer Biol Ther 2002;1:293–6.

107. Sato N, Fukushima N, Maitra A, et al. Discovery of novel targets for aberrant methylation in pancreatic carcinoma using high-throughput microarrays. Cancer Res 2003;63:3735–42.

108. Matsubayashi H, Canto M, Sato N, et al. DNA methylation alterations in the pancreatic juice of patients with suspected pancreatic disease. Cancer Res 2006; 66:1208–17.

109. Polyak K, Li Y, Zhu H, et al. Somatic mutations of the mitochondrial genome in human colorectal tumours. Nat Genet 1998;20:291–3.
110. Jones JB, Song JJ, Hempen PM, et al. Detection of mitochondrial DNA mutations in pancreatic cancer offers a "mass"-ive advantage over detection of nuclear DNA mutations. Cancer Res 2001;61:1299–304.
111. Maitra A, Cohen Y, Gillespie SE, et al. The Human MitoChip: a high-throughput sequencing microarray for mitochondrial mutation detection. Genome Res 2004;14: 812–9.
112. Fliss MS, Usadel H, Caballero OL, et al. Facile detection of mitochondrial DNA mutations in tumors and bodily fluids. Science 2000;287:2017–9.
113. Sanchez-Cespedes M, Parrella P, Nomoto S, et al. Identification of a mononucleotide repeat as a major target for mitochondrial DNA alterations in human tumors. Cancer Res 2001;61:7015–9.
114. Kuroki-Suzuki S, Kuroki Y, Nasu K, et al. Pancreatic cancer screening employing noncontrast magnetic resonance imaging combined with ultrasonography. Jpn J Radiol 2011;29:265–71.
115. Canto MI, Goggins M, Hruban RH, et al. Screening for early pancreatic neoplasia in high-risk individuals: a prospective controlled study. Clin Gastroenterol Hepatol 2006;4:766–81 [quiz 665].
116. Canto MI, Goggins M, Yeo CJ, et al. Screening for pancreatic neoplasia in high-risk individuals: an EUS-based approach. Clin Gastroenterol Hepatol 2004;2:606–21.
117. Ikeda M, Sato T, Morozumi A, et al. Morphologic changes in the pancreas detected by screening ultrasonography in a mass survey, with special reference to main duct dilatation, cyst formation, and calcification. Pancreas 1994;9:508–12.
118. American Gastroenterological Association. Medical position statement: epidemiology, diagnosis, and treatment of pancreatic ductal adenocarcinoma. Gastroenterology 1999;117:1463–84.
119. Canto MI. Screening and surveillance approaches in familial pancreatic cancer. Gastrointest Endosc Clin N Am 2008;18:535–53, x.
120. Bronstein YL, Loyer EM, Kaur H, et al. Detection of small pancreatic tumors with multiphasic helical CT. Am J Roentgenol 2004;182:619–23.
121. Vargas R, Nino-Murcia M, Trueblood W, et al. MDCT in pancreatic adenocarcinoma: prediction of vascular invasion and resectability using a multiphasic technique with curved planar reformations. Am J Roentgenol 2004;182:419–25.
122. Diehl SJ, Lehmann KJ, Sadick M, et al. Pancreatic cancer: value of dual-phase helical CT in assessing resectability. Radiology 1998;206:373–8.
123. Lu DS, Reber HA, Krasny RM, et al. Local staging of pancreatic cancer: criteria for unresectability of major vessels as revealed by pancreatic-phase, thin-section helical CT. Am J Roentgenol 1997;168:1439–43.
124. Canto MI, Schulick RD, Goggins MG, et al. Preoperative detection of familial pancreatic neoplasms by endoscopic ultrasonography (EUS), multidetector computed tomography (CT), and/or magnetic resonance cholangiopancreatography (MRCP). Gastrointest Endosc 2008;67:AB225.
125. Vasen HF, Wasser M, van Mil A, et al. Magnetic resonance imaging surveillance detects early-stage pancreatic cancer in carriers of a p16-Leiden mutation. Gastroenterology 2011;140:850–6.
126. Poley JW, Kluijt I, Gouma DJ, et al. The yield of first-time endoscopic ultrasonography in screening individuals at a high risk of developing pancreatic cancer. Am J Gastroenterol 2009;104:2175–81.
127. Brentnall TA. Cancer surveillance of patients from familial pancreatic cancer kindreds. Med Clin North Am 2000;84:707–18.

128. Tanaka M, Chari S, Adsay V, et al. International consensus guidelines for manage-
     ment of intraductal papillary mucinous neoplasms and mucinous cystic neoplasms
     of the pancreas. Pancreatology 2006;6:17–32.
129. Emerson RE, Randolph ML, Cramer HM. Endoscopic ultrasound-guided fine-needle
     aspiration cytology diagnosis of intraductal papillary mucinous neoplasm of the
     pancreas is highly predictive of pancreatic neoplasia. Diagn Cytopathol 2006;34:
     457–62.
130. Ludwig E, Olson SH, Bayuga S, et al. Feasibility and yield of screening in relatives
     from familial pancreatic cancer families. Am J Gastroenterol 2011;106:946–54.
131. Verna EC, Hwang C, Stevens PD, et al. Pancreatic cancer screening in a prospective
     cohort of high-risk patients: a comprehensive strategy of imaging and genetics. Clin
     Cancer Res 2010;16:5028–37.

Pancreatic Cancer: Radiologic Imaging

R. Brooke Jeffrey, MD

KEYWORDS

- Pancreas • Cancer • Adenocarcinoma • Imaging
- Multidetector computed tomography (MDCT)
- Fluorodeoxyglucose positron emission tomography (FDG-PET)

CLINICAL OVERVIEW

Each year in the United States, more than 40,000 patients are diagnosed with pancreatic cancer and a nearly equal number will die from their disease.[1] Pancreatic cancer is now the fourth most common cause of cancer death in the United States.[2] In recent years, there have been impressive gains in our knowledge of both the underlying risk factors and the molecular biology of this disease.[3–5] In addition, refinements in surgical management have led to considerable reduction in overall postoperative mortality.[6,7] Nevertheless, there are few long-term survivors of pancreatic cancer because of the preclinical dissemination of this disease via lymphatic and perineural spread.[8]

The only treatment that has been shown to prolong survival is surgical resection with negative margins (R0 resection); with this treatment, a mean survival of 24 months can be anticipated, compared to 12 months for patients with disease deemed unresectable.[8,9] It is important to stress, however, that even surgery with negative margins fails to result in long-term survival: only 3% to 16% of patients undergoing R0 resection are alive after 5 years.[10] There are many reasons for this; one often-cited factor is the propensity of pancreatic carcinoma to spread via the celiac and mesenteric neural plexi. Perineural invasion often results in dissemination of tumor before the onset of clinical symptoms. Standard surgical resection will fail to eliminate perineural spread of ductal adenocarcinoma, and this most likely contributes to the overall poor prognosis of the disease.[11–13]

Despite the dismal outlook for patients with pancreatic carcinoma, radiologic imaging plays a critical role in selecting either medical or surgical therapy for patients, depending on the likelihood of resectability. Accurate preoperative staging Is therefore a crucial step in identifying the small number of patients who may potentially benefit from pancreaticoduodenectomy. Conversely, identifying patients with either

The author has nothing to disclose.

Department of Radiology, Stanford University Medical Center, 300 Pasteur Drive, Stanford, CA 94305, USA

E-mail address: bjeffrey@stanford.edu

Gastroenterol Clin N Am 41 (2012) 159–177
doi:10.1016/j.gtc.2011.12.012
0889-8553/12/$ – see front matter © 2012 Published by Elsevier Inc.

distant or locally advanced disease is another important goal of imaging so that these patients are not subjected to a fruitless major surgical intervention. Finally, it is essential to distinguish a pancreatic adenocarcinoma from an ampullary tumor, given the far better prognosis associated with the latter.[14]

Although a variety of imaging techniques, such as multidetector computed tomography (MDCT), magnetic resonance imaging (MRI), endoscopic ultrasound (EUS), and fluorodeoxyglucose positron emission tomography (FDG-PET) have all been used in the initial diagnostic assessment of pancreatic lesions, in general, MDCT is the mainstay of diagnosis.[15–17] This is due in large part to the high spatial resolution of its three-dimensional (3D) data sets that are indispensable in determining the local extent of tumor infiltration.[18–21]

MDCT AND MRI TECHNIQUE

Patients with pancreatic carcinomas frequently present with vague symptoms that are often misdiagnosed clinically as other intra-abdominal abnormalities. Not infrequently, a pancreatic mass may be detected on a screening abdominal ultrasound or CT scan of the abdomen. It is important to emphasize that, in many instances, these screening studies are not adequate to assess local invasion. Therefore, a dedicated pancreatic-protocol MDCT study, which will improve the accuracy of local staging by obtaining the highest resolution possible, is indicated. A dedicated pancreatic protocol MDCT has four critical components, and attention to detail is essential to achieving optimal results. These components include (1) neutral oral contrast administration to distend the stomach and duodenal sweep, (2) intravenous contrast injection via a rapid bolus, (3) optimized biphasic MDCT scan acquisition, and (4) postprocessing with a combination of two-dimensional (2D) and 3D volumetric image displays to highlight extrapancreatic extension along blood vessels and peripancreatic tissues.

To begin the pancreatic protocol, the patient ingests 750 to 1000 mL of a neutral oral contrast, such as water, to distend the stomach and duodenum immediately before scan acquisition. Gastroduodenal distension allows better depiction of invasion of these structures and also highlights the region of the ampulla of Vater. It is important to not miss an underlying ampullary carcinoma or misconstrue it as a ducal adenocarcinoma because of the far better prognosis associated with ampullary tumors (**Fig. 1**). Ampullary carcinomas, particularly of the gastrointestinal type, may be associated with a 40% 5-year survival, which is substantially greater than survival for patients with ductal adenocarcinoma.[14]

After the ingestion of neutral contrast, an intravenous bolus is administered with a rapid 4- to 5-mL/s injection of 150 mL of nonionic contrast via power injector. This rapid bolus causes intense enhancement of the normal pancreas, which will highlight the differences in vascular perfusion between the typically hypovascular ductal adenocarcinoma and the normal pancreatic parenchyma (**Figs. 2** and **3**). A late arterial-phase acquisition, typically 35 seconds from the onset of intravenous contrast injection, is optimal to obtain the initial breath-held images of the pancreas and upper abdomen. Late arterial-phase images improve conspicuity of underlying pancreatic lesions and also demonstrate hypervascular lesions, such as neuroendocrine tumors and their hypervascular liver metastasis[22–24] (**Fig. 4**). The late arterial phase also optimally enhances the splanchnic vasculature, which enables detection of subtle perivascular infiltration of the underlying tumor[22–24] (**Fig. 5**). It is important that the entire pancreas and upper abdomen are scanned with a breath-held acquisition, as late arterial-phase images may demonstrate flow phenomena associated with subtle liver metastasis that will not be evident on portal-venous phase images alone. These

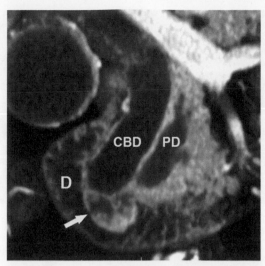

Fig. 1. Ampullary carcinoma resulting in "double-duct" sign on coronal 3D volume-rendered MDCT image. Note distention of duodenum (D) from ingested neutral oral contrast that allows visualization of an ampullary mass (*arrow*). The mass obstructs both common bile duct (CBD) and pancreatic duct (PD).

phenomena include thin peripheral enhancement around subtle hypodense metastasis and perfusion abnormalities such as a transient hepatic attenuation defect associated with hepatic metastasis.

After the late arterial-phase acquisition, an additional scan is acquired during the portal-venous phase, typically 60 to 70 seconds after the onset of intravenous injection. These venous-phase images may more optimally demonstrate small hypodense liver metastasis in some patients and improve overall visualization of a portal venous system, which will allow for assessment of venous encasement or obstruction (**Fig. 6**). Often, peripancreatic and perisplenic varices are optimally seen in this phase, which is a clue to underlying splenic or portal vein occlusion or both.

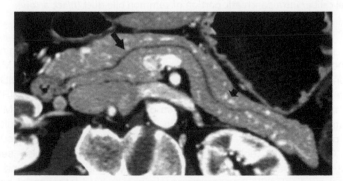

Fig. 2. Normal pancreas and pancreatic duct on curved-planar reformation on late arterial-phase MDCT scan. Note normal pancreatic duct visualized throughout its entirety (*long black arrow*) and numerous well opacified intrapancreatic blood vessels within parenchyma (*short black arrow*).

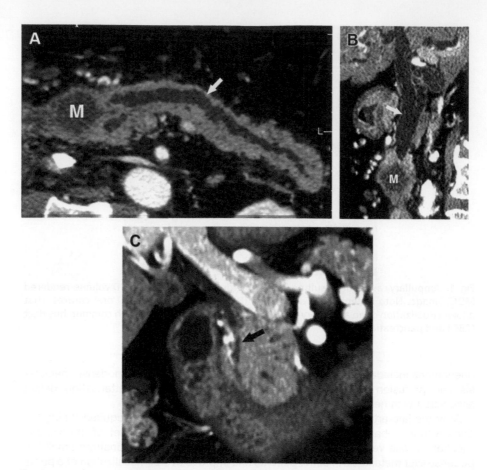

Fig. 3. Hypodense pancreatic carcinoma obstructing both pancreatic and common bile ducts on MDCT. (*A*) Curved-planar reformation along pancreatic duct demonstrating upstream dilatation of pancreatic duct (*white arrow*) due to obstructing hypodense mass (M). (*B*) Curved-planar reformation along common bile duct in same patient showing dilatation (*arrow*) by a hypodense mass (M) in head of pancreas. (*C*) In another patient, coronal volume rendered image demonstrates normal caliber intra-pancreatic portion of common bile duct (*black arrow*).

MRI has proven to be comparable to MDCT in accuracy of staging ductal adenocarcinoma.[25] Although it has slightly less spatial resolution than MDCT, the excellent contrast resolution of MRI makes it an attractive alternative to MDCT when patients are allergic to iodinated contrast. Unlike noncontrast CT, MRI without intravenous contrast may yield useful images of the pancreas, and thus MRI is very helpful in patients with renal insufficiency (**Fig. 7**). Its superior contrast resolution may also be of particular value in assessing neuroendocrine tumors and subtle liver metastasis. Optimal MRI technique involves a combination of pulse sequences, including fat-suppressed T1-weighted imaging, T2-weighted images, and gadolinium-enhanced gradient-echo images, to obtain breath-held late-arterial and portal-venous phase acquisitions through the upper abdomen and pancreas (**Fig. 8**). Diffusion-weighted imaging is a relatively new MRI technique that may be particularly valuable in the detection of liver metastasis because of restricted diffusion of these

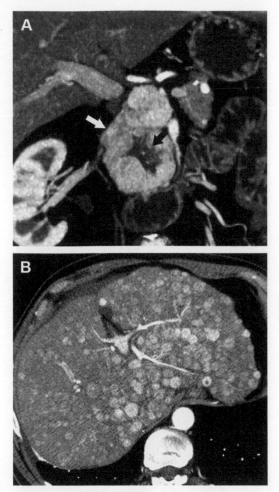

Fig. 4. Hypervascular neuroendocrine tumors in two different patients on MDCT. (*A*) Late arterial-phase coronal image of pancreas demonstrating large, hypervascular mass (*white arrow*) with central necrosis (*black arrow*). (*B*) Axial late arterial-phase image in different patient demonstrating innumerable hypervascular liver metastases from pancreatic neuroendocrine tumor.

solid lesions. In addition, newer hepatic-specific contrast agents may prove to be a valuable contribution to the overall assessment of liver metastasis.

One considerable advantage of MDCT is that the thin collimation scans (0.6 mm) result in isotropic data sets with resolution comparable in all three planes. These high-resolution data sets enable the performance of unique imaging displays in both 2D and 3D that greatly facilitate depiction of extrapancreatic spread of carcinoma.[19–21] Curved-planar reformations depict, in two dimensions, a tubular structure coursing through the 3D data set. Curved-planar reformations of the pancreatic and common bile ducts highlight subtle dilatation from underlying obstructing lesions[19] (see **Fig. 9**). hese types of displays have proven to be highly effective in visualizing tumor spread along blood vessels (**Fig. 10**). 3D imaging,

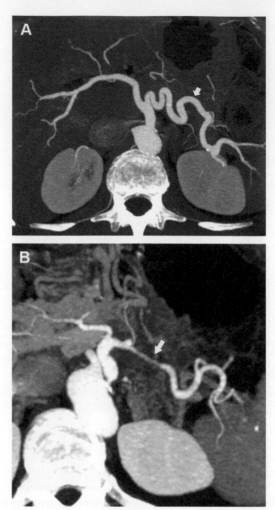

Fig. 5. Celiac axis during late arterial phase MDCT in two patients. (*A*) Axial maximum-intensity image of celiac axis showing normal splenic artery (*black arrow*) and splenic artery (*white arrow*). (*B*) Axial maximum-intensity image in another patient with pancreatic carcinoma, and demonstrates arterial narrowing of splenic artery by arterial encasement (*white arrow*).

particularly with volume-rendered displays, has been gaining widespread utilization with pancreatic-protocol MDCT[26,27] (**Fig. 11**). These are often used in an interactive display as the interpreting radiologist scrolls through a 3D volume data set to perceive subtle peripancreatic soft-tissue infiltration. Ray-casting techniques, such as maximum-intensity projections, allow depiction of peripancreatic vasculature that highlights areas of venous encasement and peripancreatic varices, as well as arterial anomalies and areas of narrowing (see **Fig. 5**). Minimum-intensity displays are often very useful in the depiction of low-attenuation structures such as the pancreatic and common bile ducts and cystic pancreatic masses[21] (**Fig. 12**).

Images of fluid-filled structures, such as the pancreatic and common bile ducts, used for MR cholangiopancreatography (MRCP) are created with heavily T2-weighted

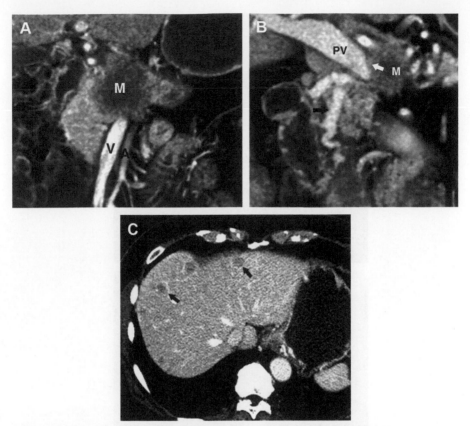

Fig. 6. Pancreatic carcinoma obstructing portal vein. (*A*) Late arterial-phase, coronal volume-rendered MDCT image demonstrating hypodense mass (M) in neck of pancreas. A, superior mesenteric artery; V, superior mesenteric vein. (*B*) Portal-venous-phase, coronal volume-rendered image demonstrating peripancreatic varices (*arrows*) due to marked narrowing of portal vein (PV) by mass (M). (*C*) Axial portal venous image demonstrates multiple hypodense liver metastases (*arrows*).

sequences and are some of the most important displays of pancreatic MRI[28,29] (see **Fig. 7**). These displays often highlight subtle areas of ductal narrowing and are particularly useful for evaluating pancreatic cystic lesions. Because MRI lacks ionizing radiation, it is often the technique of choice in follow-up examinations for patients with suspected cystic lesions of low malignant potential.

MDCT AND MRI FINDINGS IN PANCREATIC ADENOCARCINOMA

Late arterial-phase pancreatic images highlight the underlying differences in vascular perfusion of the normal pancreas compared to the hypovascular nature of underlying adenocarcinomas.[30] In 90% to 95% of patients with ductal adenocarcinoma, a hypoattenuating mass will be identified on an image acquired during this phase.[20,31] In addition to the primary finding of a hypoattenuating mass, secondary findings are often critically important, and include dilatation of either the pancreatic (**Fig. 13**) or common bile duct, or both (the "double-duct sign") (see **Fig. 3**). Subtle degrees of ductal dilatation along the course of the pancreatic duct are often highlighted by the curved-planar reformations in the 3D volumetric data set.

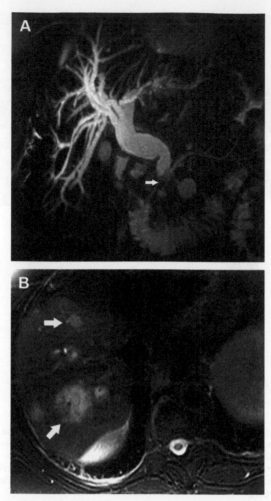

Fig. 7. Noncontrast MRI scans in two different patients with pancreatic carcinoma. (*A*) MRCP coronal image demonstrating marked dilatation of intra- and extrahepatic bile ducts from mass (*arrow*) in head of pancreas. (*B*) Axial T2-weighted image of liver in another patient showing multiple hyperintense liver metastases (*arrows*).

However, the remaining 5% to 10% of adenocarcinomas will not show an attenuation difference on late pancreatic arterial-phase images and are therefore referred to as "isodense" carcinomas[20,31] (see **Figs. 9** and **12**). This appears particularly to be true of small (<20 mm) ductal adenocarcinomas.[32] Because small pancreatic lesions may not deform the outer contour of the gland, the only clue, in many cases, to an underlying pancreatic mass is upstream dilatation of the pancreatic duct.[20,30,33] When ductal obstruction is chronic, distal pancreatic atrophy can be appreciated as another important secondary finding. On MRI, pancreatic adenocarcinomas generally appear as low-signal lesions, particularly on T1-weighted fat-suppression acquisition.[29] On T2-weighted sequences, there is often little contrast difference between the tumor and the underlying pancreas; however, the T2-weighted sequence is still useful in identifying slightly hyperintense areas of increased signal in

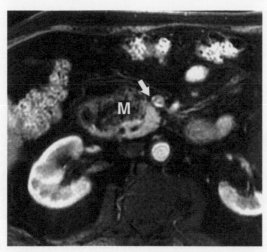

Fig. 8. Gadolinium-enhanced MRI in patient with resectable pancreatic carcinoma in head of gland. Note hypointense mass (M) with preserved fat plane (*arrow*) adjacent to mesenteric vessels, indicating lack of vascular enhancement.

the liver, which indicate underlying liver metastasis. To date, the most useful sequence for demonstrating an underlying pancreatic mass is often gadolinium-enhanced gradient-echo images that are breath held through both arterial- and venous-phase image acquisition.[25] Similar to the pharmacokinetics of iodinated contrast media with MDCT, the majority of pancreatic neoplasms on MRI will appear hypointense relative to the normal pancreas.[25] As previously mentioned, heavily T2-weighted images are particularly useful to highlight obstruction of both the pancreatic and common bile ducts with MRCP images.

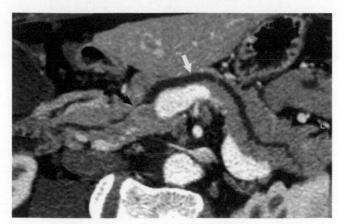

Fig. 9. Curved-planar reformation on MDCT of pancreatic duct in patient with isodense carcinoma. Note subtle upstream dilatation of pancreatic duct (*white arrow*) due to stricturing of duct (*black arrow*) by isodense mass.

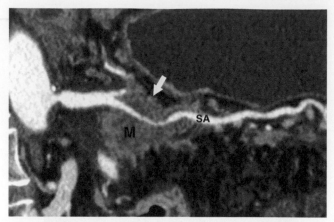

Fig. 10. Curved-planar reformation on MDCT of splenic artery in patient with unresectable pancreatic carcinoma. Note hypodense mass (M) in pancreas that narrows splenic artery (SA). Also note large tumor extension encasing splenic artery (*arrow*).

MDCT AND MRI STAGING OF PANCREATIC ADENOCARCINOMA

The patient's suitability for pancreaticoduodenectomy (Whipple resection) is the most critical determination for a patient with newly diagnosed pancreatic carcinoma. A preoperative pancreatic-protocol MDCT is often the pivotal examination that determines which therapeutic approach—medical or surgical—will be followed.[34,35] Endoscopic ultrasound is also often used as an important adjunct to the initial screening pancreatic-protocol MDCT and may help to clarify cases of subtle vascular or nodal involvement, as well as provide tissue sampling for confirmation of ductal adenocarcinoma.[36,37]

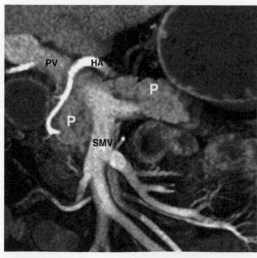

Fig. 11. 3D coronal volume-rendered MDCT image of normal pancreas (P) and surrounding vasculature. HA, hepatic artery; PV, portal vein; SMV, superior mesenteric vein.

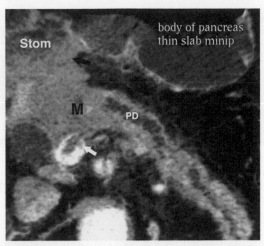

Fig. 12. Isodense pancreatic carcinoma invading portal vein and stomach on MDCT. Axial minimum-display image demonstrates isodense mass (M) obstructing upstream pancreatic duct (PD). Note that mass invades into portal vein (*white arrow*) as well as stomach (STOM). Black arrow indicates extrapancreatic extension to stomach.

In addition to the two broad categories of initial assessment—unresectable and resectable cases—a third category has emerged: "borderline resectability."[38,39] This category refers to pancreatic carcinomas that impinge but do not invade or occlude the superior mesenteric vein (SMV) or portal vein.[40] In general, classification schemes have tended to favor specificity over sensitivity in the assessment of preoperative MDCT staging to avoid denying the potential survival benefit of resection. It should be stressed, however, that the survival benefit of surgery is seen only in patients with R0 resection, that is, patients whose pathology shows negative margins. The benefits of surgery are far less in patients who have positive margins, and therefore it is equally important to decline surgery for those patients who have little chance of survival benefit.

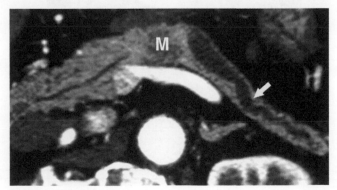

Fig. 13. Hypodense pancreatic carcinoma obstructing pancreatic duct on MDCT. Note hypodense mass (M) on curved-planar reformation that obstructs distal pancreatic duct (*arrow*) and causes distal atrophy of gland.

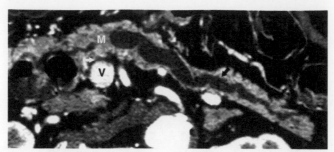

Fig. 14. Resectable pancreatic carcinoma on MDCT. Curved-planar reformation along pancreatic duct reveals obstruction of distal pancreatic duct (*black arrow*) by small isodense mass (M). Note preserved fat plane (*arrow*) around superior mesenteric vein (V) indicating lack of vascular encasement. Patient underwent successful Whipple's resection.

Resectable lesions, as defined by the National Comprehensive Cancer Network criteria, are localized to the pancreas and demonstrate no radiographic evidence of either distant metastasis or extrapancreatic organ invasion.[41](**Fig. 14**). The images for these cases demonstrate a clear fat plane demarcating the tumor from the surrounding peripancreatic vasculature, specifically the celiac axis, hepatic artery, and superior mesenteric artery (SMA). In addition, no radiographic evidence of portal-vein abutment, tumor thrombus, or venous encasement is seen.

Tumors considered unresectable have evidence of distant metastasis to the liver or peritoneal cavity; or SMA, hepatic artery, splenic artery, or celiac artery encasement greater than half the circumference of the vessel in its short axis (>180° circumferential involvement)[41](see **Fig. 10**; **Figs. 15** and **16**). Other criteria include portal-vein occlusion or direct tumor invasion, or circumferential encasement involving proximal jejunal vessels.[41]

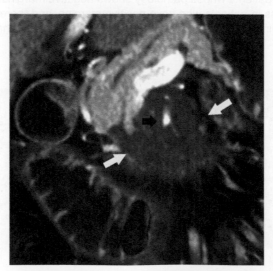

Fig. 15. Arterial encasement of SMA indicating nonresectable pancreatic carcinoma on MDCT. Coronal 3D volume-rendered image shows hypodense tumor in uncinate process of pancreas (*white arrows*) circumferentially encasing SMA (*black arrow*).

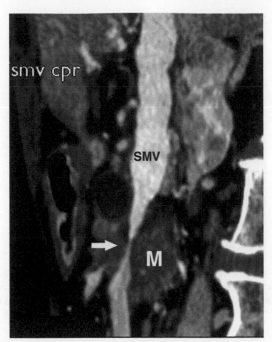

Fig. 16. Circumferential encasement of SMV indicating nonresectability on MDCT. Curved-planar reformation along SMV (*white arrow*) demonstrates high-grade stenosis of superior mesenteric vein (SMV) by hypodense mass (M).

Tumors of "borderline resectability" include those meeting the following criteria: no evidence of distant metastasis; short-segment venous involvement of the SMV–portal vein confluence that may involve impinging and narrowing in the lumen but without encasement of associated arteries; or short-segment venous occlusion, tumor invasion or involvement of the gastroduodenal artery up to the hepatic artery without extension to the celiac axis[41] (**Fig. 17**).

Notably, the criteria do not include metastasis to the lymph nodes and overall nodal status because of the low sensitivity and specificity of cross-sectional imaging with MDCT and MRI in confirming or excluding micrometastasis to lymph nodes.[42] However, if there is obvious lymphadenopathy beyond the extent of Whipple resection (primarily involving the celiac axis), these cases should be considered unresectable. Endoscopic ultrasound fine-needle aspiration biopsy of these lymph nodes is an important adjunct in confirming their unresectable status.

As reflected in the aforementioned criteria, arterial encasement greater than half the circumference of the artery in short axis is a critical finding that confirms unresectability.[41] The superior spatial resolution of MDCT has proven to be quite reliable in establishing perivascular spread. Assessing the degree of involvement is crucial because involvement of less than 180° of arterial circumference may place the patient in the category of borderline resectability.

Although arterial encasement is universally regarded as a criterion for nonresectability, the status of the portal vein and SMV has been the subject of much debate in the surgical oncology literature. Ishikawa and colleagues have attempted to correlate the actual appearance of the tumor abutment along the SMV–portal vein confluence

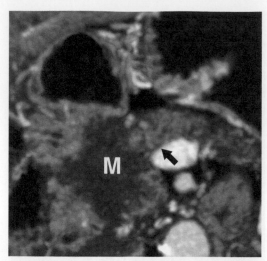

Fig. 17. Borderline resectable pancreatic carcinoma on MDCT. Axial 3D volume-rendered image demonstrates ill-defined hypodense mass (M) in head of pancreas causing focal flattening of SMV (*arrow*) without encasement; at surgery the lesion was unresectable.

to the ability to perform an R0 resection. Ishikawa and colleagues defined four different types of tumor abutment: smooth mass effect, unilateral focal mass effect with narrowing, bilateral mass effect with narrowing, and circumferential encasement with narrowing and collaterals.[43] In the work of both Ishikawa and coworkers and Chun and coworkers, R0 resections were possible in the majority of patients with either smooth or focal unilateral narrowing.[40] However, patients with bilateral narrowing and mass effect on the SMV–portal vein confluence rarely benefit from surgical resection because of the high probability of obtaining positive margins.[40]

OVERALL ACCURACY OF MDCT STAGING FOR PANCREATIC CARCINOMA

MDCT is most reliable for staging in patients with extensive locally advanced disease or clear-cut evidence of hepatic and peritoneal metastasis. It is less reliable in demonstrating microscopic peritoneal and hepatic surface implants in patients who appear to have resectable disease based on traditional MDCT criteria.[34–37] An analysis of published reports evaluating the accuracy of thin-section MDCT in predicting resectability of pancreatic carcinoma at surgery shows sensitivities ranging from 88% to 93%.[44–47] These studies have largely relied on defining unresectability as tumor involvement greater than 180° of the circumference of a peripancreatic artery or vein.[44–47] More recently, Klauss and colleagues have proposed an "invasion score" that incorporates the length of contact of the pancreatic tumor with the adjacent artery and vein, and they achieved a sensitivity of 94% with a specificity of 89%.[48] It is possible that refinements to these scoring systems will result in improved preoperative staging for pancreatic carcinoma.

PITFALLS IN THE DIAGNOSIS OF PANCREATIC ADENOCARCINOMA

Both focal and autoimmune pancreatitis may produce discrete mass lesions that at times mimic ductal adenocarcinoma[49,50] and cause secondary changes, such as upstream dilatation of the pancreatic or common bile ducts. A history of repeated bouts of pancreatitis and the presence of calcifications within the duct or parenchyma are important clues to the presence of chronic calcific pancreatitis. Often, chronic pancreatitis causes a long, smooth narrowing of both the pancreatic and common bile ducts, which may be clearly depicted on MRCP or curved-planar images on MDCT or both. However, focal chronic pancreatitis, particularly when involving the head of the gland, may be indistinguishable from ductal adenocarcinoma. Preoperative biopsy may

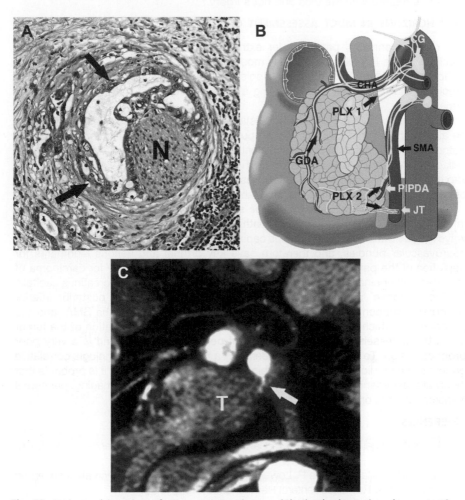

Fig. 18. Perineural invasion of pancreatic carcinoma. (*A*) Histologic section demonstrating adenocarcinoma cells (*arrows*) infiltrating perineural space around extrapancreatic nerve fascicle (N). (*B*) Schematic drawing of most common extrapancreatic pathways of perineural invasion. Pathways include along neural plexus surrounding gastroduodenal artery (GDA), plexus capitalis I (PLX-1), and plexus capitalis II (PLX-2), which extends along posterior inferior pancreaticoduodenal artery (PIPDA) and jejunal trunk (JT). CG, celiac ganglion; SMA, superior mesenteric artery. (*C*) Axial scan of tumor (T) in head of pancreas showing soft-tissue infiltration along perineural plexus of PLX-2 with encasement of PIPDA (*arrow*). (**Figs. 18**A and B *from* Deshmukh SD, Willmann JK, Jeffrey RB. Pathways of extrapancreatic perineural invasion by pancreatic adenocarcinoma: evaluation with 3D volume-rendered MDCT imaging. AJR Am J Roentgenol 2010;194(3):668–74; with permission.)

not demonstrate the underlying cancer, as there is often a component of pancreatitis associated with ductal adenocarcinoma, particularly on the periphery of the tumor. The smooth narrowing of the duct within the area of the mass, demonstrated on MRI, may be an important clue to underlying focal chronic pancreatitis.[49]

Autoimmune pancreatitis most often involves a large segment of the gland with lymphoplasmocytic infiltration. It is important to recognize this disorder preoperatively by its characteristic elevated serum IgG4, as patients with autoimmune pancreatitis should be treated with steroids and not surgery.[50]

NEW HORIZONS IN MDCT ASSESSMENT OF PANCREATIC ADENOCARCINOMA

The role of perineural pathways for extrapancreatic extension of carcinoma in a preclinical state is well known.[51] This mode of spread undoubtedly leads to dissemination beyond the bed of the Whipple resection and thus in many instances precludes R0 resections from effecting a cure or even long-term survival in these patients.

Perineural invasion is quite characteristic of ductal adenocarcinoma, though it may be also seen in some patients with ampullary cancers and cholangiocarcinomas.[26] Pathologists and anatomists have long identified the neural pathways extending from the celiac and mesenteric plexus to enervate the pancreas. Retrograde extension of cancer into the perineural space along the nerve fascicles appears to be promoted by a number of neurotrophic growth factors that are elaborated in ductal adenocarcinoma.[52]

On MDCT, perineural invasion can be suggested when there is direct soft-tissue infiltration along a known perineural pathway.[26,51] The most common neural pathways include the plexus pancreaticus capitalis 1 and 2. These pathways extend along neurovascular bundles, and therefore have key arterial and venous landmarks for depiction of the pathways[26] (**Fig. 18**). The most common pathway for carcinoma of the head and uncinate process of the gland is along the plexus pancreaticus capitalis 2. The anatomic landmarks for this neural plexus include the posterior inferior pancreaticoduodenal artery, which is the first arterial branch of the SMA, and the jejunal trunk, which extends into the SMV. Direct soft-tissue infiltration of the tumor along these vessels is an important sign of perineural invasion and is a very poor prognostic sign. To date there have been only a few radiologic–pathologic correlative papers in the medical literature describing perineural pathways, but it is probable that as greater experience is gathered, particularly with 3D volumetric imaging, perineural invasion may become an important criterion for nonresectability.[26]

REFERENCES

1. Jemal A, Siegel R, Xu J, Ward E. Cancer statistics, 2010. CA Cancer J Clin 2010; 60:277–300.
2. Raimondi S, Maisonneuve P, Lowenfels AB. Epidemiology of pancreatic cancer: an overview. Nat Rev Gastroenterol Hepatol 2009;6:699–708.
3. Ghiorzo P, Gargiulo S, Nasti S, et al. Predicting the risk of pancreatic cancer: on CDKN2A mutations in the melanoma-pancreatic cancer syndrome in Italy. J Clin Oncol 2007;25:5336–7.
4. Whelan AJ, Bartsch D, Goodfellow PJ. Brief report: a familial syndrome of pancreatic cancer and melanoma with a mutation in the CDKN2 tumor-suppressor gene. N Engl J Med 1995;333:975–7.
5. Ferrone CR, Levine DA, Tang LH, et al. BRCA germline mutations in Jewish patients with pancreatic adenocarcinoma. J Clin Oncol 2009;27:433–8.
6. Crist DW, Sitzmann JV, Cameron JL. Improved hospital morbidity, mortality, and survival after the Whipple procedure. Ann Surg 1987;206:358–65.

7. Sohn TA, Yeo CJ, Cameron JL, et al. Resected adenocarcinoma of the pancreas—616 patients: results, outcomes, and prognostic indicators. J Gastrointest Surg 2000;4:567–79.
8. Berger HG, Rau G, Gansauge F, et al. Treatment of pancreatic cancer: challenge of the facts. World J Surg 2003;27:10075–84.
9. Howard TJ, Krug JE, Yu J, et al. A margin-negative R0 resection accomplished with minimal postoperative complications is the surgeon's contribution to long-term survival in pancreatic cancer. J Gastrointest Surg 2006;10:1338–45.
10. Geer RJ, Brennan MF. Prognostic indicators for survival after resection of adenocarcinoma of the pancreas. Am J Surg 1993;165:68.
11. Kayahara M, Nagakawa T, Futagami F, et al. Lymphatic flow and neural plexus invasion associated with carcinoma of the body and tail of the pancreas. Cancer 1996;78(12):2485–91.
12. Yi SQ, Miwa K, Ohta T, et al. Innervation of the pancreas from the perspective of perineural invasion of pancreatic caner. Pancreas 2003;27(3):225–9.
13. Mitsunaga S, Hasebe T, Kinoshita T, et al. Detail histologic analysis of nerve plexus invasion in invasive ductal carcinoma of the pancreas and its prognostic impact. Am J Surg Pathol 2007;31(11):1636–44.
14. Allema JH, Reinders ME, van Gulik TM, et al. Results of pancreaticoduodenectomy for ampullary carcinoma and analysis of prognostic factors for survival. Surgery 1995;117(3):247–53.
15. Shami VM, Mahajan A, Loch MM, et al. Comparison between endoscopic ultrasound and magnetic resonance imaging for the staging of pancreatic cancer. Pancreas 2011;40(4):567–70.
16. Kinney T. Evidence-based imaging of pancreatic malignancies. Surg Clin North Am 2010;90(2):235–49.
17. Grassetto G, Rubello D. Role of FDG-PET/CT in diagnosis, staging, response to treatment, and prognosis of pancreatic cancer. Am J Clin Oncol 2011;34(2):111–4.
18. Vargas R, Nino-Murcia M, Trueblood W, et al. MDCT in pancreatic adenocarcinoma: prediction of vascular invasion and resectability using a multiphasic technique with curved planar reformations. AJR Am J Roentgenol 2004;182(2):419–25.
19. Nino-Murcia M, Jeffrey RB, Beaulieu CF, et al. Multidetector CT of the pancreas and bile duct system: value of curved planar reformations. AJR Am J Roentgenol 2001;176(3):689–93.
20. Prokesch RW, Chow LC, Beaulieu CF, et al. Isoattenuating pancreatic adenocarcinoma at multi-detector row CT: secondary signs. Radiology 2002;224(3):764–8.
21. Salles A, Nino-Murcia M, Jeffrey RB. CT of pancreas: minimum intensity projections. Abdom Imaging 2008;33(2):207–13.
22. Kaneko OF, Lee DM, Wong J, et al. Performance of multidetector computed tomographic angiography in determining surgical resectability of pancreatic head adenocarcinoma. J Comput Assist Tomogr 2010;34(5):732–8.
23. Zamboni GA, Kruskal JB, Vollmer CM, et al. Pancreatic adenocarcinoma: value of multidetector CT angiography in preoperative evaluation. Radiology 2007;245(3):770–8.
24. Manak E, Merkel S, Klein P, et al. Resectability of pancreatic adenocarcinoma: assessment using multidetector-row computed tomography with multiplanar reformations. Abdom Imaging 2009;34(1):75–80.
25. Schima W, Ba-Ssalamah A, Goetzinger P, et al. State-of-the-art magnetic resonance imaging of pancreatic cancer. Top Magn Reson Imaging 2007;18:421–9.

26. Deshmukh SD, Willmann JK, Jeffrey RB. Pathways of extrapancreatic perineural invasion by pancreatic adenocarcinoma: evaluation with 3D volume-rendered MDCT imaging. AJR Am J Roentgenol 2010;194(3):668–74.

27. Pham DT, Hura SA, Willmann JK, et al. Evaluation of periampullary pathology with CT volumetric oblique coronal reformations. AJR Am J Roentgenol 2009;193(3): W202–8.

28. Park HS, Lee JM, Choi HK, et al. Preoperative evaluation of pancreatic cancer: comparison of gadolinium-enhanced dynamic MRI with MR cholangiopancreatography versus MDCT. J Magn Reson Imaging 2009;30(3):586–95.

29. Mehmet Erturk S, Ichikawa T, Sou H, et al. Pancreatic adenocarcinoma: MDCT versus MRI in the detection and assessment of locoregional extension. J Comput Assist Tomogr 2006;30(4):583–90.

30. Hollett MD, Jorgensen MJ, Jeffrey RB. Quantitative evaluation of pancreatic enhancement during dual-phase helical CT. Radiology 1995;195(2):359–61.

31. Kim JH, Park SH, Yu ES, et al. Visually isoattenuating pancreatic adenocarcinoma at dynamic-enhanced CT: frequency, clinical and pathologic characteristics, and diagnosis at imaging examinations. Radiology 2010;257(1):87–96.

32. Yoon SH, Lee JM, Cho JY, et al. Small (< 20 mm) pancreatic adenocarcinomas: analysis of enhancement patterns and secondary signs with multiphasic multidetector CT. Radiology 2011;259(2):442–52.

33. Goodman M, Willmann JK, Jeffrey RB. Incidentally discovered solid pancreatic masses: imaging and clinical observations. Abdom Imaging 2011. [Epub ahead of print].

34. Horton KM, Fishman EK. Multidetector CT angiography of pancreatic carcinoma. AJR Am J Roentgenol 2002;178:827–31.

35. Brennan DDD, Zamboni GA, Raptopoulos VD, et al. Comprehensive preoperative assessment of pancreatic adenocarcinoma with 64-section volumetric CT. Radiographics 2007;27:1653–66.

36. Yoshinaga S, Suzuki H, Oda I, et al. Role of endoscopic ultrasound-guided fine needle aspiration (EUS-FNA) for diagnosis of solid pancreatic masses. Dig Endosc 2011; 23(Suppl 1):29–33.

37. Yasuda I, Iwashita T, Doi S, et al. Role of EUS in the early detection of small pancreatic cancer. Dig Endosc 2011; 23(Suppl 1):22–5.

38. Springett GM, Hoffe SE. Borderline resectable pancreatic cancer: on the edge of survival. Cancer Control 2008;15(4):295–307.

39. Lal A, Christians K, Evans DB. Management of borderline resectable pancreatic cancer. Surg Oncol Clin N Am 2010;19(2):359–70.

40. Chun YS, Milestone BN, Watson JC, et al. Defining venous involvement in borderline resectable pancreatic cancer. Ann Surg Oncol 2010;17(11):2832–8.

41. Callery MP, Chang KJ, Fishman EK, et al. Pretreatment assessment of resectable and borderline resectable pancreatic cancer: expert consensus statement. Ann Surg Oncol 2009;16:1727–33.

42. Sai M, Mori H, Kiyonaga M, et al. Peripancreatic lymphatic invasion by pancreatic carcinoma: evaluation with multi-detector row CT. Abdom Imaging 2010;35(2): 154–62.

43. Ishikawa O, Ohigashi H, Imaoka S, et al. Preoperative indications for extended pancreatectomy for locally advanced pancreas cancer involving the portal vein. Ann Surg 1992;215:231–6.

44. Lehmann KJ, Diehl SJ, Lachmann R, et al. Value of dual-phase-helical CT in the preoperative diagnosis of pancreatic cancer—a prospective study. Röfo 1998;168: 211–6.

45. Li H, Zeng MS, Zhou KR, et al. Pancreatic adenocarcinoma: the different CT criteria for peripancreatic major arterial and venous invasion. J Comput Assist Tomogr 2005;29: 170–5.
46. Tamm EP, Loyer EM, Faria S, et al. Staging of pancreatic cancer with multidetector CT in the setting of preoperative chemoradiation therapy. Abdom Imaging 2006;31:568–74.
47. Nakayama Y, Yamashita Y, Kadota M, et al. Vascular encasement by pancreatic cancer: correlation of CT findings with surgical and pathologic results. J Comput Assist Tomogr 2001;25:337–42.
48. Klauss M, Mohr A, von Tengg-Kobligk H, et al. A new invasion score for determining the resectability of pancreatic carcinomas with contrast-enhanced multidetector computed tomography. Pancreatology 2008;8:204–10.
49. Lee H, Lee JK, Kang SS, et al. Is there any clinical or radiologic feature as a preoperative marker for differentiating mass-forming pancreatitis from early-stage pancreatic adenocarcinoma? Hepatogastroenterology 2007;54(79):2134–40.
50. Lo RS, Singh RK, Austin AS, et al. Autoimmune pancreatitis presenting as a pancreatic mass mimicking malignancy. Singapore Med J 2011;52(4):e79–81.
51. Makino I, Kitagawa H. Ohta T, et al. Nerve plexus invasion in pancreatic cancer: spread patterns on histopathologic and embryological analyses. Pancreas 2008; 37(4):358–65.
52. Ceyhan GO, Schäfer KH, Kerscher AG, et al. Nerve growth factor and artemin are paracrine mediators of pancreatic neuropathy in pancreatic adenocarcinoma. Ann Surg 2010;251(5):923–31.

The Role of Endoscopic Ultrasonography in the Diagnosis and Management of Pancreatic Cancer

Mohamed O. Othman, MD[a], Michael B. Wallace, MD, MPH[b],*

KEYWORDS

- Endoscopic ultrasonography • Elastography
- Fine needle aspiration • Pancreatic cancer

According to the American Cancer Society, 43,140 new cases and 36,800 deaths from pancreatic cancer were expected in 2010.[1] The incidence of pancreatic adenocarcinoma in the United States decreased by 19% in males and 5% in females from 2002 to 2005 compared with the incidence in the period between 1977 and 1981. Interestingly, the incidence of pancreatic endocrine neoplasms increased over the same time periods by 106% in men and 125% in women.[2] The 5-year survival rate for pancreatic cancer is 5%, which is the lowest among gastrointestinal malignancies.[3] Recently, it was suggested that endoscopic ultrasound (EUS) evaluation of pancreatic cancer was an independent predictor of survival improvement in patients with locoregional pancreatic cancer.[4] In this article, we focus on the role of EUS in the evaluation and management of pancreatic cancer, including updates on novel approaches using EUS in the regional treatment of pancreatic cancer.

THE ROLE OF EUS IN DIAGNOSIS OF PANCREATIC CANCER

EUS has an integral role in the diagnosis of pancreatic cancer given its high sensitivity for detecting pancreatic neoplasms and the access it affords to perform fine needle aspiration (FNA) of the suspected lesions. The sensitivity of EUS for detecting pancreatic lesions ranges from 85% to 99% in most published series.[5-8] The sensitivity and accuracy of EUS are slightly higher than the sensitivity and accuracy

Disclosures: Dr Wallace has received research grants from Olympus, Cook, Boston Scientific, US Endoscopy, Mauna Kea Technologies, and American BioOptics. Dr Othman has nothing to disclose.
[a] Division of Gastroenterology, Department of Internal Medicine, Texas Tech HSC at El Paso4800 Alberta Avenue, El Paso, TX 79905, USA
[b] Division of Gastroenterology, Department of Internal Medicine, Mayo Clinic Florida, 4500 San Pablo Road, Jacksonville, FL 32224, USA
* Corresponding author.
E-mail address: wallace.michael@mayo.edu

Gastroenterol Clin N Am 41 (2012) 179–188
doi:10.1016/j.gtc.2011.12.014
0889-8553/12/$ – see front matter © 2012 Elsevier Inc. All rights reserved.

of computed tomography (CT) in detecting small pancreatic lesions.[8-10] Magnetic resonance imaging (MRI) has similar accuracy to CT scanning in detecting pancreatic cancer and vascular invasion.[11,12]

Pancreatic lesions usually appear on EUS as hypoechoic lesions with an irregular border. TNM staging of pancreatic tumors by EUS is feasible and accurate. If the tumor is limited to the pancreas, it is either a T1 or T2 lesion. Lesions smaller than 2 cm are T1; lesions larger than 2 cm are T2. If the tumor extends beyond the pancreas, then it is either a T3 or T4 lesion. Tumors extending to the celiac artery or superior mesenteric artery are considered T4 lesions, whereas tumors involving any of the surrounding structures of the pancreas, such as the portal vein, duodenum, or ampulla of Vater, without involvement of the celiac artery or superior mesenteric artery are classified as T3 tumors. The distinction of a T3 from a T4 tumor is important given that tumors extending to the celiac or superior mesenteric arteries (T4) are generally not surgically resectable for cure. If malignant lymph nodes are seen around the pancreas, such as the peripancreatic, celiac, or gastrohepatic lymph nodes, then the lesion is an N1 lesion. Occasionally, distant metastasis can be seen by EUS and, in this case, the lesion is an M1 lesion, which is also inoperable.[13] Soriano and colleageus[14] compared the accuracy of CT, MRI, and EUS in assessing TNM staging of pancreatic cancer using surgical diagnosis as the gold standard. CT had the highest accuracy for T-staging at 74%; MRI accuracy was 68% and EUS, 62%. However, EUS had the highest accuracy for N-staging (65%) with accuracy of CT and MRI for assessing N-staging at 62% and 61%, respectively. In a prospective study by Soriano and colleagues, CT had the greatest accuracy in detecting vascular invasion (83%) in comparison with EUS and MRI.[14] Similar results were seen in another trial by Tian and co-workers,[15] in which they found that helical CT had the highest accuracy in detecting vascular invasion of pancreatic cancer, and EUS had the highest accuracy of assessing lymph node metastases.[15] It is worth stressing that, although CT is more accurate in assessing T-staging of pancreatic cancer, EUS is still more sensitive and accurate in pancreatic lesions less than 3 cm in size.

FNA can be done with a variety of dedicated needles, most typically 22 gauge. Other needles available are the 25-gauge, 19-gauge, and core biopsy needles.[16] The number of passes needed to obtain sufficient tissue for diagnosis is higher in pancreatic cancer than in other lesions, and varies from 4 to 7 passes among the studies.[6,17,18] Combining cytologic and histologic analyses of the specimen can decrease the number of passes to 2.[19] There is a growing body of evidence that the 25-gauge needle may be superior to the 22-gauge needle in the diagnosis of pancreatic cancer.[20,21] Perhaps this is because less blood is aspirated with the 25-gauge needle, improving the cytologic assessment of the specimen. In addition, the 25-gauge needle is easier to use in areas with tough angulation, as in the case of lesions sampled from a duodenal sweep. On-site cytologic interpretation has been shown in many studies to improve yield and reduce the number of passes needed.[22-25]

LIMITATIONS OF EUS

Gastroenterologists should be aware of clinical scenarios in which pancreatic cancer can be missed or difficult to assess by EUS examinations. Varadarajulu and assocaites,[26] in a prospective study of 282 patients with pancreatic masses, found that the sensitivity of EUS-FNA in detecting pancreatic cancer in the setting of chronic pancreatic was 73% compared with 91% in patients without chronic pancreatitis. In another trial by Fritscher-Ravens and colleagues,[27] the sensitivity of EUS-FNA in detecting pancreatic cancer in patients with chronic pancreatitis was 54%, compared with 85% in patients without chronic pancreatitis. The No Endosonographic Detection of Tumor (NEST) study evaluated 20 pancreatic cancers missed by 9 experienced endosonographers. Twelve patients (60%) had chronic pancreatitis, 3 patients (15%) had a diffusely infiltrating tumor, 2 patients (10%) had a prominent ventral portion of the pancreas, and 1 patient had a recent episode of chronic pancreatitis.[28] On the other hand, false-positive results of EUS occur in 1% of the patients. Most of these patients have chronic pancreatitis on a surgical specimen as well.[29] Other limitations of EUS-FNA are related to the quality of specimen collected by FNA. Tumor necrosis or excessive blood on the specimen can obscure the diagnosis of pancreatic cancer. The cytopathologist's experience and the manner in which the specimens are handled can affect the overall accuracy of EUS-FNA in detection of pancreatic cancer.

NEWER EUS TECHNOLOGIES FOR THE DETECTION OF PANCREATIC CANCER

Newer technologies have emerged to improve the diagnostic accuracy of EUS, especially in the setting of chronic pancreatitis or in other situations in which cytology results are borderline or inconclusive. In this part of the review, we discuss the role of EUS elastography, contrast-enhanced EUS, and other new technology designed to improve the diagnostic accuracy of EUS.

EUS Elastography

EUS elastography is based on the premise that the compression of tissue produces a smaller strain (displacement) in hard tissue than it does in soft tissue.[30] Measuring this strain during EUS might aid in differentiating tissues with different strains, as in the case of chronic pancreatitis and pancreatic cancer. First-generation elastography used a qualitative method that entailed coloring tissues with different strains in different colors, in which blue represents the hardest tissue and red represented the softest tissue. The second generation of EUS elastography enabled quantitative measurement of the tissue strain thorough software programs.[31] It is worth mentioning that real-time EUS elastography is only available in the Pentax echoendoscopes system (Pentax Medical Company, Montvale, NJ).

In the last 4 years, a stream of studies evaluating the efficacy of EUS elastrography have been published. Saftoiu and associates evaluated 43 patients with either chronic pancreatitis or pancreatic cancer who were assessed with real-time EUS elastography. The diagnostic accuracy of EUS to differentiate benign from malignant lesions was 89.7%. Although the results were promising, there was no gold standard surgical diagnosis in the series.[32] Iglesias-Garcia and colleagues published their experience with EUS elastography in 2009. The authors evaluated 130 patients with solid pancreatic masses. The sensitivity, specificity, and diagnostic accuracy of EUS elastography for differentiating benign from malignant pancreatic lesions was 100%, 85.5%, and 94%, respectively.[33] These studies and others used the first-generation elastography, which showed promising results in improving the sensitivity and specificity of EUS in differentiating solid pancreatic masses.[34-36] However, first-generation elastography was criticized for its subjective nature; color interpretation of the tissue strain pattern was operator dependent.

The development of second-generation EUS elastography minimized this pitfall by quantitatively measuring the tissue strain. Iglesias-Garcia and co-workers evaluated the usefulness of quantitative EUS elastography in 86 patients with solid pancreatic masses. The sensitivity, specificity, and diagnostic accuracy of quantitative EUS elastography was higher than first-generation EUS elastography with values of 100%, 96.3%, and 98.7%, respectively.[37] Shrader and associates reached 100% sensitivity and specificity in differentiating benign from malignant lesions in tissues with blue color (hard tissue), as it appears on EUS elastography histogram. However, they could not reach the same results when evaluating areas with red or green colors, which represent softer tissue.[38] Although quantitative EUS elastography minimized the bias of qualitative evaluation, it is still unclear if it has a role in minimizing the bias of calculating the strain of the normal surrounding tissue around the lesion. In addition, further research is needed to develop pressure gauges so that the amount of the pressure applied by the echoendoscope in producing the tissue strain can be controlled.[39]

Contrast-Enhanced EUS

Contrast-enhanced (CE)-EUS utilizes the injection of a contrast agent through the blood stream. The contrast agent contains microbubbles that can be detected by EUS in the small, low-velocity vasculature of pancreatic tumors. Unlike the contrast agents used in CT or MRI, ultrasound contrast agents are confined to the blood stream and do not diffuse to the extracellular space.[40] The contrast agent is injected during the EUS examination and allows for real-time evaluation of the area of interest. The use of harmonic EUS can enhance the ability to detect the contrast agent in the microvasculature of the pancreatic tumor.[41] So far, there are 3 generations of the contrast agent injected during EUS. The most commonly used first-generation agents are Albunex (Nycomed, Oslo), Levovist (Schering, Berlin, Germany), and Echovist (Schering, Berlin, Germany). Second-generation agents are able to pass through the lung vasculature to the systemic circulation, which results in longer perfusion time. In addition, second-generation contrast agents can produce stronger backscatter that is easier to visualize by EUS. There are 3 second-generation contrast agents currently approved in Europe: Optison (Amersham Health, Amersham, England), Sonovue (Braco, Milano, Italy), Luminity (Lantheus Medical Imaging, North Billerica, Massachusetts). None of these agents are approved in United States. Definity (Lantheus Medical Imaging, North Billerica, Massachusetts) is a second-generation contrast agent that is US Food and Drug Administration approved in cardiac echography and was recently used as contrast agent in one of the CE-EUS pilot trials done in the United States through an investigational new drug waiver application.[42] Several studies evaluated the second-generation contrast agents in CE-EUS. In a pilot study by Napoleon and associates of 35 patients with solid pancreatic lesions, the sensitivity, specificity, and accuracy of CE-EUS for differentiating pancreatic adenocarcinoma were 89%, 88%, and 88.5%, respectively. These results were significantly higher than the evaluation with EUS with FNA alone.[43] In a larger trial (156 patients) by Sakamoto and collegues[44] utilizing Levovist as a contrast agent, CE-EUS had significantly higher sensitivity for detecting pancreatic tumors in comparison with CE-CT and power Doppler EUS (80% vs 50% and 11%, respectively). In a recent study that utilized Sonazoid (Daiichi-Sankyo, Tokyo, Japan), a second-generation contrast agent, the overall accuracy of CE-EUS in T-staging of pancreatic cancer was 92.4%.[45] It is possible that, in the future, CE-EUS will have a complementary role with EUS-FNA in evaluating pancreatic lesions. Other potential applications for CE-EUS include differentiating benign from malignant intraductal papillary mucinous neoplasms, although there are not enough data published on this topic yet.[40] In conclusion, CE-EUS technology is very promising and might be integrated into the clinical practice of EUS in the near future.

Detection of Chromosomal Abnormalities in Fine Needle Aspirates

There are situations in which FNA is inconclusive for diagnosis of pancreatic cancer, and new methods for detection of chromosomal abnormalities in the fine needle aspirates were recently introduced in the hope of improving the diagnostic accuracy of FNA. Kubiliun and co-workers[46] performed fluorescence *in situ* hybridization analysis on FNA specimens when cytology results were inconclusive or not available. Fluorescence *in situ* hybridization analysis had the sensitivity for detecting pancreatic cancer of 74% in this setting, and the combination of cytology and fluorescence *in situ* hybridization analysis had a sensitivity of 85%.[46] Mishra and colleagues[47] measured the telomerase activity in the FN aspirate of 40 patients with pancreatic cancer. The addition of telomerase measurement to the cytology results increased the sensitivity for detecting pancreatic cancer from 85% to 98% with specificity of 100%. However, telomerase was not expressed in all pancreatic cancers, only 31 from 40 cases in this study. K-ras mutation was found in 74% of pancreatic cancer patients in 1 study.[48] In a study of 101 patients with pancreatic cancer or chronic pancreatitis, the sensitivity and specificity of K-ras mutation for detecting pancreatic cancer were 70% and 100%, respectively.[49] The drawback of detecting chromosomal abnormalities in FNA specimens is that not all pancreatic cancers express the same mutation. Detection of more than 1 abnormality is needed to slightly increase the sensitivity, albeit with a significant increase in the cost.

THERAPEUTIC USES OF EUS IN PANCREATIC CANCER

EUS has evolved from a merely diagnostic procedure for staging of pancreatic cancer to an interventional procedure for different treatment modalities of pancreatic cancer. In this section, we discuss the utility of EUS-guided fiducial insertion and EUS delivery of antitumor agents. The role of EUS in celiac plexus neurolysis is discussed elsewhere in this edition.

EUS-Guided Fiducial Insertion

Sterotactic body radiotherapy delivers a controlled amount of radiation to the organ of interest without irradiating the surrounding organ. Bony organs or fiducials are used as a landmark for the organ of interest (**Fig. 1***A–C*).[50] Recent data indicate that sterotactic body radiotherapy can delay tumor progression in advanced pancreatic cancer.[51] EUS insertion of fiducial implants to guide sterotactic body radiotherapy was proven feasible and effective. In a prospective study by Park and co-workers,[52] EUS-guided fiducial insertion was successful in 88% of the 57 patients included in the study. The endoscopists in this trial back-loaded the fiducials into a 19-gauge needle, fixed the fiducials to the tip of the needle with bone wax, and then, after choosing the correct placement, they flushed the needle with sterile water instead of pushing the stylets, which prevented coiling of the fiducials. Sanders and associates[53] had a success rate of 90% for EUS fiducial insertion in a prospective study of 51 patients. The endoscopists in this study used a pushing stylet technique for fiducial insertion. DiMaio and colleageus[54] evaluated the EUS-guided fiducial insertion with a 22-gauge needle in various gastrointestinal sites (9 pancreatic cancer patients) and they had a success rate of 97%.

EUS Delivery of Antitumor Agents

EUS-guided local delivery of various anti-tumor agents is currently under investigation. In a phase I clinical trial of EUS-guided injection of allogeneic mixed lymphocyte culture in pancreatic cancer patients (stage II to stage IV), there were no procedure-related complications.[55] Two of the 8 patients included in this study had partial response to the single injection. ONYX-015 is a gene-deleted replication-selective adenovirus, which selectively targets malignant pancreatic tissue. A phase I/II trial

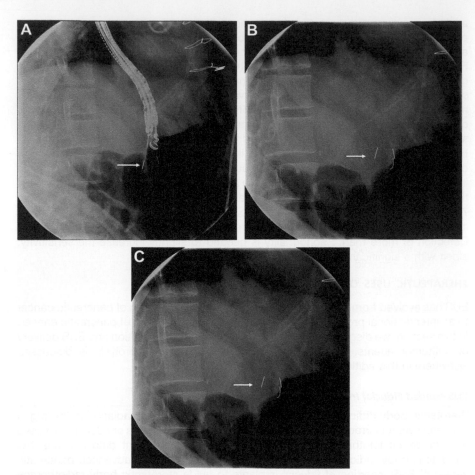

Fig. 1. EUS-guided fiducial placement for radiotherapy or proton therapy guidance. (*A, B*) EUS endoscopic placing fiducial markers (Visicoil, Santa Barbara, CA) in a borderline resectable pancreatic body tumor. (*C*) Final placement of 3 markers. At least 3 markers should be placed, typically at least 1 to 2 cm apart to allow for precise registration of tumor with markers. *Arrows* indicate the fiducial marker in the tumor (tumor not seen on radiograph).

delivered ONYX-015 locally under EUS guidance for 8 sessions in 21 patients. The local treatment was given in combination with gemcitabine. Two patients had duodenal perforation in this study. Only 2 patients had partial regression of the disease.[56] Another strategy is the injection of immature dendritic cells, which induce T-cell immune response against malignant cells. Irisawa and co-workers[57] successfully delivered dendritic cells into the tumors of 7 patients with unresectable pancreatic cancer, without any procedure-related complications. Median survival in the cohort was 9.9 months.[57] Tumor necrosis factor-α is a potent antitumor cytokine, naturally released by the macrophage.[58] Local injection of tumor necrosis factor-α showed promising results in solid tumor and soft tissue sarcoma.[59,60] EUS-guided local injection of tumor necrosis factor-α for pancreatic and esophageal cancer is currently under investigation.[61]

SUMMARY

EUS with FNA is highly sensitive and specific for diagnosing pancreatic cancer. However, in certain situations, such as in patients with chronic pancreatitis, this high sensitivity and specificity can significantly diminish. The use of new technology, such as EUS elastography, CE-EUS, and gene mutations detection in FNA specimens, can help to differentiate chronic pancreatitis from pancreatic cancer. EUS has evolved from a diagnostic procedure to a therapeutic intervention in pancreatic cancer. EUS-guided fiducial insertion and EUS-guided delivery of antitumor agents, in addition to celiac plexus neurolysis, are the main therapeutic applications of EUS in pancreatic cancer.

REFERENCES

1. Cancer Facts and Figures 2010. American Cancer Society, 2010. Available at: http://www.cancer.org/acs/groups/content/@epidemiologysurveilance/documents/document/acspc-026238.pdf. Accessed December 8, 2011.
2. Zhou J, Enewold L, Stojadinovic A, et al. Incidence rates of exocrine and endocrine pancreatic cancers in the United States. Cancer Causes Control 2010;21:853–61.
3. Saif MW. Pancreatic neoplasm in 2011: an update. JOP 2011;12:316–21.
4. Ngamruengphong S, Li F, Zhou Y, et al. EUS and survival in patients with pancreatic cancer: a population-based study. Gastrointest Endosc 2010;72:78–83.
5. Chang KJ, Nguyen P, Erickson RA, et al. The clinical utility of endoscopic ultrasound-guided fine-needle aspiration in the diagnosis and staging of pancreatic carcinoma. Gastrointest Endosc 1997;45:387–93.
6. Eloubeidi MA, Jhala D, Chhieng DC, et al. Yield of endoscopic ultrasound-guided fine-needle aspiration biopsy in patients with suspected pancreatic carcinoma. Cancer 2003;99:285–92.
7. Siddiqui AA, Brown LJ, Hong SK, et al. Relationship of pancreatic mass size and diagnostic yield of endoscopic ultrasound-guided fine needle aspiration. Dig Dis Sci 2011;56:3370–5.
8. Agarwal B, Abu-Hamda E, Molke KL, et al. Endoscopic ultrasound-guided fine needle aspiration and multidetector spiral CT in the diagnosis of pancreatic cancer. Am J Gastroenterol 2004;99:844–50.
9. Legmann P, Vignaux O, Dousset B, et al. Pancreatic tumors: comparison of dual-phase helical CT and endoscopic sonography. AJR Am J Roentgenol 1998;170:1315–22.
10. Bronstein YL, Loyer EM, Kaur H, et al. Detection of small pancreatic tumors with multiphasic helical CT. AJR Am J Roentgenol 2004;182:619–23.
11. Koelblinger C, Ba-Ssalamah A, Goetzinger P, et al. Gadobenate dimeglumine-enhanced 3.0-T MR imaging versus multiphasic 64-detector row CT: prospective evaluation in patients suspected of having pancreatic cancer. Radiology 2011;259:757–66.
12. Arslan A, Buanes T, Geitung JT. Pancreatic carcinoma: MR, MR angiography and dynamic helical CT in the evaluation of vascular invasion. Eur J Radiol 2001;38:151–9.
13. van Hemel BM, Lamprou AA, Weersma R, et al. Procedure-related, false-positive cytology results during EUS-guided FNA in patients with esophageal cancer. Gastrointest Endosc 2010;71:1130–3.
14. Soriano A, Castells A, Ayuso C, et al. Preoperative staging and tumor resectability assessment of pancreatic cancer: prospective study comparing endoscopic ultrasonography, helical computed tomography, magnetic resonance imaging, and angiography. Am J Gastroenterol 2004;99:492–501.

15. Tian YT, Wang CF, Wang GQ, et al. [Prospective evaluation of the clinical significance of ultrasonography, helical computed tomography, magnetic resonance imaging and endoscopic ultrasonography in the assessment of vascular invasion and lymph node metastasis of pancreatic carcinoma]. Zhonghua zhong liu za zhi [Chinese Journal of Oncology] 2008;30:682–5.

16. Othman MO, Raimondo M. Endoscopic ultrasound fine needle aspiration of pancreatic lesions: Is a smaller needle safer and better? Dig Liver Dis 2011;43:587–8.

17. Erickson RA, Sayage-Rabie L, Beissner RS. Factors predicting the number of EUS-guided fine-needle passes for diagnosis of pancreatic malignancies. Gastrointest Endosc 2000;51:184–90.

18. LeBlanc JK, Ciaccia D, Al-Assi MT, et al. Optimal number of EUS-guided fine needle passes needed to obtain a correct diagnosis. Gastrointest Endosc 2004;59:475–81.

19. Moller K, Papanikolaou IS, Toermer T, et al. EUS-guided FNA of solid pancreatic masses: high yield of 2 passes with combined histologic-cytologic analysis. Gastrointest Endosc 2009;70:60–9.

20. Fabbri C, Polifemo AM, Luigiano C, et al. Endoscopic ultrasound-guided fine needle aspiration with 22- and 25-gauge needles in solid pancreatic masses: a prospective comparative study with randomisation of needle sequence. Dig Liver Dis 2011;43: 647–52.

21. Sakamoto H, Kitano M, Komaki T, et al. Prospective comparative study of the EUS guided 25-gauge FNA needle with the 19-gauge Trucut needle and 22-gauge FNA needle in patients with solid pancreatic masses. J Gastroenterol Hepatol 2009;24:384–90.

22. Hikichi T, Irisawa A, Bhutani MS, et al. Endoscopic ultrasound-guided fine-needle aspiration of solid pancreatic masses with rapid on-site cytological evaluation by endosonographers without attendance of cytopathologists. J Gastroenterol 2009;44: 322–8.

23. Savoy AD, Raimondo M, Woodward TA, et al. Can endosonographers evaluate on-site cytologic adequacy? A comparison with cytotechnologists. Gastrointest Endosc 2007;65:953–7.

24. Jhala NC, Eltoum IA, Eloubeidi MA, et al. Providing on-site diagnosis of malignancy on endoscopic-ultrasound-guided fine-needle aspirates: should it be done? Ann Diagn Pathol 2007;11:176–81.

25. Klapman JB, Logrono R, Dye CE, et al. Clinical impact of on-site cytopathology interpretation on endoscopic ultrasound-guided fine needle aspiration. Am J Gastroenterol 2003;98:1289–94.

26. Varadarajulu S, Tamhane A, Eloubeidi MA. Yield of EUS-guided FNA of pancreatic masses in the presence or the absence of chronic pancreatitis. Gastrointest Endosc 2005;62:728–36.

27. Fritscher-Ravens A, Brand L, Knofel WT, et al. Comparison of endoscopic ultrasound-guided fine needle aspiration for focal pancreatic lesions in patients with normal parenchyma and chronic pancreatitis. J Gastroenterol 2002;97:2768–75.

28. Bhutani MS, Gress FG, Giovannini M, et al. The No Endosonographic Detection of Tumor (NEST) study: a case series of pancreatic cancers missed on endoscopic ultrasonography. Endoscopy 2004;36:385–9.

29. Siddiqui AA, Kowalski TE, Shahid H, et al. False-positive EUS-guided FNA cytology for solid pancreatic lesions. Gastrointest Endosc 2011;74:535–40.

30. Ophir J, Cespedes I, Ponnekanti H, et al. Elastography: a quantitative method for imaging the elasticity of biological tissues. Ultrasonic Imaging 1991;13:111–34.

31. Saftoiu A. State-of-the-art imaging techniques in endoscopic ultrasound. World J Gastroenterol 2011;17:691–6.

32. Saftoiu A, Vilmann P, Gorunescu F, et al. Neural network analysis of dynamic sequences of EUS elastography used for the differential diagnosis of chronic pancreatitis and pancreatic cancer. Gastrointest Endosc 2008;68:1086–94.

33. Iglesias-Garcia J, Larino-Noia J, Abdulkader I, et al. EUS elastography for the characterization of solid pancreatic masses. Gastrointest Endosc 2009;70:1101–8.

34. Giovannini M, Hookey LC, Bories E, et al. Endoscopic ultrasound elastography: the first step towards virtual biopsy? Preliminary results in 49 patients. Endoscopy 2006;38:344–8.

35. Janssen J, Schlorer E, Greiner L. EUS elastography of the pancreas: feasibility and pattern description of the normal pancreas, chronic pancreatitis, and focal pancreatic lesions. Gastrointest Endosc 2007;65:971–8.

36. Hirche TO, Ignee A, Barreiros AP, et al. Indications and limitations of endoscopic ultrasound elastography for evaluation of focal pancreatic lesions. Endoscopy 2008;40:910–7.

37. Iglesias-Garcia J, Larino-Noia J, Abdulkader I, et al. Quantitative endoscopic ultrasound elastography: an accurate method for the differentiation of solid pancreatic masses. Gastroenterology 2010;139:1172–80.

38. Schrader H, Wiese M, Ellrichmann M, et al. Diagnostic value of quantitative EUS elastography for malignant pancreatic tumors: relationship with pancreatic fibrosis. Ultraschall Med 2011 May 31 [Epub ahead of print].

39. Saftoiu A, Vilman P. Endoscopic ultrasound elastography: a new imaging technique for the visualization of tissue elasticity distribution. J Gastrointestin Liver Dis 2006;15:161–5.

40. Giovannini M. Contrast-enhanced and 3-dimensional endoscopic ultrasonography. Gastroenterol Clin North Am 2010;39:845–58.

41. Claudon M, Cosgrove D, Albrecht T, et al. Guidelines and good clinical practice recommendations for contrast enhanced ultrasound (CEUS): update 2008. Ultraschall Med 2008;29:28–44.

42. Romagnuolo J, Hoffman B, Vela S, et al. Accuracy of contrast-enhanced harmonic EUS with a second-generation perflutren lipid microsphere contrast agent (with video). Gastrointest Endosc Jan 2011;73:52–63.

43. Napoleon B, Alvarez-Sanchez MV, Gincoul R, et al. Contrast-enhanced harmonic endoscopic ultrasound in solid lesions of the pancreas: results of a pilot study. Endoscopy 2010;42:564–70.

44. Sakamoto H, Kitano M, Suetomi Y, et al. Utility of contrast-enhanced endoscopic ultrasonography for diagnosis of small pancreatic carcinomas. Ultrasound Med Biol 2008;34:525–32.

45. Imazu H, Uchiyama Y, Matsunaga K, et al. Contrast-enhanced harmonic EUS with novel ultrasonographic contrast (Sonazoid) in the preoperative T-staging for pancreaticobiliary malignancies. Scand J Gastroenterol 2010;45:732–8.

46. Kubiliun N, Ribeiro A, Fan YS, et al. EUS-FNA with rescue fluorescence *in situ* hybridization for the diagnosis of pancreatic carcinoma in patients with inconclusive on-site cytopathology results. Gastrointest Endosc 2011;74:541–7.

47. Mishra G, Zhao Y, Sweeney J, et al. Determination of qualitative telomerase activity as an adjunct to the diagnosis of pancreatic adenocarcinoma by EUS-guided fine-needle aspiration. Gastrointest Endosc 2006;63:648–54.

48. Takahashi K, Yamao K, Okubo K, et al. Differential diagnosis of pancreatic cancer and focal pancreatitis by using EUS-guided FNA. Gastrointest Endosc Jan 2005;61:76–9.

49. Salek C, Benesova L, Zavoral M, et al. Evaluation of clinical relevance of examining K-ras, p16 and p53 mutations along with allelic losses at 9p and 18q in EUS-guided fine needle aspiration samples of patients with chronic pancreatitis and pancreatic cancer. World J Gastroenterol 2007;13:3714–20.

50. Timmerman RD, Kavanagh BD, Cho LC, et al. Stereotactic body radiation therapy in multiple organ sites. J Clin Oncol 2007;25:947–52.
51. Koong AC, Christofferson E, Le QT, et al. Phase II study to assess the efficacy of conventionally fractionated radiotherapy followed by a stereotactic radiosurgery boost in patients with locally advanced pancreatic cancer. Int J Radiat Oncol Biol Physics 2005;63:320–3.
52. Park WG, Yan BM, Schellenberg D, et al. EUS-guided gold fiducial insertion for image-guided radiation therapy of pancreatic cancer: 50 successful cases without fluoroscopy. Gastrointest Endosc 2010;71:513–8.
53. Sanders MK, Moser AJ, Khalid A, et al. EUS-guided fiducial placement for stereotactic body radiotherapy in locally advanced and recurrent pancreatic cancer. Gastrointest Endosc 2010;71:1178–84.
54. DiMaio CJ, Nagula S, Goodman KA, et al. EUS-guided fiducial placement for image-guided radiation therapy in GI malignancies by using a 22-gauge needle (with videos). Gastrointest Endosc 2010;71:1204–10.
55. Chang KJ, Nguyen PT, Thompson JA, et al. Phase I clinical trial of allogeneic mixed lymphocyte culture (cytoimplant) delivered by endoscopic ultrasound-guided fine-needle injection in patients with advanced pancreatic carcinoma. Cancer 2000;88: 1325–35.
56. Hecht JR, Bedford R, Abbruzzese JL, et al. A phase I/II trial of intratumoral endoscopic ultrasound injection of ONYX-015 with intravenous gemcitabine in unresectable pancreatic carcinoma. Clin Cancer Res 2003;9:555–61.
57. Irisawa A, Takagi T, Kanazawa M, et al. Endoscopic ultrasound-guided fine-needle injection of immature dendritic cells into advanced pancreatic cancer refractory to gemcitabine: a pilot study. Pancreas 2007;35:189–90.
58. Wallach D, Varfolomeev EE, Malinin NL, et al. Tumor necrosis factor receptor and Fas signaling mechanisms. Annu Rev Immunol 1999;17:331–67.
59. McLoughlin JM, McCarty TM, Cunningham C, et al. TNFerade, an adenovector carrying the transgene for human tumor necrosis factor alpha, for patients with advanced solid tumors: surgical experience and long-term follow-up. Ann Surg Oncol 2005;12825–30.
60. Senzer N, Mani S, Rosemurgy A, et al. TNFerade biologic, an adenovector with a radiation-inducible promoter, carrying the human tumor necrosis factor alpha gene: a phase I study in patients with solid tumors. J Clin Oncol 2004;22:592–601.
61. Chang KJ, Lee JG, Holcombe RF, et al. Endoscopic ultrasound delivery of an antitumor agent to treat a case of pancreatic cancer. Nat Clin Pract Gastroenterol Hepatol 2008;5:107–11.

Pancreatic Cancer: Medical Management (Novel Chemotherapeutics)

David Páez, MD[a,b],
Melissa J. Labonte, PhD[a], Heinz-Josef Lenz, MD[a,*]

KEYWORDS
- Chemoradiation • Chemotherapy • Pancreatic adenocarcinoma
- Treatment

Pancreatic adenocarcinoma (PC) is the fourth leading cause of cancer death[1] and is associated with an extremely poor prognosis: The 5-year survival probability is less than 5% for all stages combined.[1–3] The only chance for cure or longer survival is surgical resection; however, only approximately 10% to 20%[1,4] of patients with pancreatic cancer have resectable disease, and even though surgical techniques have improved, most patients who undergo complete resection experience a recurrence. Adjuvant systemic therapy is used to reduce the recurrence rate and improve the outcome of resected pancreatic tumors.[5–7] There is also a potential role for radiation therapy as part of the treatment for locally advanced disease, although its use in both the adjuvant and neoadjuvant settings remains controversial.[8–13]

The majority of patients with PC (80%) present with a locally advanced tumor or metastatic disease, and thus palliative systemic therapy, and, in some cases, chemoradiotherapy (CRT) remain the only options for almost all of these patients.[4] Although the use of gemcitabine has been shown to improve survival compared with best supportive care, PC has been relatively resistant to all systemic therapies, including hormonal therapy[14–16] and cytotoxic chemotherapy.[17] In the last decade, drug development has included a focus on the combination of cytotoxic agents, but this approach has so far not led to a major impact in the clinic. Newer drugs have assessed the efficacy of targeted therapies through the inhibition of important pathways that are involved in the proliferation, invasion, and metastasis of pancreatic tumor cells.

There is growing evidence that the exceptionally poor prognosis in PC is caused by the tumor's characteristic abundant desmoplastic stroma that plays a critical role in

Disclosure: David Páez is the recipient of a fellowship from the Instituto de Salud Carlos III (CM08/00065).
[a] Division of Medical Oncology, University of Southern California/Norris Comprehensive Cancer Center, Keck School of Medicine, 1441 Eastlake Avenue, NOR 5322, Los Angeles, CA 90033, USA
[b] Medical Oncology Department, Hospital de la Santa Creu i Sant Pau, Barcelona, Spain
* Corresponding author.
E-mail address: lenz@usc.edu

Gastroenterol Clin N Am 41 (2012) 189–209
doi:10.1016/j.gtc.2011.12.004
0889-8553/12/$ – see front matter © 2012 Elsevier Inc. All rights reserved.

Table 1				
Adjuvant phase III clinical trials in pancreatic cancer				
Study Year	No. of Patients	Protocol Treatments	Median Survival (mos)	P-Value
GITSG, 1985[22]	49	CRT (5-FU bolus) Surgery alone	20 11	.01
EORTC, 1999[24,25]	218	CRT (5-FU CI) Surgery alone	17.1 12.6	.049
ESPAC1, 2001[26,27]	541	CT (5-FU bolus) CRT (5-FU bolus) CRT+CT Surgery alone	19.7 (CT) 14 (non CT) 15.1 (CRT) 16.1 (non CRT)	.005
RTOG 97-04, 2008[29,30]	451	5-FU+CRT Gemcitabine+CRT	16.9 20.5	.09
CONKO-001, 2007[33,34]	179 175	Gemcitabine Observation	22.8 20.2	.005
ESPAC-3, 2010[36]	1088	5-FU Gemcitabine	23 23.6	.39

Abbreviations: CI, continuous infusion; CRT, chemoradiotherapy; CT, chemotherapy; EORTC, European Organization for Research and Treatment of Cancer; ESPAC, European Study Group for Pancreatic Cancer; GITSG, Gastrointestinal Tumor Study Group; RTOG, Radiation Therapy Oncology Group; 5-FU, 5-fluorouracil.

tumor cell growth, invasion, metastasis, and chemoresistance.[18] Carefully designed clinical trials that include translational analysis will provide a better understanding of the tumor biology and its relation to the host stromal cells. Future drug development will involve testing new targeted agents, investigating the efficacy of different combinations strategies, and looking for predictive and prognostic biomarkers.

TREATMENT OF RESECTABLE DISEASE
Adjuvant Chemoradiation

Surgical resection is the only curative treatment for patients with PC, yet only 10% to 15% of patients have a resectable tumor at the time of diagnosis. Moreover, after surgery, the 5-year survival is less than 20%.[19-21] In this context, adjuvant chemotherapy, with or without radiotherapy, is the recommended approach after surgery to improve both locoregional control and overall survival (OS).

Several trials have analyzed the efficacy of CRT after pancreaticoduodenectomy (**Table 1**). The Gastrointestinal Tumor Study Group (GITSG) was the first to document that adjuvant CRT after surgical resection prolonged survival.[22] In this study, radiation was administered in combination with bolus 5-fluorouracil (5-FU) and was followed by maintenance 5-FU. Although the study was terminated prematurely because of a low rate of accrual, a survival advantage was demonstrated for the patients who received the combination treatment in comparison with patients who were treated with surgery alone. A subsequent nonrandomized study by the GITSG confirmed the support for the use of adjuvant CRT, rather than either radiation therapy alone or surgery alone, for patients with resectable disease.[23]

The European Organization for Research and Treatment of Cancer conducted a trial in which 218 patients with pancreatic and nonpancreatic periampullary adenocarcinoma were randomized to either observation alone or to a combination of radiotherapy and 5-FU (administered as a continuous infusion) after potentially curative resection.[24] No additional postradiation chemotherapy was administered. The preliminary analysis did not find a significant benefit to adjuvant chemoradiation; however, a subsequent statistical reanalysis demonstrated a significant survival improvement with the combination treatment for patients with pancreatic head cancers.[25]

In contrast, the controversial results of the European Study Group for Pancreatic Cancer (ESPAC-1) suggested a detrimental effect on survival with adjuvant CRT compared with adjuvant chemotherapy or surgery alone.[26,27] In this 4-arm trial, 541 patients were randomized, based on a 2×2 factorial design, to one of the following arms: (1) Observation, (2) concomitant CRT alone with 500 mg/m^2 of 5-FU IV bolus during the first 3 days of radiation therapy and repeated after a planned 2-week break, (3) chemotherapy alone with leucovorin, 20 mg/m^2 bolus plus 5-FU, 425 mg/m^2 administered for 5 consecutive days and repeated every 28 days for 6 cycles, or (4) CRT followed by chemotherapy. No difference was found in survival between patients assigned to CRT (median survival, 15.5 months) versus observation (median survival, 16.1 months; $P = .24$). A trend to a survival advantage for those patients treated with chemotherapy alone (median survival, 17.4 months) versus observation alone (15.9 months; $P = .19$) was described. Despite criticisms of the study design, including criticism of the enrollment criteria and radiation therapy techniques, the authors concluded that adjuvant CRT did not offer any OS advantage, whereas a potential benefit existed for adjuvant chemotherapy alone after surgical resection.[28]

To determine if the addition of gemcitabine to adjuvant 5-FU chemoradiation improved survival for patients with resected PC, 451 patients were randomized to either 5-FU (250 mg/m^2 per day) or gemcitabine (1000 mg/m^2 weekly) for 3 weeks before CRT and for 12 weeks after CRT therapy (Intergroup/RTOG 97-04 phase III trial). Chemoradiation with a continuous infusion of 250 mg/m^2 per day 5-FU during radiation therapy was the same for all patients. In this phase III trial, patients with pancreatic head tumors had a median survival of 20.5 months in the gemcitabine groups versus a 16.9 months in the 5-FU group ($P = .09$).[29] Grade 4 hematologic toxicity was reported in 1% of the fluorouracil group and 14% of the gemcitabine group ($P<.001$) without a difference in febrile neutropenia or infection. Although the survival improvement was not significant, the authors concluded that the addition of gemcitabine to adjuvant fluorouracil-based chemoradiation was associated with a survival benefit for patients with resected PC. A long-term follow-up of this trial was recently published. The 5-year results of this study demonstrate that the previously observed improvement in 3-year OS with the addition of gemcitabine to adjuvant fluorouracil-based CRT for patients with pancreatic head tumors was not seen at 5 years: OS was 22% with gemcitabine versus 18% with 5-FU. A trend toward significance in improvement of OS in the gemcitabine arm was seen on a multivariate analysis ($P = .08$).[30]

Several institutions have prospectively or retrospectively demonstrated the utility of adjuvant CRT compared with surgery alone. The Johns Hopkins Hospital–Mayo Clinic Collaborative Study recently reported a large collaborative analysis of 1092 patients who underwent resection with curative intent. Compared with the OS for those undergoing surgery alone, the OS was longer for recipients of CRT (median OS 21.1 vs 15.5 months; $P>.001$). In the multivariate analysis, after adjusting for different variables, OS remained superior for patients treated with adjuvant CRT compared with those who received surgery alone.[31]

The European Organization for Research and Treatment of Cancer's phase II trial assessed the toxicity of gemcitabine followed by gemcitabine concurrent with radiation. The results showed that adjuvant gemcitabine followed by the combination of gemcitabine and radiation (50.4 Gy) was feasible and only slightly more toxic than gemcitabine alone, pointing to a further evaluation of this multimodal approach in a phase III trial.[32]

Adjuvant Chemotherapy

To test the hypothesis that gemcitabine after resection improves disease-free survival, the CONKO-001 study randomized 368 (354 were elegible for intent-to-treat-analysis) patients with completely resected PC to 6 cycles of gemcitabine or surgery alone. The study demonstrated a significant improvement in its primary endpoint of disease-free survival for patients receiving postoperative gemcitabine (13.4 vs 6.9 months; $P<.001$) but without an improvement in OS (22.1 vs 20.2 months; $P = .06$).[33] However, the recently reported 5-year results demonstrated a significant improvement in OS with a median and 5-year survival rate of 22.8 months and 21% in the gemcitabine arm and 20.2 months and 9% in the surgery alone arm ($P = .005$).[34]

The ESPAC-3 phase III randomized trial was designed to determine whether fluorouracil or gemcitabine is superior in terms of OS as adjuvant treatment after resection of PC. A total of 1088 patients were randomized to receive either gemcitabine or 5-FU plus folinic acid. In contrast with the findings for nonresected advanced PC,[35] there was no significant difference in OS between patients treated with postoperative adjuvant 5-FU plus folinic acid and patients who were treated with gemcitabine. However, gemcitabine showed a superior toxicity profile with fewer treatment-related serious adverse events (7.5%) compared with 14% of patients receiving 5-FU plus folinic acid ($P<.001$). The lower toxicity and the ease of administration of gemcitabine in a weekly treatment schedule led to consideration of this treatment as the standard of care for most patients[36] (see **Table 1**).

Although a growing body of literature indicates a benefit of adjuvant treatment in localized PC after a potentially curative resection, the vast majority of tumors recur and the patients succumb to their disease a short time after diagnosis.

To summarize, strong evidence from randomized trials suggest that adjuvant chemotherapy (gemcitabine or 5-FU) is the standard treatment option. However, there remains controversy regarding the role of adjuvant CRT. Future clinical trials exploring different adjuvant chemotherapy or chemoradiation schedules, as well as the integration of novel cytotoxic and targeted agents, could elucidate which is the best option to improve the outcome for patients with resected PC. The ESPAC-4 trial is evaluating the addition of the oral fluropyrimidine, capecitabine, to gemcitabine after resection of localized PC. The RTOG0848 trial will analyze whether both erlotinib and fluoropyrimidine-based chemoradiation improves the survival of patients treated with gemcitabine as adjuvant treatment for patients with resected head of PC.

Preoperative Chemoradiation

Neoadjuvant, or preoperative, therapy has been used to improve survival in resectable PC. There are several reasons to consider a neoadjuvant approach, such as:

1. Early treatment of micrometastasis disease;
2. Extension of potentially curative treatment to patients with borderline disease;
3. Increasing the rates of negative margin resections and decrease local failure rates; and
4. Improving the selection of patients for whom resection will not offer a survival benefit.

To date, several single-institution studies have demonstrated that patients who undergo resection after neoadjuvant therapy have a significantly improved survivals compared with those treated with surgery and adjuvant therapy.[37,38] However, data from randomized, prospective, phase III trials comparing neoadjuvant with adjuvant strategies are not available. The first multicenter, randomized, controlled trial comparing neoadjuvant CRT and surgery with surgery alone has been recruiting patients since June 2003 but, because of the unreasonably slow recruitment, the study will be finished before reaching the initially planned 254 patients.[39]

A rigorous meta-analysis of 56 phase I and II trials studying the effect of neoadjuvant therapy was completed. Interestingly, for patients with resectable tumors who received neoadjuvant therapy, resection frequencies and survival after neoadjuvant therapy were similar to those patients with primarily resected tumors treated with adjuvant therapy, showing no advantage of neoadjuvant therapy for patients with resectable tumors. However, among patients with initially staged unresectable tumors, one third were resected after neoadjuvant therapy, with survival comparable with those patients with initially resectable tumors.[40]

Recently, a large pancreatic series from the California Cancer Surveillance Program for Los Angeles County retrospectively identified 458 patients with nonmetastatic PC who underwent definitive pancreatic resection and received systemic chemotherapy. In contrast with the conclusions of the meta-analysis, patients who received neoadjuvant therapy presented a lower rate of lymph node positivity (45%) and improved OS (34 months) compared with the adjuvant group of patients (65% [$P = .11$] and 19 months [$P = .003$], respectively). In the multivariate analysis, neoadjuvant therapy remained an independent predictor of improved survival ($P = .013$). The authors suggested that this strategy should be considered an acceptable alternative to the initial surgery treatment in operable PC.[41]

To summarize, although neoadjuvant CRT can be administered safely, the recommended practice for resectable disease outside the clinical trial setting should be surgery followed by adjuvant chemotherapy with or without radiation.

TREATMENT OF LOCALLY ADVANCED DISEASE

Thirty percent of patients with PC present with a locally advanced unresectable primary tumor. Locally advanced PC is most commonly described by T4 lesions, in which the primary tumor involves branches of the celiac axis or the superior mesenteric artery. The standard treatment for locally advanced PC can involve CRT, which has been highly debated over the last 30 years, or chemotherapy alone.[42]

Several prospective, randomized trials have shown a benefit with chemoradiation compared with best supportive care, radiation, or chemotherapy alone in the management of locally advanced disease (Table 2).

Only 1 randomized trial, including 31 patients, compared CRT (continuous infusion of 5-FU at 200 mg/m^2 per day concomitantly with a planned total dose of 50.4 Gy) with best supportive care. The study results demonstrated a significant benefit of CRT for OS ($P<.001$) and quality of life ($P<.001$).[43]

The earliest trial, published in 1969 by the GITSG, included patients randomized to receive either 35 to 40 Gy radiation plus 5-FU or the same radiation therapy plus a placebo. Although this study included patients with different types of GI cancers, the median survival in the combined modality arm was significantly higher than in the radiation therapy only arm (10.4 vs 6.3 months).[44] In 1981, Moertel and colleagues[44] published a study in which 194 patients with locally advanced PC were randomized to receive a split-course radiation schedule, either alone (60 Gy) or combined with 5-FU (500 mg/m^2 on the first 3 days of each 20 Gy radiation). The combined modality arms (60Gy plus 5-FU or 40Gy plus 5-FU) showed an improved median time-to-tumor progression, as well as improved OS (9.7 and 9.3 vs 5.3 months in the radiotherapy

Table 2
Randomized clinical trials in locally advanced pancreatic cancer

Study Year	No. of Patients	Protocol Treatments	Median Survival (mos)	P-Value
CRT vs best supportive care				
Shinchi, 2002[43]	31	CRT (50.8 Gy + 5-FU)	13	<.01
		Best supportive care	6.4	
CRT vs RT				
Moertel, 1981[45]	194	RT (60 Gy)	5.3	<.01
		CRT (40 Gy + 5-FU)	9.7	
		CRT (60 Gy + 5-FU)	9.3	
Cohen, 2005[46]	108	RT(59.4 Gy)	7.1	.16
		CRT (50.4 Gy + 5-FU + MMC)	8.4	
CRT vs CT				
GITSG, 1988[47]	43	CT (5-FU + streptomycin + MMC)	7.4	NA
		CRT (54 Gy + 5-FU)	9.7	
Hazel, 1981[48]	30	CT (5-FU + lomustine)	7.8	NA
		CRT (46 Gy + 5-FU)	7.3	
Klaasen, 1985[49]	91	CT (5-FU)	8.2	NA
		CRT (40 Gy + 5-FU)	8.3	
Chauffert, 2007[50]	119	CT (gemcitabine)	13	.03
		CRT (60 Gy + 5-FU + cisplatin)	8.6	
Loherer, 2008[51]	74	CT (gemcitabine)	9.2	.044
		CRT (50.4 Gy + gemcitabine)	11	

Abbreviations: CRT, chemoradiotherapy; CT, chemotherapy; Gy, Gray; GITSG, Gastrointestinal Tumor Study Group; MMC, mitomycin; NA, not available; RT, radiotherapy; 5-FU, 5-fluorouracil.

arm; $P<.01$).[45] A study comparing standard radiotherapy (59.4 Gy) with CRT using mitomycin and 5-FU showed no difference between the 2 arms (8.4 months for CRT vs 7.1 months for radiotherapy; $P<.16$).[46] In both trials, higher hematologic and digestive toxicities were presented in the CRT arms.

Several randomized trials compared CRT to chemotherapy alone. In the first 3 trials, published before 1990, CRT (doses ranging from 40 to 54 Gy) was compared with different chemotherapy regimens, including 5-FU; lomustine and 5-FU; and streptomycin, mitomycin and 5-FU.[47-49] Only the GITSG study, using mitomycin and 5-FU, showed a significant improvement in median survival (9.7 vs 7.4 months) for the chemoradiation arm, with a higher 1-year survival rate (41% vs 19% in the chemotherapy group; $P<.02$). Therefore, the use of different chemotherapy agents with radiation therapy failed to demonstrate a survival advantage compared with 5-FU, which tends to have less toxicity.

The clinical benefits of gemcitabine in the metastatic setting and its radiosensitizing properties have merited the exploration of this agent's use in locally advanced PC. In the recent French FFCD-SFRO study, CRT was delivered to a total dose of 60 Gy concurrently with cisplatin (20 mg/m² during weeks 1 and 5 of radiotherapy) and 5-FU (continuous infusion at 300 mg/m² per day). The patients in the chemotherapy arm were treated with gemcitabine (1000 mg/m² per week). In contrast with the initial hypothesis of the trial, OS was shorter in the CRT arm. Higher grade 3 to 4 toxicity rates were observed in the CRT arm compared with the chemotherapy arm (66% vs 40%, respectively).[50]

The ECOG phase III trial (E4201), comparing gemcitabine (600 mg/m^2 weekly) plus radiotherapy (50.4 Gy) followed by weekly gemcitabine (1000 mg/m^2 weekly, 3 of 4 weeks) with gemcitabine alone, was prematurely closed owing to low recruitment. With 74 patients included, a higher median OS was observed in the CRT arm (11 vs 9.2 months; $P<.044$).[51]

Two meta-analyses[52,53] that included most of the studies previously mentioned compared CRT with exclusive radiotherapy and CRT with chemotherapy alone in patients with locally advanced PC. Although, there is a significant variability between the different studies analyzed, the main conclusions of the meta-analyses were that:

1. CRT increase OS compared with radiotherapy alone; and
2. OS was not significantly different between CRT and chemotherapy alone.

Two retrospective studies have shown a potential survival improvement of induction chemotherapy before CRT.[54,55] This strategy may improve selection of those patients who benefit from CRT after a short course of chemotherapy. The phase III trial LAP07 being conducted by the Groupe Cooperateur Multidisciplinaire en Oncologie (GERCOR) may help to clarify the role of induction chemotherapy. In this ongoing study, patients with a controlled tumor after the first 4 months of induction chemotherapy are randomly assigned between CRT and 2 additional cycles of chemotherapy.

In conclusion, the optimal treatment for locally advanced PC remains controversial. CRT increases OS when compared with exclusive radiotherapy or best supportive care, but survival does not change for patients treated with CRT when compared with patients treated with chemotherapy with gemcitabine. The addition of CRT after 3 to 4 months of induction chemotherapy is a promising approach that has to be validated in prospective trials.

TREATMENT OF METASTATIC AND RECURRENT DISEASE
Single Agent

The standard treatment for patients with advanced metastatic or recurrent PC is systemic chemotherapy. However, responses rates (RR) to the current available drugs are low and treatment should be considered palliative. For many years, the most active chemotherapeutic agent used in the treatment for patients with advanced PC has been 5-FU. In different phase II studies, patients treated with 5-FU achieved a RR from 0% to 20% with a median survival of 4 to 5 months. The modulation of 5-FU with other agents, such as leucovorin, did not show clear evidence of increased RR in phase II studies.[56–59] Many subsequent studies were developed to evaluate different 5-FU combinations; however, in randomized phase III studies, the survival of patients treated with 5-FU alone was not different from that of patients treated with more aggressive and more toxic chemotherapeutic regimens.

In 1997, a randomized phase III clinical trial compared gemcitabine with 5-FU in 126 patients with advanced metastatic PC who had not received prior systemic therapy[35] (Table 3). Patients were randomized to receive gemcitabine (800 mg/m^2 as a 30-minute intravenous injection weekly for 3 consecutive weeks followed by 1 week of rest) or 5-FU (600 mg/m^2 once a week). Although the RR was 5.4% for gemcitabine and 0% for 5-FU, a positive clinical benefit response (a combination of performance status, analgesic usage, and measurements of pain) was experienced by 23.8% of gemcitabine-treated patients compared with 4.8% of 5-FU–treated patients ($P = .002$). There was an overall disease control rate (partial response plus stable disease) of 45% with gemcitabine versus 19% with 5-FU. The median times-to-tumor progression were 3.8 and 1.9 months and the median survival durations were 5.7 and

Table 3
Randomized phase III clinical trials comparing chemotherapy regimens in advanced pancreatic cancer

Study, Year	No. of Patients	Protocol Treatments	Median Survival (mos)	P-Value
Burris, 1997[35]	126	Gemcitabine	5.7	.002
		5-FU	4.4	
Poplin, 2009[63]	832	Gemcitabine	4.8	.04
		Gemcitabine FDR	6.2	
		Gemcitabine + Oxaliplatin	5.7	
Berlin, 2002[64]	327	Gemcitabine	5.4	.09
		Gemcitabine + 5-FU	6.7	
Herrmann, 2007[66]	319	Gemcitabine	6.2	.23
		Gemcitabine + Capecitabine	7.1	
Cunningham, 2009[67]	533	Gemcitabine	8.2	.08
		Gemcitabine + Capecitabine	8.3	
Heinemann, 2006[70]	195	Gemcitabine	6	.15
		Gemcitabine + Cisplatin	7.5	
Colucci, 2010[71]	400	Gemcitabine	8.3	.38
		Gemcitabine + Cisplatin	7.2	
Louvet, 2005[73]	326	Gemcitabine	7.1	.13
		Gemcitabine + Oxaliplatin	9	
Oettle, 2005[76]	565	Gemcitabine	6.3	.84
		Gemcitabine + Pemetrexed	6.2	
Abou-Alfa, 2006[78]	349	Gemcitabine	6.2	.52
		Gemcitabine + Exatecan	6.7	
Conroy, 2011[82]	342	Gemcitabine	6.8	<.001
		FOLFIRINOX	11.1	

Abbreviations: FDR, fixed-dose rate; 5-FU, 5-fluorouracil.

4.4 months for gemcitabine and 5-FU–treated patients, respectively ($P = .002$). The survival rate at 12 months was 18% for gemcitabine patients and 2% for 5-FU patients. Because of these results, gemcitabine was approved as first-line treatment of metastatic PC in the United States and many other countries and currently is considered the standard agent for the treatment of this disease.

Other trials have explored alternative schedules for administering gemcitabine. It was postulated that a prolonged administration schedule would result in increased intracellular levels of its active metabolite, gemcitabine triphosphate.[60] The administration of gemcitabine using a fixed-dose-rate (FDR) infusion increased the maximum tolerated dose to 1500 mg/m² administered as 10 mg/m² per minute.[61] Promising phase II studies showed that patients treated with the FDR had a higher RR (11.6% vs 4.1%), longer median survival (8 vs 5 months), and 1-year survival (23.8% vs 7.3%) compared with patients treated on the conventional schedule.[62] However, in a large, randomized, phase III study, this strategy did not show survival benefits.[63]

Combination Chemotherapy

Numerous clinical trials have tested the safety, tolerability, and efficacy of gemcitabine in combination with other drugs compared with single-agent gemcitabine. The most frequently studied combinations were gemcitabine with different fluoropyrimidines schedules. Although the combination regimens have been associated with modest increases in RR, median survivals, and 1-year survivals, no differences were observed with regard to RR and OS in most of the randomized phase III trials.[64]

An initially promising approach was the combination of gemcitabine with the oral fluorpyrimidine, capecitabine. To explore the therapeutic potential and tolerance of this combination more precisely, Scheithauer and colleageus[65] randomized 83 patients to treatment with biweekly gemcitabine (2200 mg/m^2 given as a 30-min intravenous infusion on day 1) or the same treatment plus oral capecitabine (2500 mg/m^2 given from days 1 to 7). This study showed that this combination was well-tolerated and demonstrated a trend toward better survival.[65] Two subsequent, large, phase III, randomized, controlled trials were conducted with this combination.[66,67] The first study published by Herrmann and colleagues did not demonstrate a clear OS improvement but reported a trend toward better survival in patients with good performance status who recieved gemcitabine plus capecitabine. In the second study, using a higher dose of capecitabine, the authors reported that the gemcitabine plus capecitabine combination was associated with a median survival of 7.1 months compared with 6.2 months in the gemcitabine alone arm ($P = .08$). Cunningham and associates[67] performed a meta-analysis combining these 3 trials' data. The analysis revealed that the gemcitabine plus capecitabine combination produced a modest survival benefit over gemcitabine alone [hazard ratio (HR), 0.86 (95% confidence interval, 0.75–0.98); $P = .02$].

It is known that there is a synergistic activity between gemcitabine and platinating agents owing to a decreased ability of the cell to repair DNA damage induced by cisplatin in the presence of gemcitabine. In preliminary studies, cisplatin in combination with gemcitabine has demonstrated a reasonable tolerability profile. Different phase II trials suggested an improvement in the RR and median survivals of patients treated with gemcitabine in combination with cisplatin.[68,69] A German, multicenter, phase III clinical trial comparing gemcitabine plus cisplatin with single-agent gemcitabine included 195 patients with advanced or locally advanced PC. The gemcitabine plus cisplatin combination regimen was associated with a prolonged median progression-free survival (PFS; 5.3 vs 3.1 months; $P = .053$). In addition, the median OS was superior for patients treated in the gemcitabine plus cisplatin arm as compared with patients treated with gemcitabine alone (7.5 vs 6.0 months), an advantage that did not, however, attain significance ($P = .15$).[70] More recently, 400 patients were enrolled in a phase III trial, conducted by the Gruppo Italiano Pancreas 1; however, the addition of weekly cisplatin to gemcitabine failed to demonstrate any improvement as first-line treatment of advanced PC.[71]

The combination of gemcitabine and oxaliplatin (GemOx) has also been studied, with promising results in an initial phase II trial. In patients with metastatic disease, the combination achieved a RR of 30.3% and a median OS of 8.7 months.[72] In a subsequent phase III intergroup study, conducted by GERCOR and the Italian Group for the Study of Gastrointestinal Tract Cancer, the combination of a biweekly regimen of oxaliplatin (100 mg/m^2) plus gemcitabine (1000 mg/m^2 administered as a 10-mg/m^2 FDR infusion) was tested.[73] The GemOx combination was superior to single-agent gemcitabine, increasing PFS from 3.7 to 5.8 months and OS from 7.1 to 9.0 months. The pooled analysis of the GERCOR/Italian Group for the Study of Gastrointestinal Tract Cancer intergroup study and the German multicenter study indicates that the combination of gemcitabine with a platinum analog, such as oxaliplatin or cisplatin, significantly improves PFS and OS compared with single-agent gemcitabine in advanced PC.[74] However, recent results contradicted this conclusion. The ECOG 6201 compared standard gemcitabine with both FDR infusion gemcitabine and the gemcitabine plus oxaliplatin combination in 832 patients. Neither FDR gemcitabine nor GemOx resulted in substantially improved survival or symptom benefit over standard gemcitabine in patients with advanced PC.[63]

On the basis of phase II data that demonstrated single-agent pemetrexed activity in PC with a RR of 5.7%, median survival of 6.5 months, and 1-year survival of 28%,[75] the synergy between gemcitabine and pemetrexed was explored in a phase III study. Unfortunately, the addition of pemetrexed to gemcitabine did not improve the primary endpoint of OS.[76]

With the intention of identifying a promising gemcitabine-based regimen to explore in a formal phase III study, the CALGB 89904 phase II study randomized 3 different gemcitabine-based combinations (docetaxel plus gemcitabine, irinotecan plus gemcitabine, and cisplatin plus gemcitabine) or FDR-infusion gemcitabine in patients with advanced PC. The conclusion of this study was that FDR gemcitabine and all of the combination arms had similar antitumor activity in metastatic PC and did not offer a significant benefit compared with standard gemcitabine therapy. Therefore, the authors suggested that none of these approaches (with a similar median OS times ranged from 6.4 to 7.1 months) can be recommended for routine clinical use for patients with this disease.[77]

Other gemcitabine-based combinations that have been tested in phase II and III studies with unsuccessful results include the topoisomerase inhibitor exatecan,[78] the COX-2 inhibitor celecoxib,[79] and the anti-androgen drug flutamide.[80]

Several studies have evaluated 3 or more drug combination regimens in PC. Reni and co-workers[81] enrolled a total of 104 patients in a randomized, controlled, multicenter, phase III trial of gemcitabine in combination with epirubicin and cisplatin (PEFG regimen) compared with gemcitabine alone. More patients assigned to the PEFG group (60%) were progression free at 4 months than those assigned to gemcitabine alone (28%). However, because of its higher rates of grades 3 and 4 hematologic toxicities (mainly neutropenia and thrombocytopenia), and criticism of the sample size and the study design (PFS as the primary endpoint), the PEFG regimen has not been universally accepted.[81]

More recently, the results of a randomized phase III trial comparing the FOLFIRINOX regimen (oxaliplatin, irinotecan, fluorouracil, and leucovorin) with gemcitabine in advanced PC have been published. Median OS increased from 6.8 to 11.1 months ($P<.001$). Interestingly, almost half of the patients in the FOLFIRINOX group were alive after 1 year and the RR was 31.6%. The FOLFIRINOX regimen was quite toxic: 46% of the patients had grade 3 or 4 neutropenia and 5.4% had grade 3 or 4 febrile neutropenia. Therefore, for patients with a good performance status, normal bilirubin, and a good supportive care system, FOLFIRINOX may be a viable option. This trial provided many valuable insights that can be incorporated in future trials of treatments for advanced PC.[82]

New Approaches

During the last few years, a better understanding of the biological mechanisms of disease and an increasing number of new drugs have made possible the identification and validation of new targeted agents in PC. The different targeted agents that have been tested in PC include epidermal growth factor receptor (EGFR) inhibitors, vascular endothelial growth factor (VEGF) inhibitors, farnesyl transferase inhibitors, and matrix metalloproteinase inhibitors (**Table 4**).

Table 4
Randomized phase III clinical trials comparing chemotherapy and biologic agents in advanced pancreatic carcinoma

Study, Year	No. of Patients	Protocol Treatments	Median Survival (mos)	P-Value
Moore, 2007[87]	569	Gemcitabine	5.9	.038
		Gemcitabine + Erlotinib	6.2	
Philip, 2010[90]	735	Gemcitabine	6	.23
		Gemcitabine + Cetuximab	6.5	
Kindler, 2010[96]	535	Gemcitabine	5.9	.9
		Gemcitabine + Bevacizumab	5.8	
Van Cutsem, 2009[99]	301	Gemcitabine + Erlotinib	6	.2
		Gemcitabine + Erlotinib + Bevacizumab	7.1	
Bramhall, 2002[100]	239	Gemcitabine	5.5	.9
		Gemcitabine + Marimastat	5.5	
Moore, 2003[101]	277	Gemcitabine	6.7	.001
		BAY 12-9566	3.7	
Van Cutsem, 2009[102]	688	Gemcitabine	6.1	.7
		Gemcitabine + Tipifarnib	6.4	

Inhibitors of the EGFR

EGFR type 1 is a receptor tyrosine kinase that, when activated, leads to downstream signaling cascades, including the Ras/Raf/MEK/ERK and the PI3K/Akt/mTOR pathways. These signaling pathways result in the activation of genes involved in cellular proliferation and resistance to apoptosis, thus leading to tumor growth.[83] EGFR has been found to be overexpressed in PC[84] and this overexpression may be associated with tumor aggressiveness and the poor prognosis.[85]

Erlotinib is an orally administered small-molecule inhibitor of the intracellular EGFR, tyrosine kinase domain. Preliminary data showed an inhibition of tumor growth and a synergy with gemcitabine.[86] The combination of gemcitabine with erlotinib was evaluated in the phase III study PA.3, conducted by the National Cancer of Canada Trials Group, in which 569 patients with locally advanced (25%) or metastatic (75%) PC received either standard-dose gemcitabine plus erlotinib or gemcitabine plus placebo. The addition of erlotinib to gemcitabine resulted in a significant improvement in survival (HR, 0.82; 95% CI, 0.69–0.99; $P = .038$), with improvement in the median survival from 5.91 to 6.24 months. The 1-year survival rate was greater with the addition of erlotinib (23% vs 17%) and PFS improved significantly in the gemcitabine plus erlotinib group (HR, 0.77; $P = .004$). Severe adverse event rates were similar in the 2 treatment groups, with the exception of rash (6% vs 1%), and diarrhea (6% vs 2%), which were more frequent in the erlotinib group.[87] EGFR gene copy number and *KRAS* mutation status were not identified as predictive markers of a survival benefit from the combination of erlotinib with gemcitabine. However, patients treated with erlotinib who developed a grade 2 or greater rash had a significantly better outcome; median survival increased as rash severity increased (median survival, 10.5 months; 1-year survival rate, 43%; $P<.0001$).[88]

Cetuximab, a monoclonal antibody that has shown activity in a variety of different tumors, belongs to the second clinically relevant class of agents that inhibit EGFR.[89] The promising results of the initial phase II trial led to the design of an open label phase III study by the Southwest Oncology Group, in which the combination of cetuximab plus gemcitabine was compared with gemcitabine alone. A total of 735 patients were randomized and the results showed no difference in objective RR and PFS between the 2 arms of the study.[90] Other trials exploring the combination of cetuximab plus gemcitabine and platinum agents have failed to demonstrate any significant clinical benefit.[91,92]

Inhibitors of the VEGF

VEGF and its tyrosine kinase receptors, flt-1 (VEGFR-1) and KDR (VEGFR-2), are involved in angiogenesis and other signal transduction pathways that promote cell growth.[93] Bevacizumab, a monoclonal antibody against VEGF, has been successfully used in the treatment of colon and lung cancers.[94,95] A total of 52 patients were enrolled in a phase II trial of bevacizumab plus gemcitabine. The results showed a 21% partial RR and 46% stable disease with a median PFS of 5.4 months and a median OS of 8.8 months.[96] However, the randomized, phase III trial conducted by the Cancer and Leukemia Group B, with 535 patients, revealed no benefit from the addition of bevacizumab to gemcitabine.[97]

After preliminary evidence of activity in PC, axitinib, an orally active selective inhibitor of VEGF1, 2, and 3, and aflibercept (also known as VEGF-trap), a soluble VGF receptor with high anti-angiogenesis activity, were combined with gemcitabine and tested in phase II-III trials, with unsuccessful results (97, ESMO GI 2010; Abst O–0006).[98]

Because of the molecular complexity of PC and the multiple genes involved, several trials combined different targeted agents in an attempt to achieve greater efficacy. Kindler and colleagues[99] conducted a phase II trial testing the efficacy of gemcitabine combined with bevacizumab and erlotinib compared with gemcitabine combined with bevacizumab and cetuximab. The median survival was 7.2 months in the erlotinib arm and 7.8 months in the cetuximab arm. However, the results from the large, randomized, phase III AVITA study demonstrated a nonsignificant trend to improvement in survival with the addition of bevacizumab to gemcitabine and erlotinib.[100]

Other targeted agents

The matrix metalloproteinase inhibitors are a group of closely related proteases that are dysregulated in the majority of human neoplasms, including PC. The increased activity of these enzymes leads to extracellular matrix breakdown and facilitates tumor growth, progression, invasion, generation of blood vessels, and metastasis. Matrix metalloproteinase inhibitors, marimastat, and BAY12-9566, have both been tested in phase III trials and the results revealed no improvement in outcomes.[101,102]

Mutations in the oncogene RAS are the most frequently occurring genetic abnormality in PC. These mutations lead to a constitutive activation of the KRAS protein, resulting in the activation of downstream signaling pathways. Because RAS must be farnesylated to become active (a post-translational modification mediated by the enzyme farnesyltransferase), inhibitors of this enzyme have been explored as potential RAS inhibitors. A large, phase III trial testing the effect of the addition of the farnesyl transferase inhibitor, tipifarnib, to gemcitabine failed to demonstrate significant activity.[103]

Insulin-like growth factor (IGF)-1 and its receptor, IGF-1R, lead to the activation of the PI3K/Akt pathway, providing anti-apoptotic signals through the main mediator, mammalian target of rapamycin (mTOR). The oral mTOR inhibitor everolimus, administered as a single agent, has shown minimal clinical activity in metastatic PC patients resistant to gemcitabine.[104] Interestingly, inhibition of mTOR activates

PI3K/Akt by up-regulating IGF-1R signaling. A constitutive overexpression of IGF-1 and IGF-1R is implicated in PC; therefore, it has been suggested that therapy with a combination of mTOR inhibitors and IGF-1/IGF-1R inhibitors may improve the clinical outcome. In theory, this would neutralize the feedback effects of mTOR inhibition on IGF-1 signaling.[105] There are currently several phase I and II trials investigating the combination of a humanized monoclonal antibody against IGF-1R with other chemotherapeutics. However, because IGF-1 and its receptor IGF-1R are ubiquitously expressed throughout the body, there are difficulties in targeting this pathway. Moreover, when using antibodies against IGF-1R, the structurally similar insulin receptor might also be blocked, leading to hyperglycemia as a severe side effect.

The Notch signaling pathway is mechanistically associated with the molecular characteristics of cancer stem cells in PC. Cancer stems cells are known to be highly drug resistant and responsible for tumor recurrence and metastasis; therefore, it is likely that targeted inactivation of Notch signaling would be useful for overcoming drug resistance and the elimination of cancer stem cells.[106] Curcumin, a plant-derived dietary ingredient with potent nuclear factor-κB, has tumor inhibitory properties through inactivation of the Notch pathway. In a phase II trial, oral curcumin was well tolerated and, despite its limited absorption, had biological activity in some patients with PC.[107]

There is growing evidence that the stroma surrounding tumors, characteristically dense in PC, blocks drug penetration and contributes to tumor survival.[108] Recent studies have shown that interactions between the tumor and its microenvironment play a critical role in tumor invasion, metastasis, and chemoresistance. In this context, the role of the hedgehog (Hh) pathway in the biology of PC is an emerging area of investigation. Paracrine Hh signaling from neoplastic cells to stromal cells promotes stromal desmoplasia and the survival and proliferation signal feedback from the stroma to the tumor cells. The addition of Hh inhibitors to chemotherapy as well as biologic drugs might introduce novel synergistic treatment options. Combining gemcitabine with the Hh inhibitor IPI-926, a specific smoothened homolog inhibitor, reduced tumor size and significantly improved survival in a PC gemcitabine-resistant xenograft mouse model.[109] Current clinical studies including an Hh inhibitor and the associated translational analyses will help to elucidate the role of the Hh pathway in the biology of PC.

Preclinical and clinical studies have shown that albumin-bound paclitaxel (nab-paclitaxel) delivered more paclitaxel to the tumor without increasing toxic side effects. The albumin in nab-paclitaxel binds to albumin receptors in tumor blood vessels and is released into the tumor microenvironment. Secreted protein acid rich in cysteine is a protein highly expressed in PC, especially in the stroma, that actively binds the albumin in nab-paclitaxel and further concentrates the drug in the tumor.[110] Results from a phase I/II trial of nab-paclitaxel in combination with gemcitabine in metastatic PC showed a partial response in 23 out of 58 evaluable patients and a median PFS of 7.9 months.[111]

Several other targeted therapies with biological rationale and preclinical activity have been explored in PC. The oral multi-kinase inhibitor, sunitinib, has shown modest activity in phase II trials in patients with progressive metastatic PC who were treated after earlier gemcitabine-based therapy.[112]

To date, however, only the gemcitabine plus erlotinib combination, and recently the FOLFIRINOX regimen, have been associated with relatively small but statistically significant improvements in OS when compared directly with gemcitabine alone in the randomized setting. Although several meta-analyses have suggested a benefit associated with combination chemotherapy, whether this benefit is clinically meaningful remains unclear, particularly in light of the enhanced toxicity associated with combination regimens. Future directions will involve testing of new targeted agents, understanding the pharmacodynamics of our current targeted agents, searching for predictive markers, and exploring the efficacy of combining targeted agents.

SUMMARY

Pancreatic adenocarcinoma is the fourth leading cause of cancer death and has an extremely poor prognosis: The 5-year survival probability is less than 5% for all stages. The only chance for cure or longer survival is surgical resection; however, only 10% to 20% of patients have resectable disease. Although surgical techniques have improved, most who undergo complete resection experience a recurrence. Adjuvant systemic therapy reduces the recurrence rate and improves outcomes. There is a potential role for radiation therapy as part of treatment for locally advanced disease, although its use in both the adjuvant and neoadjuvant settings remains controversial. Palliative systemic treatment is the only option for patients with metastatic disease. To date, however, only the gemcitabine plus erlotinib combination, and recently the FOLFIRINOX regimen, have been associated with relatively small but statistically significant improvements in OS when compared directly with gemcitabine alone. Although several meta-analyses have suggested a benefit associated with combination chemotherapy, whether this benefit is clinically meaningful remains unclear, particularly in light of the enhanced toxicity associated with combination regimens. There is growing evidence that the exceptionally poor prognosis in PC is caused by the tumor's characteristic abundant desmoplastic stroma that plays a critical role in tumor cell growth, invasion, metastasis, and chemoresistance. Carefully designed clinical trials that include translational analysis will provide a better understanding of the tumor biology and its relation to the host stromal cells. Future directions will involve testing of new targeted agents, understanding the pharmacodynamics of our current targeted agents, searching for predictive and prognostic biomarkers, and exploring the efficacy of different combinations strategies.

REFERENCES

1. Jemal A, Siegel R, Ward E, et al. Cancer statistics. CA Cancer J Clin 2009;59:225–49.
2. Heinemann V, Boeck S, Hinke A, et al. Metaanalysis of randomized trials: evaluation of benefit from gemcitabine-based combination chemotherapy applied in advanced pancreatic cancer. BMC Cancer 2008;8:82.
3. Sultana A, Tudur Smith C, Cunningham D, et al. Meta-analyses of chemotherapy for locally advanced and metastatic pancreatic cancer: results of secondary end points analyses. Br J Cancer 2008;99:6–13.
4. Yip D, Karapetis C, Strickland A, et al. Chemotherapy and radiotherapy for inoperable advance pancreatic cancer. Cochrane Database Syst Rev 2002;3:CD002093.
5. Oettle H, Post S, Neuhaus P, et al. Adjuvant chemotherapy with gemcitabine vs observation in patients undergoing curative-intent resection of pancreatic cancer: a randomized controlled trial. JAMA 2007297:267–77.
6. Neoptolemos JP, Buchler M, Stocken DD, et al. ESPAC-3(v2): a multicenter, international, open-label, randomized, controlled Phase III trial of adjuvant 5-fluorouracil/folinic acid (5-FU/FA) versus gemcitabine (GEM) in patients with resected pancreatic ductal adenocarcinoma. J Clin Oncol 2009;18S:Abstract 4505.
7. Neoptolemos JP, Stocken DD, Tudur Smith C, et al. Adjuvant 5-fluorouracil and folinic acid vs observation for pancreatic cancer: composite data from the ESPAC-1 and -3(v1) trials. Br J Cancer 2009;100:246–50.

8. Klinkenbijl JH, Jeekel J, Sahmoud T, et al. Adjuvant radiotherapy and 5-fluorouracil after curative resection of cancer of the pancreas and periampullary region: phase III trial of the EORTC gastrointestinal tract cancer cooperative group. Ann Surg 1999;230:776–82.

9. Neoptolemos JP, Dunn JA, Stocken DD, et al. Adjuvant chemoradiotherapy and chemotherapy in resectable pancreatic cancer: a randomised controlled trial. Lancet 2001;358:1576–85.

10. Neoptolemos JP, Stocken DD, Friess H, et al. A randomized trial of chemoradiotherapy and chemotherapy after resection of pancreatic cancer. N Engl J Med 2004;350:1200–10.

11. Yip D, Karapetis C, Strickland A, et al. Chemotherapy and radiotherapy for inoperable advanced pancreatic cancer. Cochrane Database Syst Rev 2006;3:CD002093.

12. Sultana A, Tudur Smith C, Cunningham D, et al. Systematic review, including meta-analyses, on the management of locally advanced pancreatic cancer using radiation/combined modality therapy. Br J Cancer 2007;96:1183–90.

13. Marten A, Schmidt J, Ose J, et al. A randomized multicentre Phase II trial comparing adjuvant therapy in patients with interferon a-2b and 5-FU alone or in combination with either external radiation treatment and cisplatin (CapRI) or radiation alone regarding event-free survival: CapRI-2. BMC Cancer 2009;9:160.

14. Keating JJ, Johnson PJ, Cochrane AM, et al. A prospective randomised controlled trial of tamoxifen and cyproterone acetate in pancreatic carcinoma. Br J Cancer 1989;60:789–92.

15. Taylor OM, Benson EA, McMahon MJ. Clinical trial of tamoxifen in patients with irresectable pancreatic adenocarcinoma. The Yorkshire gastrointestinal tumour group. Br J Surg 1993;80:384–6.

16. Negi SS, Agarwal A, Chaudhary A. Flutamide in unresectable pancreatic adenocarcinoma: a randomized, double-blind, placebo-controlled trial. Invest New Drugs 2006;24:189–94.

17. Sultana A, Smith CT, Cunningham D, et al. Meta-analyses of chemotherapy for locally advanced and metastatic pancreatic cancer. J Clin Oncol 2006;25:2607–15.

18. Pilarsky C, Ammerpohl O, Sipos B, et al. Activation of Wnt signalling in stroma from pancreatic cancer identified by gene expression profiling. J Cell Mol Med 2008;12:2823–35.

19. Trede M, Schwall G, Saeger HD. Survival after pancreatoduodenectomy. 118 consecutive resections without an operative mortality. Ann Surg 1990;211:447–58.

20. Geer RJ, Brennan MF. Prognostic indicators for survival after resection of pancreatic adenocarcinoma. Am J Surg 1993;165:68–72.

21. Crist DW, Sitzmann JV, Cameron JL. Improved hospital morbidity, mortality, and survival after the Whipple procedure. Ann Surg 1987;206:358–65.

22. Kalser MH, Ellenberg SS. Pancreatic cancer. Adjuvant combined radiation and chemotherapy following curative resection. Arch Surg 1985;120:899–903.

23. Gastrointestinal Tumor Study Group. Further evidence of effective adjuvant combined radiation and chemotherapy following curative resection of pancreatic cancer. Cancer 1987;59:2006–10.

24. Klinkenbijl JH, Jeekel J, Sahmoud T, et al. Adjuvant radiotherapy and 5-fluorouracil after curative resection of cancer of the pancreas and periampullary region: phase III trial of the EORTC gastrointestinal tract cancer cooperative group. Ann Surg 1999;230:776–82.

25. Garofalo MC, Regine WF, Tan MT. On statistical reanalysis, the EORTC trial is a positive trial for adjuvant chemoradiation in pancreatic cancer. Ann Surg 2006;244:332–3.

26. Neoptolemos JP, Stocken DD, Friess H, et al. A randomized trial of chemoradiotherapy and chemotherapy after resection of pancreatic cancer. N Engl J Med 2004;350:1200–10.

27. Neoptolemos JP, Dunn JA, Stocken DD, et al. Adjuvant chemoradiotherapy and chemotherapy in resectable pancreatic cancer: a randomised controlled trial. Lancet 2001;358:1576–85.

28. Yeo TP, Hruban RH, Leach SD, et al. Pancreatic cancer. Curr Probl Cancer 2002;26:176–275.

29. Regine WF, Winter KA, Abrams RA, et al. Fluorouracil vs gemcitabine chemotherapy before and after fluorouracil-based chemoradiation following resection of pancreatic adenocarcinoma: a randomized controlled trial. JAMA 2008;299:1019–26.

30. Regine WF, Winter KA, Abrams R, et al. Fluorouracil-based Chemoradiation with Either Gemcitabine or Fluorouracil Chemotherapy after Resection of Pancreatic Adenocarcinoma: 5-Year Analysis of the U.S. Intergroup/RTOG 9704 Phase III Trial. Ann Surg Oncol 2001;18:1319–26.

31. Hsu CC, Herman JM, Corsini MM, et al. Adjuvant chemoradiation for pancreatic adenocarcinoma: the Johns Hopkins Hospital-Mayo Clinic collaborative study. Ann Surg Oncol 2010;17:981–90.

32. Van Laethem JL, Hammel P, Mornex F, et al. Adjuvant gemcitabine alone versus gemcitabine-based chemoradiotherapy after curative resection for pancreatic cancer: a randomized EORTC-40013-22012/FFCD-9203/GERCOR phase II study. J Clin Oncol 2010;28:4450–6.

33. Oettle H, Post S, Neuhaus P, et al. Adjuvant chemotherapy with gemcitabine vs observation in patients undergoing curative-intent resection of pancreatic cancer: a randomized controlled trial. JAMA 2007;297:267–77.

34. Neuhaus P, Riess H, Post S, et al. CONKO-001: final results of the randomized, prospective, multicenter phase III trial of adjuvant chemotherapy with gemcitabine versus observation in patients with resected pancreatic cancer (PC). J Clin Oncol 2008;26(Suppl LBA4504).

35. Burris HA 3rd, Moore MJ, Andersen J, et al. Improvements in survival and clinical benefit with gemcitabine as first-line therapy for patients with advanced pancreas cancer: a randomized trial. J Clin Oncol 1997;15:2403–13.

36. Neoptolemos JP, Stocken DD, Bassi C, et al. Adjuvant chemotherapy with fluorouracil plus folinic acid vs gemcitabine following pancreatic cancer resection: a randomized controlled trial. JAMA 2010;304:1073–81.

37. Evans DB, Varadhachary GR, Crane CH, et al. Preoperative gemcitabine-based chemoradiation for patients with resectable adenocarcinoma of the pancreatic head. J Clin Oncol 2008;26:3496–502.

38. Varadhachary GR, Wolff RA, Crane CH, et al. Preoperative gemcitabine and cisplatin followed by gemcitabine-based chemoradiation for resectable adenocarcinoma of the pancreatic head. J Clin Oncol 2008;26:3487–95.

39. Brunner TB, Grabenbauer GG, Meyer T, et al. Primary resection versus neoadjuvant chemoradiation followed by resection for locally resectable or potentially resectable pancreatic carcinoma without distant metastasis. A multi-centre prospectively randomised phase II-study of the Interdisciplinary Working Group Gastrointestinal Tumours (AIO, ARO, and CAO). BMC Cancer 2007;7:41.

40. Gillen S, Schuster T, Meyer Zum Büschenfelde C, et al. Preoperative/neoadjuvant therapy in pancreatic cancer: a systematic review and meta-analysis of response and resection percentages. PLoS Med 2010;7:e1000267.

41. Artinyan A, Anaya DA, McKenzie S, et al. Neoadjuvant therapy is associated with improved survival in resectable pancreatic adenocarcinoma. Cancer 2011;117: 2044–9.
42. Huguet F, Girard N, Guerche CS, et al. Chemoradiotherapy in the management of locally advanced pancreatic carcinoma: a qualitative systematic review. J Clin Oncol 2009;27:2269–77.
43. Shinchi H, Takao S, Noma H, et al. Length and quality of survival after external-beam radiotherapy with concurrent continuous 5-fluorouracil infusion for locally unresectable pancreatic cancer. Int J Radiat Oncol Biol Phys 2002;53:146–50.
44. Moertel CG, Childs DS Jr, Reitemeier RJ, et al. Combined 5-fluorouracil and supervoltage radiation therapy of locally unresectable gastrointestinal cancer. Lancet 1969;2:865–7.
45. Moertel CG, Frytak S, Hahn RG, et al. Therapy of locally unresectable pancreatic carcinoma: a randomized comparison of high dose (6000 rads) radiation alone, moderate dose radiation (4000 rads + 5-fluorouracil), and high dose radiation + 5-fluorouracil: The Gastrointestinal Tumor Study Group. Cancer 1981;48:1705–10.
46. Cohen SJ, Dobelbower R, Lipsitz S, et al. A randomized phase III study of radiotherapy alone or with 5-fluorouracil and mitomycin-C in patients with locally advanced adenocarcinoma of the pancreas: Eastern Cooperative Oncology Group study E8282. Int J Radiat Oncol Biol Phys 2005;62:1345–50.
47. Gastrointestinal Tumor Study Group. Treatment of locally unresectable carcinoma of the pancreas: Comparison of combined-modality therapy (chemotherapy plus radiotherapy) to chemotherapy alone. J Natl Cancer Inst 1988;80:751–5.
48. Hazel JJ, Thirlwell MP, Huggins M, et al. Multi-drug chemotherapy with and without radiation for carcinoma of the stomach and pancreas: A prospective randomized trial. J Can Assoc Radiol 1981;32:164–5.
49. Klaassen DJ, MacIntyre JM, Catton GE, et al. Treatment of locally unresectable cancer of the stomach and pancreas: a randomized comparison of 5-fluorouracil alone with radiation plus concurrent and maintenance 5-fluorouracil: An Eastern Cooperative Oncology Group study. J Clin Oncol 1985;3:373–8.
50. Chauffert B, Mornex F, Bonnetain F, et al. Phase III trial comparing intensive induction chemoradiotherapy (60 Gy, infusional 5-FU and intermittent cisplatin) followed by maintenance gemcitabine with gemcitabine alone for locally advanced unresectable pancreatic cancer. Definitive results of the 2000-01 FFCD/SFRO study. Ann Oncol 2008;19:1592–9.
51. Loehrer PJ, Powell Me, Cardenes HR, et al. A randomized phase III study of gemcitabine in combination with radiation therapy versus gemcitabine alone in patients with localized, unresectable pancreatic cancer: E4201. J Clin Oncol 2008; 26(Suppl):214s.
52. Yip D, Karapetis C, Strickland A, et al. Chemotherapy and radiotherapy for inoperable advanced pancreatic cancer. Cochrane Database Syst Rev 2006;3: CD002093.
53. Sultana A, Tudur SC, Cunningham D, et al. Systematic review, including meta-analyses, on the management of locally advanced pancreatic cancer using radiation/combined modality therapy. Br J Cancer 2007;96:1183–90.
54. Krishnan S, Rana V, Janjan NA, et al. Induction chemotherapy selects patients with locally advanced, unresectable pancreatic cancer for optimal benefit from consolidative chemoradiation therapy. Cancer 2007;110:47–55.
55. Huguet F, Andre T, Hammel P, et al. Impact of chemoradiotherapy after disease control with chemotherapy in locally advanced pancreatic adenocarcinoma in GERCOR phase II and III studies. J Clin Oncol 2007;25:326–31.

56. Glimelius B, Hoffman K, Sjoden PO, et al. Chemotherapy improves survival and quality of life in advanced pancreatic and biliary cancer. Ann Oncol 1996;7:593–600.

57. Palmer KR, Kerr M, Knowles G, et al. Chemotherapy prolongs survival in inoperable pancreatic carcinoma. Br J Surg 19954;81:882–5.

58. Mallinson CN, Rake MO, Cocking JB, et al. Chemotherapy in pancreatic cancer: results of a controlled, prospective, randomised, multicentre trial. BMJ 1980; 281:1589–91.

59. Crown J, Casper ES, Botet J, et al. Lack of efficacy of high-dose leucovorin and fluorouracil in patients with advanced pancreatic adenocarcinoma. J Clin Oncol 1991;9:1682–6.

60. Hochster HS. Newer approaches to gemcitabine-based therapy of pancreatic cancer: fixed-dose-rate infusion and novel agents. Int J Radiat Oncol Biol Phys 2003;56:24–30.

61. Brand R, Capadano M, Tempero M. A phase I trial of weekly gemcitabine administered as a prolonged infusion in patients with pancreatic cancer and other solid tumors. Invest New Drugs 1997;15:331–41.

62. Tempero M, Plunkett W, Ruis Van Haperen V, et al. Randomized phase II comparison of dose-intense gemcitabine: thirty-minute infusion and fixed dose rate infusion in patients with pancreatic adenocarcinoma. J Clin Oncol 2003;21: 3402–8.

63. Poplin E, Feng Y, Berlin J, et al. Phase III, randomized study of gemcitabine and oxaliplatin versus gemcitabine (fixed-dose rate infusion) compared with gemcitabine (30-minute infusion) in patients with pancreatic carcinoma E6201: a trial of the Eastern Cooperative Oncology Group. J Clin Oncol 2009;27:3778–85.

64. Berlin JD, Catalano P, Thomas JP, et al. Phase III study of gemcitabine in combination with fluorouracil versus gemcitabine alone in patients with advanced pancreatic carcinoma: Eastern Cooperative Oncology Group Trial E2297. J Clin Oncol 2002; 20:3270–5.

65. Scheithauer W, Schüll B, Ulrich-Pur H, et al. Biweekly high-dose gemcitabine alone or in combination with capecitabine in patients with metastatic pancreatic adenocarcinoma: a randomized phase II trial. Ann Oncol 2003;14:97–104.

66. Herrmann R, Bodoky G, Ruhstaller T, et al. Gemcitabine plus capecitabine compared with gemcitabine alone in advanced pancreatic cancer: a randomized, multicenter, Phase III trial of the Swiss group for Clinical Cancer Research and the Central European Cooperative Oncology Group. J Clin Oncol 2007;25:2212–7.

67. Cunningham D, Chau I, Stocken DD, et al. Phase III randomized comparison of gemcitabine versus gemcitabine plus capecitabine in patients with advanced pancreatic cancer. J Clin Oncol 2009;27:5513–8.

68. Philip PA, Zalupski MM, Vaitkevicius VK, et al. Phase II study of gemcitabine and cisplatin in the treatment of patients with advanced pancreatic carcinoma. Cancer 2001.92:569–77.

69. Colucci G, Giuliani F, Gebbia V, et al. Gemcitabine alone or with cisplatin for the treatment of patients with locally advanced and/or metastatic pancreatic carcinoma: a prospective, randomized phase III study of the Gruppo Oncologia dell'Italia Meridionale. Cancer 2002;94:902–10.

70. Heinemann V, Quietzsch D, Gieseler F, et al. Randomized phase III trial of gemcitabine plus cisplatin compared with gemcitabine alone in advanced pancreatic cancer. J Clin Oncol 2006;24:3946–52.

71. Colucci G, Labianca R, Costanza V, et al. Randomized Phase III Trial of Gemcitabine Plus Cisplatin Compared With Single-Agent Gemcitabine As First-Line Treatment of Patients With Advanced Pancreatic Cancer: The GIP-1 Study J Clin Oncol 2010;28:1645–51.

72. Louvet C, Andre T, Lledo G, et al. Gemcitabine combined with oxaliplatin in advanced pancreatic adenocarcinoma: final results of a GERCOR multicenter Phase II study. J Clin Oncol 2002;20:1512–8.

73. Louvet C, Labianca R, Hammel P, et al. Gemcitabine in combination with oxaliplatin compared with gemcitabine alone in locally advanced or metastatic pancreatic cancer: results of a GERCOR and GISCAD phase III trial. J Clin Oncol 2005;23:3509–16.

74. Heinemann V, Labianca R, Hinke A, et al. Increased survival using platinum analog combined with gemcitabine as compared to single-agent gemcitabine in advanced pancreatic cancer: pooled analysis of two randomized trials, the GERCOR/GISCAD intergroup study and a German multicenter study. Ann. Oncol 2007;18:1652–9.

75. Miller KD, Picus J, Blanke C, et al. Phase II study of the multi-targeted antifolate LY231514 (ALIMTA, MTA, pemetrexed disodium) in patients with advanced pancreatic cancer. Ann Oncol 2000;11:101–3.

76. Oettle H, Richards D, Ramanathan RK, et al. A phase III trial of pemetrexed plus gemcitabine versus gemcitabine in patients with unresectable or metastatic pancreatic cancer. Ann Oncol 2005;16:1639–45.

77. Kulke MH, Tempero MA, Niedzwiecki D, et al. Randomized phase II study of gemcitabine administered at a fixed dose rate or in combination with cisplatin, docetaxel, or irinotecan in patients with metastatic pancreatic cancer: CALGB 89904. J Clin Oncol 2009;27:5506–12.

78. Abou-Alfa GK, Letourneau R, Harker G, et al. Randomized phase III study of exatecan and gemcitabine compared with gemcitabine alone in untreated advanced pancreatic cancer. J Clin Oncol 2006;24:4441–7.

79. Dragovich T, Burris H 3rd, Loehrer P, et al. Gemcitabine plus celecoxib in patients with advanced or metastatic pancreatic adenocarcinoma: results of a phase II trial. Am J Clin Oncol 2008;31:157–62.

80. Negi SS, Agarwal A, Chaudhary A. Flutamide in unresectable pancreatic adenocarcinoma: a randomized, double-blind, placebo-controlled trial. Invest New Drugs 2006;24:189–94.

81. Reni M, Cordio S, Milandri C, et al. Gemcitabine versus cisplatin, epirubicin, fluorouracil, and gemcitabine in advanced pancreatic cancer: a randomised controlled multicentre phase III trial. Lancet Oncol 2005;6:369–76.

82. Conroy T, Desseigne F, Ychou M, et al. FOLFIRINOX versus gemcitabine for metastatic pancreatic cancer. N Engl J Med 2011;364:1817–25.

83. Xiong HQ. Molecular targeting therapy for pancreatic cancer. Cancer Chemother Pharmacol 2004;54(Suppl 1):S69–S77.

84. Fjallskog ML, Lejonklou MH, Oberg KE, et al. Expression of molecular targets for tyrosine kinase receptor antagonists in malignant endocrine pancreatic tumors. Clin. Cancer Res 2003;9:1469–73.

85. Ueda S, Ogata S, Tsuda H, et al. The correlation between cytoplasmic overexpression of epidermal growth factor receptor and tumor aggressiveness: poor prognosis in patients with pancreatic ductal adenocarcinoma. Pancreas 2004;29:e1–e8.

86. Bruns CJ, Solorzano CC, Harbison MT, et al. Blockade of the epidermal growth factor receptor signaling by a novel tyrosine kinase inhibitor leads to apoptosis of endothelial cells and therapy of human pancreatic carcinoma. Cancer Res 2000;60:2926–35.

87. Moore MJ, Goldstein D, Hamm J, et al. Erlotinib plus gemcitabine compared with gemcitabine alone in patients with advanced pancreatic cancer: a phase III trial of the National Cancer Institute of Canada Clinical Trials Group. J Clin Oncol 2007;25: 1960–6.

88. da Cunha Santos G, Dhani N, Tu D, et al. Molecular predictors of outcome in a phase 3 study of gemcitabine and erlotinib therapy in patients with advanced pancreatic cancer: National Cancer Institute of Canada Clinical Trials Group Study PA.3. Cancer 2010;116:5599–607.

89. Jonker DJ, O'Callaghan CJ, Karapetis CS, et al. Cetuximab for the treatment of colorectal cancer. N Engl J Med 2007;357:2040–8.

90. Philip PA, Benedetti J, Corless CL, et al. Phase III study comparing gemcitabine plus cetuximab versus gemcitabine in patients with advanced pancreatic adenocarcinoma: Southwest Oncology Group-directed intergroup trial S0205. J Clin Oncol 2010;28:3605–10.

91. Cascinu S, Berardi R, Labianca R, et al. Cetuximab plus gemcitabine and cisplatin compared with gemcitabine and cisplatin alone in patients with advanced pancreatic cancer: a randomised, multicentre, Phase II trial. Lancet Oncol 2008;9:39–44.

92. Merchan JR, Ferrell A, Macintyre J, et al. Phase II Study of Gemcitabine, Oxaliplatin, and Cetuximab in Advanced Pancreatic Cancer. Am J Clin Oncol 2011. [Epub ahead of print].

93. Korc M. Pathways for aberrant angiogenesis in pancreatic cancer. Mol Cancer 2003;2:8.

94. Hurwitz H, Fehrenbacher L, Novotny W, et al. Bevacizumab plus irinotecan, fluorouracil, and leucovorin for metastatic colorectal cancer. N Engl J Med 2004;350:2335–42.

95. Sandler A, Gray R, Perry MC, et al. Paclitaxel–carboplatin alone or with bevacizumab for non-small-cell lung cancer. N Engl J Med 2006;355:2542–50.

96. Kindler HL, Friberg G, Singh DA, et al. Phase II trial of bevacizumab plus gemcitabine in patients with advanced pancreatic cancer. J Clin Oncol 2005;23:8033–40.

97. Kindler H, Niedzwiecki D, Hollis D, et al. Gemcitabine plus bevacizumab compared with gemcitabine plus placebo in patients with advanced pancreatic cancer: phase III trial of the Cancer and Leukemia Group B (CALGB 80303). J Clin Oncol 2010;28: 3617–22.

98. Kindler HL, Niedzwiecki D, Hollis D, et al. Efficacy of gemcitabine plus axitinib compared with gemcitabine alone in patients with advanced pancreatic cancer: an open-label randomised Phase II study. Lancet 2008;371:2101–8.

99. Kindler HL, Gangadhar T, Karrison T, et al. Final analysis of a randomized Phase II study of bevacizumab (B) and gemcitabine (G) plus cetuximab (C) or erlotinib (E) in patients (pts) with advanced pancreatic cancer (PC). J Clin Oncol 2008;26:Abstract 4502.

100. Van Cutsem E, Vervenne WL, Bennouna J, et al. Phase III trial of bevacizumab in combination with gemcitabine and erlotinib in patients with metastatic pancreatic cancer. J Clin Oncol 2009;27:2231–7.

101. Bramhall SR, Schulz J, Nemunaitis J, et al. A double-blind placebo-controlled, randomised study comparing gemcitabine and marimastat with gemcitabine and placebo as first line therapy in patients with advanced pancreatic cancer. Br J Cancer 2002;87:161–7.

102. Moore MJ, Hamm J, Dancey J, et al. Comparison of gemcitabine versus the matrix metalloproteinase inhibitor BAY 12-9566 in patients with advanced or metastatic adenocarcinoma of the pancreas: a Phase III trial of the National Cancer Institute of Canada Clinical Trials Group. J Clin Oncol 2003;21:3296–302.

103. Van Cutsem E, van de Velde H, Karasek P, et al. Phase III trial of gemcitabine plus tipifarnib compared with gemcitabine plus placebo in advanced pancreatic cancer. J Clin Oncol 2004;22:1430–8.

104. Wolpin BM, Hezel AF, Abrams T, et al. Oral mTOR inhibitor everolimus in patients with gemcitabine-refractory metastatic pancreatic cancer. J Clin Oncol 2009;27: 193–8.

105. Rieder S, Michalski CW, Friess H, Kleeff J. Insulin-Like Growth Factor Signaling as a Therapeutic Target in Pancreatic Cancer. Anticancer Agents Med Chem 2011. [Epub ahead of print].

106. Wang Z, Ahmad A, Li Y, et al. Targeting notch to eradicate pancreatic cancer stem cells for cancer therapy. Anticancer Res 2011;31:1105–13.

107. Dhillon N, Aggarwal BB, Newman RA, et al. Phase II trial of curcumin in patients with advanced pancreatic cancer. Clin Cancer Res 2008;14:4491–9.

108. Garber K. Stromal depletion goes on trial in pancreatic cancer. Natl Cancer Inst 2010;102:448–50.

109. Olive KP, Jacobetz MA, Davidson CJ, et al. Inhibition of Hedgehog signaling enhances delivery of chemotherapy in a mouse model of pancreatic cancer. Science 2009;324:1457–61.

110. Gradishar WJ. Albumin-bound paclitaxel: a next-generation taxane. Expert Opin Pharmacother 2006;7:1041–53.

111. Von Hoff DD, Ramanathan R, Borad M, et al. SPARC correlation with response to gemcitabine (G) plus nab-paclitaxel (nab-P) in patients with advanced metastatic pancreatic cancer: A phase I/II study. J Clin Oncol 2009;27:15s.

112. O'Reilly EM, Niedzwiecki D, Hall M, et al. Cancer and Leukemia Group B. A Cancer and Leukemia Group B phase II study of sunitinib malate in patients with previously treated metastatic pancreatic adenocarcinoma (CALGB 80603). Oncologist 2010; 15:1310–9.

The Surgical Management of Pancreatic Cancer

Lea Matsuoka, MD, Rick Selby, MD, Yuri Genyk, MD*

KEYWORDS

• Pancreas • Cancer • Adenocarcinoma • Whipple

Surgical resection remains an important component in the treatment of pancreatic cancer. Unfortunately, only approximately 10% to 20% of patients are eligible for surgical resection at presentation.[1] Many patients with pancreatic cancer, especially cancer of the distal pancreas, present at a late stage and their disease is unresectable secondary to locally advanced or metastatic disease. The surgical approach depends on the location of the tumor: tumors of the pancreatic head require pancreaticoduo-denectomy (PD) or pylorus-preserving pancreaticoduodenectomy (PPPD), whereas tumors located in the body or tail require distal pancreatectomy and splenectomy (DP). In hopeful attempts to extend the limits of resection and improve survival, many centers have performed more aggressive resections, including extended lymphade-nectomy and vascular resections.

PANCREATICODUODENECTOMY

The standard of care for resection of cancers of the pancreatic head, neck, and uncinate process is PD (**Fig. 1**). The development of the PD procedure has been credited in the United States to Allen O. Whipple. In 1935, he described a 2-stage operation; the first operation involves a cholecystogastrostomy followed 3 to 4 weeks later by resection of the stomach, pancreas, and duodenum.[2] Dr. Whipple later described a 1-stage PD in 1941.[3] Experience with pancreatic resections began to grow, but morbidity and mortality rates at that time remained prohibitive.

Since the time of Dr. Whipple, there have been significant improvements in anesthesia, critical care, and surgical technique, which have led to decreased mortality rates and improved survival. In a recent large single-institution study, Winter and colleagues[4] evaluated the outcomes of 1175 patients who underwent PD for ductal adenocarcinoma from 1970 to 2006. Median blood loss was 800 mL and operating time was 380 minutes. Perioperative mortality rate was 2%, morbidity was 38%, length of stay was 9 days, and median survival time was 18 months. They

---

The authors have nothing to disclose.

Hepatobiliary/Pancreatic Surgery and Abdominal Transplantation Division, University of Southern California, 1510 San Pablo Street, Suite 200, Los Angeles, CA 90033, USA

* Corresponding author.

E-mail address: Yuri.Genyk@health.usc.edu

Gastroenterol Clin N Am 41 (2012) 211–221

doi:10.1016/j.gtc.2011.12.015
gastro.theclinics.com

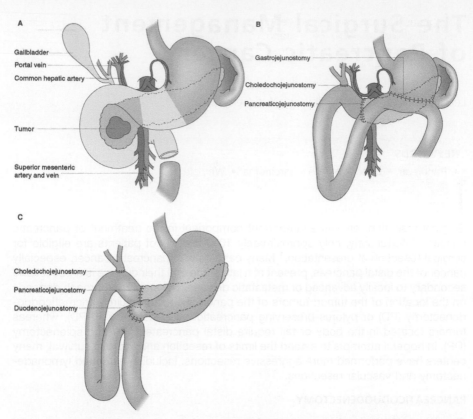

Fig. 1. Pancreaticoduodenectomy. (*A*) The tissue to be resected in a standard pancreaticoduodenectomy. (*B*) Reconstruction after a standard pancreaticoduodenectomy. (*C*) Reconstruction after a pylorus-preserving variation. (*From* Nakeeb A, Lillemoe K. Neoplasms of the exocrine pancreas. In: Muholland MW, Lillemoe KD, editors. Greenfield's surgery: scientific principles and practice. 5th edition. Philadelphia: Lippincott Williams and Wilkins; 2010; with permission.)

reported median survival in the 1970s to be 8 months, in the 1980s to be 14 months, in the 1990s to be 17 months, and in the 2000s to be 19 months. McPhee and colleagues[5] performed a national database study and also reported a low mortality rate of 5.5% in 2003, which had significantly decreased from 8.2% in 1998. Additional studies have reported morbidity rates of 42% to 47%; the most common complications being delayed gastric emptying, pancreatic fistula, and wound infections.[6,7] Pancreatic fistulas have traditionally been the Achilles' heel of PD, being a fairly common and potentially life-threatening complication. Pancreatic fistula rates vary widely in the literature, in part secondary to the lack of a universal definition. The international study group on pancreatic fistula proposed a standard definition in 2005.[8] The group defined a pancreatic fistula as any volume of drain fluid after postoperative day 3, with amylase content greater than 3 times serum. The group further classified the fistulas by grade according to clinical severity. Grade A fistulas require little change in management and are considered "transient fistulas." Grade B fistulas require a change in management, including parenteral nutrition, antibiotics, or somatostatin analogues. Grade C fistulas require a major change in management, such as additional drainage procedures, and often lead to an extended hospital stay. Hopefully, with the use of a standard definition, accurate comparisons between centers can be made, potentially leading to improvements in the rates or management of pancreatic fistulas.

In their study of 1175 patients, Winter and coworkers[4] reported the significant factors influencing survival to be tumor diameter, resection margin, lymph node status, and histologic grade. Additional studies have confirmed the importance of tumor size, lymph node status, histologic grade, and negative surgical margins.[6,9] Wagner and colleagues[9] found a significant difference between patients who received R1 resections (median survival, 11.5 months) and R0 resections (median survival, 20.1 months) and found R0 resection to be a significant independent predictor of long-term survival.[9] However, not all studies found resection margin to be a significant factor for survival.[10] This discrepancy may be, in part, because of the lack of a universal consensus on pathologic examination of PD specimens. When margins are examined, the pancreatic resection margin, bile duct margin, and stomach/duodenal margin are evaluated. The difficulty lies in assessing the soft tissue margin that abuts the superior mesenteric vessels. This soft tissue margin is the most common margin involved with the tumor.[11] Some centers circumferentially evaluate an anterior, posterior, and medial margin, whereas other centers examine the medial margin, also known as the retroperitoneal or uncinate margin. Wide variation (16%–85%) in rates of R1 resections has been reported.[11] Esposito and coworkers,[12] when comparing margin results using new, more thorough standardized pathologic reporting, found that rates of R1 resections increased from 14% to 76%.[12] The need for a standardized method of examining PD specimens and evaluating margins is imperative because the rates of local recurrence are high, and these recurrences often are located at the superior mesenteric vessels.[13] Improving the assessment of margins will lead to more accurate assessment of outcomes and surgical and adjuvant treatments. Operative blood loss has also been reported as a factor influencing survival. Kazanjian and colleagues[6] described blood loss of greater than 400 mL to be a predictor of poor survival, and Sohn and colleagues[14] reported an estimated blood loss of less than 750 mL to be a favorable prognostic indicator.

Additionally, multiple studies have supported the regionalization of complex procedures such as the PD. Luft[15] and coworkers initially supported the early regionalization for procedures such as open heart surgery, major vascular surgery, and total hip replacement.[9] In 1999, Birkmeyer and colleagues[16] published a study based on the Medicare claims database showing that hospital volumes for PD were strongly related to perioperative mortality and long-term survival. Subsequent studies looked at the effect of surgeon volume for pancreatic resections and found that higher surgeon procedure volumes correlated with lower mortality rates.[17,18] These studies suggest that regionalization of pancreatic resections may lead to decreased mortality and improved survival. The PD has become a procedure that can be performed with low mortality and acceptable morbidity rates in large centers and should be performed with the intent of achieving negative margins and minimizing blood loss.

PANCREATICODUODENECTOMY VERSUS PYLORUS-PRESERVING PANCREATICODUODENECTOMY

Dr. Watson first described the PPPD in 1944.[19] However, interest in this procedure was stimulated by Traverso and Longmire after their report of 18 patients who underwent PPPD for chronic pancreatitis and early periampullary cancers, with improved gastrointestinal function.[20] There has since been long debate over the benefits of PPPD versus PD. Proponents of PPPD claim that it allows for fewer cases of dumping syndrome, less blood loss, and shorter operating times. Proponents of PD argue that PPPD is associated with more delayed gastric emptying and question its effectiveness as an oncologic procedure. In a prospective, randomized comparison by Lin and Lin,[21] the same surgeon performed 16 PPPD and 15 PD. Both PPPD and PD were associated with low morbidity and mortality rates with no significant differences between the 2 groups. Patients also had similar operating times and blood loss. Tran and coworkers[22] subsequently published a prospective, randomized, multicenter study out of the Netherlands. In this study, 170 consecutive patients were randomly assigned to undergo either PPPD or PD for suspected pancreatic or periampullary cancer. Both groups were similar with regard to operating times, blood loss, and length of stay. Additionally, rates of delayed gastric emptying and positive resection margins were equivalent. When patients with confirmed pancreatic or periampullary adenocarcinoma were analyzed, patients who were treated with PPPD had a median disease-free survival of 15 months, whereas patients who were treated with PD had a median disease-free survival of 14 months ($P = 0.80$). The conclusion of the study was that PD and PPPD were both effective in the treatment of pancreatic cancer. A recent Cochrane review confirmed these findings.[23] The Cochrane review included all randomized, controlled trials, regardless of language. Six studies between March 2006 and January 2011 with a total of 465 patients were included. The study found no differences in morbidity, mortality, and survival for patients receiving PPPD or PD. Despite the theorized pros and cons of preserving the duodenum, the bulk of the literature shows no difference in outcomes after PPPD compared with PD.

DISTAL PANCREATECTOMY

The standard surgical therapy for pancreatic cancers of the body and tail of the pancreas is distal pancreatectomy and splenectomy. The first distal pancreatic resection was first reported in 1884 by Bilroth. In the years following, pancreatic resection was associated with high morbidity and mortality, and the wisdom of pancreatic resection was questioned. In recent years, however, there has been tremendous improvement in outcomes after DP. Lillemoe and colleagues[24] retrospectively studied 235 patients who underwent DP for a variety of benign and malignant conditions between 1994 and 1997. Mortality rate was 0.9%, operating time was 4.3 hours, and blood loss was 450 mL. Morbidity after DP was 31% and the rate of pancreatic fistula was 5%. Additional studies have reported low mortality rates and morbidity rates ranging from 20% to 50%.[5,25,26]

In the study by Lillemoe et al, 18% of the patients who underwent DP had adenocarcinoma of the pancreas diagnosed. Long-term survival rates in this subset of patients were not reported. Sperti and coworkers[27] reported on 24 patients who underwent DP for adenocarcinoma of the body and tail of the pancreas with no adjuvant radiotherapy or chemotherapy. Morbidity reported in the study was 25% and mortality 8%. Five-year survival rate for these patients was 12.5%, similar to rates reported for survival after PD for pancreatic head cancer. The authors recommended an aggressive surgical approach, supporting the resection of adjacent organs if necessary to achieve complete tumor resection.

EXTENDED RESECTION

In an attempt to extend the limits of resectability for pancreatic tumors, Fortner in the 1970s described extended PD resections, which included total pancreatectomy, extended lymph node resection, and combinations of portal vein, arterial, colon, and gastric resection and reconstruction.[28] These procedures greatly increased resectability

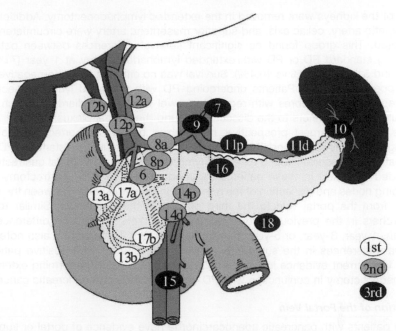

Fig. 2. Lymph node groups for tumor located in the head of the pancreas. *Open circle*, the first group; *shaded circle*, second group; *solid circle*, third group. (*From* Matsuno S. Pancreatic cancer registry in Japan. Pancreas 2004;28:220, with permission.)

rates but resulted in high postoperative morbidity and mortality rates. Since then, there has been reluctance to perform such extensive surgery. However, with improvements in anesthesia, surgical technique, and perioperative care, many centers have been exploring the utility of extended pancreatic resection.

Extended Lymphadenectomy

Regional lymph nodes typically resected with the PD specimen include anterior and posterior pancreaticoduodenal nodes, as shown as the first group of nodes in **Fig. 2**. Three prospective, randomized, controlled trials have been published that address the utility of performing PD in conjunction with extended lymphadenectomy. The first study, by Pedrazzoli and coworkers,[29] is a multicenter study that randomly assigned 40 patients to standard PD and 41 patients to PD with extended lymphadenectomy. Extended lymphadenectomy included removal of nodes from the liver hilum and along the aorta from the diaphragm to the inferior mesenteric artery and laterally to both renal hilum. Circumferential clearance of the celiac trunk and superior mesenteric artery was also included. Mean lymph nodes retrieved were significantly higher in the extended group (19.8 vs 13.3), and morbidity and mortality rates were similar. Overall survival did not differ between the 2 groups; however, when examining node-positive patients only, the authors found a longer survival rate in those patients undergoing PD with extended lymphadenectomy.

The second prospective, randomized trial involved 40 patients who underwent standard PD and were compared with 39 patients who underwent PD with extended lymphadenectomy.[30] The retroperitoneal tissue and para-aortic lymph nodes from the celiac axis superiorly to the inferior mesenteric artery inferiorly, and laterally to the hilum of the kidneys were removed in the extended lymphadenectomy. Additionally, the hepatic artery, celiac axis, and superior mesenteric artery were circumferentially dissected. This group found no significant survival differences between patients receiving standard PD or PD with extended lymphadenectomy at 1 year (71% vs 82%) and 5 years (16.5% vs 16.4%). Survival was no different for node-negative and node-positive patients. Patients undergoing PD with extended lymphadenectomy also reported lower scores with regard to bowel control and diarrhea, which was attributed by the authors to the dissection around the arterial plexus.

The third and largest prospective, randomized trial was reported by Yeo and colleagues.[31] This study randomly assigned 146 patients to receive standard PD and 148 patients to receive PD and extended lymphadenectomy and distal gastrectomy. Extended resection in these patients included a 30% to 40% gastrectomy with attending nodes and dissection of the retroperitoneal lymph nodes between the renal hilum, from the portal vein to the third portion of the duodenum. Similar to the researchers in the previous study, Yeo and coworkers[31] found no differences in median, 1-year, 3-year, or 5-year survival between the 2 groups and also noted no survival differences in the subgroups of node-negative or node-positive patients. Thus, the current evidence in the literature does not support performing extending lymphadenectomy in conjunction with PD for the treatment of pancreatic cancer.

Resection of the Portal Vein

Some patients with pancreatic adenocarcinoma have evidence of portal or superior mesenteric vein invasion diagnosed on preoperative imaging or intraoperatively. The utility of portal venous resection in conjunction with PD has been long debated. Is the benefit of portal vein resection worth the additional risk? In a study out of MD Anderson, 110 patients underwent PD with portal vein resection for pancreatic adenocarcinoma.[32] When compared with patients who underwent PD alone, similar rates of morbidity and mortality and a median survival of approximately 2 years were reported for both groups. On multivariate analysis, only the presence of nodal disease and perioperative complications significantly impacted survival. Similarly, multiple other studies have reported equivalent morbidity, mortality, and survival rates in patients who underwent PD with portal vein resection compared with patients who underwent PD alone.[33–37] Mortality rates after PD with portal vein resection range from 0% to 6%, whereas morbidity rates range from 21% to 48%.[32,33,35–40] Reported 5-year survival rates range from 8% to 23%.[33,35–40]

It is important to note that not all patients with portal vein invasion have true histologic invasion by tumor. In many cases, peritumoral inflammation mimics tumor invasion. Rates of histologically confirmed vein invasion reported in the literature range from 52% to 78%.[33,35,40] In a study by Nakagohri and coworkers,[36] only 52% of patients who underwent PD with portal vein resection had invasion on histology. The cohort of patients with histologic portal vein invasion had a higher rate of positive margins and poorer prognosis compared with patients who underwent portal vein resection without histologic invasion. The importance of achieving negative margins with PD and portal vein resection has been emphasized by various studies.[33,37,40,41] However, other studies have found no difference in survival between patients with true vascular invasion on histology compared with those without invasion.[32,35,42] It is likely that this discrepancy exists because venous invasion often is a function of the tumor's location and size rather than its aggressiveness. Differences may also exist because of variations in pathology protocols and the strong impact of other factors, such as node positivity.

PD in conjunction with portal vein resection is now accepted therapy in many specialized centers, with equivalent outcomes when compared with PD alone.

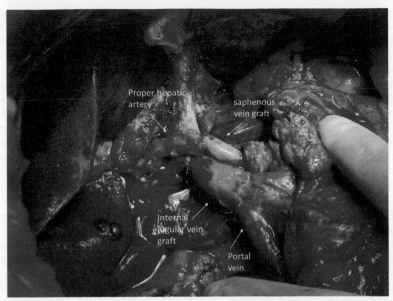

Fig. 3. Intraoperative photograph of pancreaticoduodenectomy with vascular reconstruction. Saphenous vein interposition graft was used to reconstruct the common hepatic to proper hepatic artery. Internal jugular vein interposition graft was used to reconstruct the portal vein.

Although PD with portal vein resection does not lead to improved survival over PD alone, it does increase the number of patients amenable to complete resection. These patients who are now able to undergo complete resection of their tumor have significantly improved survival compared with patients with unresectable disease.

Arterial Resection/Reconstruction

When their tumors are invading or encasing arterial vasculature, including the hepatic artery, celiac trunk, or superior mesenteric artery, patients are classified as having locally advanced, unresectable disease. Very few studies have published specific outcomes after pancreatic and arterial resection or reconstruction (**Fig. 3**). Nakao and colleagues[43] reported arterial resection of the celiac artery in 3 patients, the hepatic artery in 9 patients, and the superior mesenteric artery in 3 patients undergoing PD, total pancreatectomy, or distal pancreatectomy. Most of these patients underwent concomitant portal vein resection. The authors reported a 30-day mortality rate of 35.7% with these pancreatic combined with arterial resections and noted that this group had more advanced tumors with a higher incidence of invasion into the peripancreatic margin. Takahashi and coworkers[44] also reported a subset of 16 patients who underwent portal vein resection and arterial resection of the hepatic artery, celiac trunk, or superior mesenteric artery. Thirteen of these patients underwent total pancreatectomy and 3 patients underwent PD. Seven patients in this subset died within 6 months, resulting in a 44% mortality rate.[44] These authors concluded that the indications for arterial resection were limited and associated with a high mortality rate.

More recently, Yekebas and colleagues[42] from Germany described 13 patients who underwent pancreatic resections with associated arterial resections. Eight patients had arterial resection alone, and 5 patients had combined portal venous and arterial resections. Eight of these patients underwent total pancreatectomy, 3 underwent PD, and 2 underwent subtotal pancreatectomies. Eight patients survived more than 1 year, and 4 patients survived longer than 2 years. The authors comment that the role of en bloc arterial resection, although controversial, led to longer survival in some patients compared with palliative measures. Stitzenberg and coworkers[45] administered neoadjuvant chemoradiotherapy followed by pancreatic and arterial resection in 12 patients with pancreatic adenocarcinoma. The procedures included 6 PD, 2 subtotal pancreatectomies, 2 distal pancreatectomies, and 2 total pancreatectomies. Ten of these cases also involved celiac trunk resections and 2 involved hepatic artery resections. Mortality rate was 17%, and median survival in this group of patients was 17 months. The authors concluded that pancreatic resection with arterial resection should be performed only for select patients and may prolong survival, but it is unlikely to result in cure. The literature on pancreatic resection with arterial resection is sparse and associated with a high mortality. Although some studies seem to show improved survival in these select patients compared with that of palliative measures, arterial invasion still remains a contraindication to surgical intervention in the majority of patients.

SUMMARY

There have been significant advances made over the years in the areas of critical care, anesthesia, and surgical technique, which have led to improved mortality rates and survival after resection for pancreatic cancer. The standard of care is currently PD or PPPD for pancreatic cancers of the head, uncinate process, or neck and DP for pancreatic cancers of the body or tail. Resections are performed with the goals of negative margins and minimal blood loss, and referral to high-volume centers and surgeons is encouraged. However, 5-year survival rate after curative resection still remains at less than 20%.[14] In an effort to improve survival and extend the limits of resectability, many centers have attempted extended lymphadenectomy and portal venous and even arterial resection and reconstruction. Extended lymphadenectomy has not led to improved survival for these patients. Portal vein resection has increased the number of patients amenable to resection, with equivalent survival rates compared with those of standard resections. Portal vein invasion is thus no longer considered a contraindication to resection at many large centers. Resection and reconstruction of involved arteries have been rarely performed and are currently not considerations for most patients. It is likely that future improvements in survival lie in the realm of adjuvant therapy. As chemotherapeutic and other tumor-directed agents continue to evolve and advance, this will hopefully lead to improved survival for patients undergoing surgical resection for pancreatic cancer.

REFERENCES

1. Neoptolemos JP, Stocken DD, Friess H, et al. A randomized trial of chemoradiotherapy and chemotherapy after resection of pancreatic cancer. N Engl J Med 2004;350:1200–10.
2. Whipple AO, Parsons WB, Mullins CR. Treatment of carcinoma of the ampulla of Vater. Ann Surg 1935;102:763–79.
3. Whipple AO. The rationale of radical surgery for cancer of the pancreas and ampullary region. Ann Surg 1941;114:612–5.

4. Winter JM, Cameron JL, Campbell KA, et al. 1423 pancreaticoduodenectomies for pancreatic cancer: a single-institution experience. J Gastrointest Surg 2006;10: 1199–210; discussion 210–1.
5. McPhee JT, Hill JS, Whalen GF, et al. Perioperative mortality for pancreatectomy: a national perspective. Ann Surg 2007;246:246–53.
6. Kazanjian KK, Hines OJ, Duffy JP, et al. Improved survival following pancreaticoduodenectomy to treat adenocarcinoma of the pancreas: the influence of operative blood loss. Arch Surg 2008;143:1166–71.
7. Grobmyer SR, Pieracci FM, Allen PJ, et al. Defining morbidity after pancreaticoduodenectomy: use of a prospective complication grading system. J Am Coll Surg 2007;204:356–64.
8. Bassi C, Dervenis C, Butturini G, et al. Postoperative pancreatic fistula: an international study group (ISGPF) definition. Surgery 2005;138:8–13.
9. Wagner M, Redaelli C, Lietz M, et al. Curative resection is the single most important factor determining outcome in patients with pancreatic adenocarcinoma. Br J Surg 2004;91:586–94.
10. Butturini G, Stocken DD, Wente MN, et al. Influence of resection margins and treatment on survival in patients with pancreatic cancer: meta-analysis of randomized controlled trials. Arch Surg 2008;143:75–83; discussion.
11. Verbeke CS. Resection margins and R1 rates in pancreatic cancer—are we there yet? Histopathology 2008;52:787–96.
12. Esposito I, Kleeff J, Bergmann F, et al. Most pancreatic cancer resections are R1 resections. Ann Surg Oncol 2008;15:1651–60.
13. Heye T, Zausig N, Klauss M, et al. CT diagnosis of recurrence after pancreatic cancer: is there a pattern? World J Gastroenterol 2011;17:1126–34.
14. Sohn TA, Yeo CJ, Cameron JL, et al. Resected adenocarcinoma of the pancreas— 616 patients: results, outcomes, and prognostic indicators. J Gastrointest Surg 2000;4:567–79.
15. Luft HS, Bunker JP, Enthoven AC. Should operations be regionalized? The empirical relation between surgical volume and mortality. N Engl J Med 1979;301:1364–9.
16. Birkmeyer JD, Warshaw AL, Finlayson SR, et al. Relationship between hospital volume and late survival after pancreaticoduodenectomy. Surgery 1999;126:178–83.
17. Nathan H, Cameron JL, Choti MA, et al. The volume-outcomes effect in hepato-pancreato-biliary surgery: hospital versus surgeon contributions and specificity of the relationship. J Am Coll Surg 2009;208:528–38.
18. Eppsteiner RW, Csikesz NG, McPhee JT, et al. Surgeon volume impacts hospital mortality for pancreatic resection. Ann Surg 2009;249:635–40.
19. Watson K. Carcinoma of the ampulla of Vater. Successful radical resection. Br J Surg 1944;31:368–73.
20. Traverso LW, Longmire WP Jr. Preservation of the pylorus in pancreaticoduodenectomy a follow-up evaluation. Ann Surg 1980;192:306–10.
21. Lin PW, Lin YJ. Prospective randomized comparison between pylorus-preserving and standard pancreaticoduodenectomy. Br J Surg 1999;86:603–7.
22. Tran KT, Smeenk HG, van Eijck CH, et al. Pylorus preserving pancreaticoduodenectomy versus standard Whipple procedure: a prospective, randomized, multicenter analysis of 170 patients with pancreatic and periampullary tumors. Ann Surg 2004;240:738–45.
23. Diener MK, Fitzmaurice C, Schwarzer G, et al. Pylorus-preserving pancreaticoduodenectomy (pp Whipple) versus pancreaticoduodenectomy (classic Whipple) for surgical treatment of periampullary and pancreatic carcinoma. Cochrane Database Syst Rev 2011;5:CD006053.

24. Lillemoe KD, Kaushal S, Cameron JL, et al. Distal pancreatectomy: indications and outcomes in 235 patients. Ann Surg 1999;229:693–8; discussion 8–700.

25. Sledzianowski JF, Duffas JP, Muscari F, et al. Risk factors for mortality and intra-abdominal morbidity after distal pancreatectomy. Surgery 2005;137:180–5.

26. Fahy BN, Frey CF, Ho HS, et al. Morbidity, mortality, and technical factors of distal pancreatectomy. Am J Surg 2002;183:237–41.

27. Sperti C, Pasquali C, Pedrazzoli S. Ductal adenocarcinoma of the body and tail of the pancreas. J Am Coll Surg 1997;185:255–9.

28. Fortner JG. Regional pancreatectomy for cancer of the pancreas, ampulla, and other related sites. Tumor staging and results. Ann Surg 1984;199:418–25.

29. Pedrazzoli S, DiCarlo V, Dionigi R, et al. Standard versus extended lymphadenectomy associated with pancreatoduodenectomy in the surgical treatment of adenocarcinoma of the head of the pancreas: a multicenter, prospective, randomized study. Lymphadenectomy Study Group. Ann Surg 1998;228:508–17.

30. Farnell MB, Pearson RK, Sarr MG, et al. A prospective randomized trial comparing standard pancreatoduodenectomy with pancreatoduodenectomy with extended lymphadenectomy in resectable pancreatic head adenocarcinoma. Surgery 2005; 138:618–28; discussion 28–30.

31. Yeo CJ, Cameron JL, Lillemoe KD, et al. Pancreaticoduodenectomy with or without distal gastrectomy and extended retroperitoneal lymphadenectomy for periampullary adenocarcinoma, part 2: randomized controlled trial evaluating survival, morbidity, and mortality. Ann Surg 2002;236:355–66; discussion 66–8.

32. Tseng JF, Raut CP, Lee JE, et al. Pancreaticoduodenectomy with vascular resection: margin status and survival duration. J Gastrointest Surg 2004;8:935–49; discussion 49–50.

33. Riediger H, Makowiec F, Fischer E, et al. Postoperative morbidity and long-term survival after pancreaticoduodenectomy with superior mesenterico-portal vein resection. J Gastrointest Surg 2006;10:1106–15.

34. Harrison LE, Klimstra DS, Brennan MF. Isolated portal vein involvement in pancreatic adenocarcinoma. A contraindication for resection? Ann Surg 1996;224:342–7; discussion 7–9.

35. Muller SA, Hartel M, Mehrabi A, et al. Vascular resection in pancreatic cancer surgery: survival determinants. J Gastrointest Surg 2009;13:784–92.

36. Nakagohri T, Kinoshita T, Konishi M, et al. Survival benefits of portal vein resection for pancreatic cancer. Am J Surg 2003;186:149–53.

37. Shibata C, Kobari M, Tsuchiya T, et al. Pancreatectomy combined with superior mesenteric-portal vein resection for adenocarcinoma in pancreas. World J Surg 2001;25:1002–5.

38. Al-Haddad M, Martin JK, Nguyen J, et al. Vascular resection and reconstruction for pancreatic malignancy: a single center survival study. J Gastrointest Surg 2007;11: 1168–74.

39. Hartel M, Niedergethmann M, Farag-Soliman M, et al. Benefit of venous resection for ductal adenocarcinoma of the pancreatic head. Eur J Surg 2002;168:707–12.

40. Bachellier P, Nakano H, Oussoultzoglou PD, et al. Is pancreaticoduodenectomy with mesentericoportal venous resection safe and worthwhile? Am J Surg 2001;182: 120–9.

41. Nakao A, Takeda S, Sakai M, et al. Extended radical resection versus standard resection for pancreatic cancer: the rationale for extended radical resection. Pancreas 2004;28:289–92.

42. Yekebas EF, Bogoevski D, Cataldegirmen G, et al. En bloc vascular resection for locally advanced pancreatic malignancies infiltrating major blood vessels: perioperative outcome and long-term survival in 136 patients. Ann Surg 2008;247:300–9.
43. Nakao A, Takeda S, Inoue S, et al. Indications and techniques of extended resection for pancreatic cancer. World J Surg 2006;30:976–82; discussion 83–4.
44. Takahashi S, Ogata Y, Tsuzuki T. Combined resection of the pancreas and portal vein for pancreatic cancer. Br J Surg 1994;81:1190–3.
45. Stitzenberg KB, Watson JC, Roberts A, et al. Survival after pancreatectomy with major arterial resection and reconstruction. Ann Surg Oncol 2008;15:1399–406.

Modern Radiation Therapy Techniques for Pancreatic Cancer

Nicholas Trakul, MD, PhD, Albert C. Koong, MD, PhD,
Peter G. Maxim, PhD, Daniel T. Chang, MD*

KEYWORDS

- Pancreatic adenocarcinoma • Radiation therapy
- Intensity-modulated radiation therapy
- Image-guided radiation therapy
- Stereotactic body radiotherapy

Pancreatic ductal adenocarcinoma comprises more than 90% of pancreatic tumors. It is the 10th most common cancer diagnosis in the United States, but represents the fourth most common cause of cancer deaths, with nearly 40,000 deaths reported in 2010.[1] This disproportionate mortality rate highlights the aggressive and deadly nature of this disease. Unfortunately, despite improvements in mortality rates in other malignancies, little improvement has been observed in pancreatic adenocarcinoma.[2]

Surgery, most often pancreatoduodenectomy, remains the standard of care and offers the only chance of cure for pancreatic cancer. Unfortunately, only 20% of patients are found to be acceptable surgical candidates at the time of diagnosis.[3] Radiation therapy can be utilized in a wide range of clinical presentations of pancreatic cancer, from early stage to widely metastatic disease, and its role is evolving, along with surgery and chemotherapy, aided by advances in technology and technique.

Radiotherapy of pancreatic cancer is technically challenging for a variety of reasons. Pancreatic tumors are often difficult to clearly define, even with advanced imaging techniques like fluorodeoxyglucose positron emission tomography (^{18}F-FDG-PET) and magnetic resonance imaging (MRI), making clear designation of treatment volumes difficult. In addition, organ motion throughout the respiratory cycle can further compromise the accuracy of planned treatment delivery. Also, the proximity of radiosensitive organs, such as the bowel, liver, and kidney, to the pancreas, can result in significant normal-tissue toxicity with the delivery of tumoricidal doses of radiation outside of the target. Recent technologic advances in the

Department of Radiation Oncology, Stanford University School of Medicine and Cancer Center, 875 Blake Wilbur Drive, Stanford, CA 94305, USA
* Corresponding author.
E-mail address: dtchang@stanford.edu

Gastroenterol Clin N Am 41 (2012) 223–235
doi:10.1016/j.gtc.2011.12.011   gastro.theclinics.com
0889-8553/12/$ – see front matter © 2012 Elsevier Inc. All rights reserved.

planning and delivery of radiation therapy, such as intensity-modulated radiation therapy (IMRT), arc therapy, image-guided radiation therapy (IGRT), and stereotactic ablative body radiotherapy (SABR), allow the potential for greater tumor control with reduced treatment-related toxicity and represent significant steps forward in the field.

RADIOTHERAPY IN THE TREATMENT OF PANCREATIC ADENOCARCINOMA

Although surgery is the standard treatment that offers the only reasonable chance of cure, 5-year survival rates for patients who undergo a tumor-free margin (R0) resection are only 10% to 25%,[4] which emphasizes the importance of adjuvant treatment. There also remains the problem of how to optimally manage inoperable patients, especially those without evidence of distant spread. Unfortunately, the median survival for patients who are unable to undergo resection is on the order of 10 to12 months,[3] highlighting the need for more effective therapeutic strategies in this population. The indications for the use of radiotherapy in the treatment of pancreatic cancer are not straightforward. It has been suggested that preoperative (neoadjuvant) radiotherapy treatment may provide some benefit by improving outcomes and potentially converting inoperable cases to operable ones.[5]

Unlike with other gastrointestinal (GI) malignancies, randomized trials have not led to clear indications for the use of adjuvant chemoradiation for pancreatic cancer. Early trials from the United States found a survival benefit,[6,7] whereas European trials found little or no benefit[8,9] to chemoradiation but a significant benefit with the use of adjuvant chemotherapy alone.[10,11] All of these early trials had severe limitations, and their radiation doses and delivery have been deemed ineffective by today's standards.[12] As a consequence, the role of radiation therapy still remains controversial. Currently, a combined Radiation Therapy Oncology Group (RTOG)/European Organisation for Research and Treatment of Cancer (EORTC) trial (RTOG 0848) is testing the small-molecule kinase-inhibitor erlotinib in combination with gemcitabine and the role of adjuvant chemoradiation using modern doses (50.4 Gy), modern scheduling, and modern radiation techniques.[13]

Preoperative radiotherapy has been shown to be both feasible and effective in GI malignancies like rectal and esophageal cancer. Its use is appealing in the treatment of pancreatic cancer for the following reasons: (1) it may increase the chances of an R0 resection; (2) it may allow for the downstaging of inoperable disease, thereby leading to surgical resection and a chance for cure; (3) it allows for earlier initiation of systemic therapy, which may provide a theoretical advantage in the treatment of distant disease when the burden is low rather than 6 to 8 weeks postoperatively[14]; (4) it may spare patients an unnecessary surgery if metastatic disease is detected during the course of preoperative treatment; and (5) it increases the efficacy of radiation and chemotherapy when given with an intact vascular supply to the tumor, making it easier to identify the target.

TARGET DEFINITION AND IMAGE-GUIDED RADIATION THERAPY

Historically, radiation therapy has been guided by imaging, but a more recent collection of research and advances in technology have vastly improved our understanding and ability to utilize imaging throughout the entire treatment process, a concept that is broadly termed *image-guided radiation therapy* (IGRT). To understand the power of IGRT, one must understand how the treatment area is defined.

Conventional nomenclature refers to the visible tumor as the gross tumor volume. An internal tumor volume has been defined as the volume occupied by the tumor throughout the respiratory cycle to account for motion associated with diaphragmatic excursion. The area at risk for clinical spread of tumor, such as the draining lymph nodes and tissue adjacent to the tumor, which may have been microscopically invaded, is called the clinical treatment volume. Typically, a fourth volume, the planning treatment volume, has also been defined, which is an additional expansion to account for inaccuracies and variability in daily patient positioning. The exact amount of the expansion depends on the reproducibility of the patient positioning and the quality and frequency of imaging to verify proper alignment. The more accurately one can position the patient and confidently deliver the treatment, the less expansion required, resulting in a smaller overall volume of nearby normal tissue that is treated, which reduces treatment-related toxicity.

Multiple imaging modalities are used to diagnose and stage pancreatic cancer, many of which can assist in the delineation of these volumes, including endoscopic ultrasound, endoscopic retrograde cholangiopancreatography, magnetic resonance imaging (MRI), computed tomography (CT), and positron emission tomography (PET). Each of these imaging modalities has its limitations, such as significant interobserver variability, but altogether they provide the treating radiation oncologist with valuable information about location, size, extent of spread, and possible lymph node involvement in each individual.

Modern radiation treatment planning begins by obtaining a high-quality CT scan used to contour the tumor as well as surrounding normal tissue and organs. Even with the use of intravenous contrast, pancreatic tumors can be isodense and difficult to distinguish from surrounding normal tissue. For example, one study comparing the size of pancreatic tumors as seen on CT and the actual size of surgical specimens after resection found that the CT scan significantly undersized pancreatic tumors by a median 7 mm in most patients (84%).[15]

MRI provides excellent soft-tissue definition, but image quality is degraded by movement. Although motion artifact-reducing MRI scanners do exist, most radiation therapy departments are not equipped with them.

^{18}F-FDG-PET provides the ability to distinguish metabolically active disease and is commonly being utilized during radiotherapy simulation in an increasing number of cancer types (Fig. 1). Pancreatic tumors are generally ^{18}F-FDG avid, although the avidity can vary, and cystic tumors can result in false positivity.

At some institutions, PET and CT are obtained at the time of treatment planning for pancreatic tumors. It has been reported that PET and CT may be particularly useful in distinguishing pancreatic head tumors from the adjacent duodenum,[16] which is particularly important, as radiation dose to this area is a critical determination of toxicity during SABR treatments.[17] Additionally, the degree of PET positivity in pretreatment scans has been found to hold prognostic value, as patients with higher maximum standard uptake values displayed worse progression-free and overall survival rates.[18]

Tumors in the thorax and upper abdomen move throughout the respiratory cycle. It has been reported that pancreatic tumors can move as much as 2 to 3 cm with normal respiration.[19] Four-dimensional CT (4DCT) was developed to address the problem of organ motion during respiration. 4DCT is a type of CT scan commonly used for planning radiation treatment and creates a CT "movie" to determine how tumors move during breathing. 4DCT image processing tools are readily available and allow the determination of tumor motion extent and the design of motion-compensating treatment strategies. The main goal of 4DCT imaging is to design treatment strategies that safely reduce treatment margins, thus, sparing healthy tissue. Among these strategies is airway breathing control, which is when a patient holds his or her breath during treatment delivery to eliminate motion. With respiratory gating, radiation

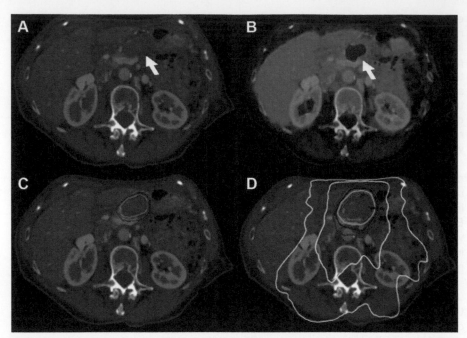

Fig. 1. The role of PET/CT in radiation treatment planning for SABR. (*A*) Contrast-enhanced CT scan shows a pancreatic tumor (*arrow*). (*B*) Overlay of ^{18}F-FDG-PET image onto CT shows tumor edge. (*C*) Target definition. GTV (*green*) and PTV (*red*) are contoured onto the treatment planning CT. (*D*) Typical SABR plan. Prescribed dose was 33 Gy in 5 fractions. Isodose lines are represented as follows: 33 Gy (*red*), 30 Gy (*green*), 25 Gy (*blue*), 20 Gy (*magenta*), 10 Gy (*yellow*), and 5 Gy (*white*).

is delivered only during specific phases of the patients' respiratory cycle. Abdominal compression devices can limit the amount of diaphragmatic excursion, reducing organ motion during breathing. And with tumor tracking, the radiation beam follows, or tracks, the tumor as it moves during the respiratory cycle.[20]

IMAGE GUIDANCE DURING TREATMENT DELIVERY

Although knowing and accounting for tumor and organ motion during the planning phase of radiotherapy is critical, this information must also be recalled during actual treatment delivery. Mechanical methods (airway breathing control, respiratory-gating, and abdominal compression) that limit motion at the time of simulation and planning are also used during the daily treatment delivery.

Verification of setup positioning is critical to ensuring accurate radiation delivery to the target. Traditionally, verification was done with megavoltage (MV) imaging using the linear accelerator (linac) as a beam source and a detector mounted at the opposite side of the linac. The quality of MV images of the patient in the actual treatment position varies, and the images are mainly used to confirm that the bony anatomy of the patient is well aligned with respect to a reference image used during treatment planning. However, with more-sophisticated radiation treatment delivery techniques available, IGRT was developed to improve upon accuracy. Modern linacs now have a kilovoltage (kV) source with a flat-panel detector mounted orthogonally to the treatment beam, which improves resolution imaging for bony-anatomy alignment. Cone-beam CT (CBCT), a method similar to conventional 3-dimensional anatomic imaging, can be performed to align patients based on soft tissue, which is otherwise impossible with MV or kV 2-dimensional imaging. Whether used alone or combined, either method will ensure accurate patient setup when a high degree of accuracy is needed.

One of the difficulties particular to treatment of the pancreas with IGRT is that bony anatomy does not necessarily reflect the position of the tumor. The farther the tumor is from the bony landmarks used to localize it radiographically, the greater the possibility for error. To compensate for this distance, gold fiducial markers are placed in or as near to the tumor as possible because they can be easily seen on x-ray imaging. Park and colleagues[21] describe a technique by which gold fiducials are placed via fine-needle aspiration under endoscopic ultrasound.[21] Revealing only a 5% complication rate, the procedure was found to be safe and effective with a median of 5 implantations and a mean of 3 fiducials seen at the time of CT simulation, which was secondary to fiducial loss or migration. Percutaneous fiducial placement has also been reported.[22]

These many imaging advances, used alone or together, can decrease uncertainty when defining treatment volumes and increase accuracy when irradiating these volumes. Delivering radiation with better conformality allows physicians to safely treat smaller volumes to higher doses, a paradigm that is reaching its apotheosis in SABR.

INTENSITY-MODULATED RADIOTHERAPY

IMRT is a highly conformal radiation delivery method that uses a device known as the multileaf collimator (MLC) to dynamically shape radiation beams into varying patterns from multiple beam angles. IMRT represents an increase in complexity over 3-dimensional conformal radiotherapy where the modulation of the beam intensity is limited. In IMRT, more than 4 complex radiation fields are divided into dozens of smaller beamlets, each with an intensity that can be modulated by moving the MLC to achieve the desired dose distribution across the target volume. The main advantage of IMRT is that it provides more precise control over the target as well as normal-tissue dose distribution. The selection of the beamlets and their individual intensity modulations are determined by computer-based iterative optimization algorithms that satisfy dose limits to defined normal structures and provide adequate radiation delivery to the target.

IMRT allows highly precise gradients of dose to be deposited within tissue, for example, creating a sharp "drop off" of dose from the edge of a tumor to a critical nearby structure (**Fig. 2**). While IMRT allows for radiation doses to be delivered more precisely, it does not eliminate dose to normal tissues. In fact, it is often the case that a larger volume of at-risk tissue is irradiated using IMRT, albeit at a lower dose (also termed a *low-dose bath*). Whether this pattern of normal-tissue dosing has a similar threshold and manner of toxicity as that seen with older forms of treatment and how organs differ in their sensitivity to this type of irradiation are topics of ongoing clinical investigation.[23]

Another drawback to the high precision of IMRT is the potential for underdosing part of the intended target, termed a *marginal miss*, if portions of at-risk regions are not properly included in the target volume. Therefore, an understanding of anatomy and lymph node drainage, proper delineation of at-risk regions, and optimal visualization of the target are crucial to the successful delivery IMRT.

IMRT can decrease toxicity compared with 3DCRT without sacrificing disease control, while safely increasing the radiation dose to the tumor. No randomized trials

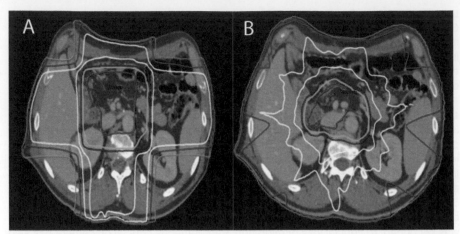

Fig. 2. A comparison of 3-dimensional conformal radiotherapy and IMRT in adjuvant radio-therapy for pancreatic cancer. (A) Three-dimensional conformal treatment plan for adjuvant radiotherapy after pancreatoduodenectomy. Prescribed dose 50.4 Gy in 28 fractions. Isodose lines are represented as follows: 50 Gy (red), 45 Gy (green), 40 Gy (blue), 30 Gy (white), 20 Gy (yellow), 10 Gy (magenta), 5 Gy (orange). (B) IMRT plan for the same patient prescribed to same dose. Isodose lines are represented as follows: 50 Gy (red), 45 Gy (green), 40 Gy (blue), 30 Gy (white), 20 Gy (yellow), 10 Gy (magenta), 5 Gy (orange). Note the higher degree of conformality at higher doses using IMRT, along with the larger area receiving low-dose radiation.

comparing IMRT and 3DCRT for pancreatic cancer have been performed, but early studies on the use of IMRT in chemoradiotherapy of pancreatic cancer have found acceptable levels of toxicity and tumor control.[24–26] A study from the University of Maryland showed significantly reduced acute gastrointestinal toxicity when patients were treated with IMRT-based chemoradiation compared with a similar group of patients treated with 3DCRT under a national protocol.[27] Dosimetric studies have also been performed that show significant sparing of the small bowel, liver, and kidneys using IMRT, with a coincident reduction in expected toxicity using radiobiological models of normal-tissue toxicity.[28] IMRT can be utilized for dose escalation, as seen in a dosimetric study by Brown and coworkers,[29] which demonstrated the ability of IMRT to deliver up to 64.8 Gy to pancreatic tumors without exceeding the radiation tolerance of liver, kidneys, small bowel, or spinal cord.

ARC THERAPY

Dynamic conformal arc therapy delivers radiation by rotating the gantry of a linac through 1 or more arcs with radiation delivered continuously. This type of treatment is analogous to positioning multiple static fields at equidistant angles around the patient. Using this technique, the MLC constantly conforms to the target shape as the gantry rotates around the patient, rapidly delivering radiation as it rotates. The concept of intensity modulation was subsequently added to arc therapy to create volumetric-modulated arc therapy (VMAT),[30–32] which further refines variations in machine dose rate and gantry speed, thereby optimizing treatment plans. VMAT algorithms were commercialized and made available under such names as RapidArc (Varian Medical Systems, Palo Alto, CA, USA) and SmartArc

(Philips, Amsterdam, The Netherlands).[33] Currently, no clinical studies have been performed using these techniques, so there is little clinical evidence that they are improving outcomes.

STEREOTACTIC ABLATIVE BODY RADIOTHERAPY

A technique born of the synthesis of all of the above-mentioned advances is SABR, also known as stereotactic body radiotherapy (SBRT). SBRT is probably best known as a promising treatment for early-stage, medically inoperable lung cancer[34] and metastatic lung lesions,[35] but its use is becoming far more widespread. SBRT has been applied to tumors in the liver, prostate, thyroid, kidney, pelvis, and pancreas.[36] SABR relies on the delivery of relatively few fractions (usually 1 to 5) of higher (ablative) doses of radiation. In contrast to conventionally fractionated radiotherapy (usually 5 fractions per week for 5–10 weeks), in which radiation doses are thought to be tumoricidal but below the threshold needed to cause irreparable damage to normal tissue, SABR doses are sufficiently high to permanently damage any tissue within the prescription dose area. Thus, a high degree of precision in both target definition and delivery are critical to delivering SABR safely and effectively.

Stereotactic radiosurgery was developed in the 1950s for the treatment of intracranial malignancies and other conditions. Stereotactic radiosurgery treatment has been successful because it can localize the tumor with great accuracy through rigid immobilization with a head frame attached to the patient's skull. The treatment of lesions outside the skull presents a more difficult problem, as targets are often in motion secondary to physiologic processes, such as respiration and normal organ hysteresis. Immobilization outside of the skull is also more difficult given the larger, irregular size of the body compared with the cranium and the inability to fix the immobilization frame to the body. Lax and colleagues[37] developed the first rigid immobilization system for the treatment of body lesions in the 1990s at the Karolinska Institute in Sweden. They used a vacuum pillow with high surface-area contact to immobilize the patient, abdominal compression to limit internal organ movement with respiration, and external reference markers to provide a stereotactic reference system. Since that time, additional improvements and modifications have been made in tumor imaging, image guidance and tumor tracking during treatment, and more rapid treatment delivery and respiratory compensation during irradiation, as described earlier.[37]

Many commercially available treatment devices are capable of delivering SABR. Common to all are advanced image guidance features for repositioning or tracking of the tumor in real time immediately before or during treatment. Treatment devices that utilize real-time tracking via orthogonal images taken during treatment include the Novalis Tx (BrainLAB AG, Feldkirchen, Germany) and Cyberknife (Accuray Inc, Sunnyvale, CA, USA). The patient is shifted during treatment to align with these images. The TomoTherapy Hi-Art System (Accuray Inc) delivers radiation slice by slice by moving the patient through the treatment machine slice-by-slice, similar to patient movement through a CT scanner. TomoTherapy differs from other forms of external-beam radiation therapy in which the entire tumor volume is irradiated at one time. The Varian Trilogy and TrueBeam (Varian Medical Systems, Palo Alto, CA, USA) as well as the Elekta Synergy (Elekta AB, Stockholm, Sweden) are linacs with a gantry-mounted CBCT scanner that allows imaging and repositioning just before treatment. Like TomoTherapy, these machines are capable of delivering modulated arc treatments (VMAT, IMAT, RapidArc).

Similar to other types of radiation delivery, respiratory motion of the tumor and day-to-day patient setup variation remain problems with SABR. However, these factors are even more important to address in SABR than in conventionally fraction-ated radiotherapy because the larger fraction sizes and fewer treatments can accentuate the consequences of a slight miss.

TECHNICAL CONSIDERATIONS

The current technique at Stanford University is to use respiratory-gated RapidArc™ for SABR treatments for patients with locally advanced unresectable pancreatic cancer. High-quality image guidance is necessary to ensure setup accuracy to minimize normal tissue radiation. Approximately 3 to 7 gold fiducial seeds are placed endoscopically in or near the tumor. The target volume is defined as the primary tumor plus a 1- to 3-mm margin for setup variability, and regional nodes are not included in the target. All normal adjacent structures are also outlined (ie, duodenum, stomach, small bowel, kidneys, liver, and spinal cord).

During treatment, kV imaging, including CBCT, is used to ensure the alignment of the fiducial markers to their respective positions as determined during the treatment planning process. Radiation is delivered using respiratory gating, in which the position of the fiducial markers will gate the beam when the markers are at the proper position, which is verified by fluoroscopy just before delivering the radiation. During fluoros-copy, the actual and intended positions of the markers can be visualized, thereby allowing adjustment of the respiratory gating system so that the beam is turned on when the markers are in the proper position and turned off otherwise (**Fig. 3**). Once marker position is verified, the treatment is delivered over 1 to 2 intensity-modulated arcs. The typical prescription dose is 33 Gy given in 5 daily fractions.

CLINICAL EVIDENCE

Studies by the Gastro-intestinal Study Group and others using conventionally fractionated external-beam radiation therapy in locally advanced pancreatic cancer

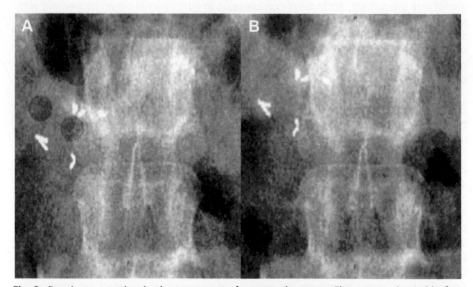

Fig. 3. Respiratory gating in the treatment of pancreatic cancer. Fluoroscopy is used before treatment delivery to track the respiratory motion of fiducial markers. During treatment, the beam is "off" during the designated portion of the respiratory cycle when the markers are outside the gating window (*A*) and "on" when the markers are inside the window (*B*).

Table 1
Selected studies using SABR to treat pancreatic cancer

Study	Patients	Dose	Local Control (%)	Distant Control (%)	Median Survival (mo)	Toxicity	Notes
Koong et al, 2004[39]	15 LA/LR	15–25 Gy × 1	80	0	11	33% grade 1–2 0% ≥ grade 3	Dose escalation
Koong et al, 2005[41]	16 LA	25 Gy × 1 (boost)	94	0	8.3	69% grade 1–2 12.5% ≥ grade 3	IMRT is given before CRT (45 Gy)
Hoyer et al, 2005[40]	22 LA	15 Gy × 3	57	13	5.4	79% ≥ grade 2 4.5% grade 4	
Didolkar et al, 2010[43]	85 LA/LR	5–10 Gy × 3	91.7	24	18.6	22.3% ≥ grade 3	
Mahadevan et al, 2010[44]	36 LA	8–12 Gy × 3	78	22	14.3	33% grade 1–2 8% grade 3	
Polistina et al, 2010[46]	23 LA	10 Gy × 3	82	NR	10.6	20% grade 1 0% ≥ grade 2	
Mahadevan et al, 2011[45]	39 LA	8–12 Gy × 3	85	46	20	41% grade 1–2 0% > grade 3	Induction gemcitabine
Rwigema et al, 2011[47]	71 LA, LR, RPM, MD	24 Gy (median) × 1 (94%) 20–24 Gy × 2–3 (6%)	71.7	NR	10.3	39.5% grade 1–2 4.2% grade 3	
Schellenberg et al, 2011[50]	20 LA	25 Gy × 1	94	15	11.8	15% grade 1–2 5% ≥ grade 3	Induction gemcitabine

Abbreviations: CRT, chemoradiotherapy; LA, locally advanced; LR, locally recurrent; MD, metastatic disease; NR, not reported; RPM, resected positive margins.

have noted a high rate of local failure (approaching 60%),[38] suggesting that dose escalation, such as that capable with SABR, may provide a benefit in the treatment of pancreatic cancer by enhancing local control.

The first experience using SABR in the treatment of pancreatic tumors was published in 2004 at Stanford University. This phase I dose escalation trial treated 15 patients with single-fraction doses of 15, 20, or 25 Gy delivered via the Cyberknife.[39] Despite a local control rate of 100% and minimal toxicity (grade 2, 20%), metastatic disease subsequently developed in all patients, and median survival was 11 months. In contrast, a phase II study from Denmark used 30 Gy in 3 fractions and reported a local control rate of only 57% and much higher toxicity, with 18% of patients experiencing "severe" GI mucositis and 4.5% experiencing gastric perforation. The differences in local control may be attributable to the fractionation scheme, resulting in a lower biologically effective dose, and the toxicity may be caused by a larger treatment volume definition that encompassed both the tumor and surrounding edema.[40] The contrast of these 2 studies shows the need for further investigations into the optimal dose, fractionation, and normal tissue constraints for this aggressive malignancy.

With the goal of improving overall outcomes, the investigators at Stanford University combined a stereotactic boost of 25 Gy delivered after a conventional course of chemoradiotherapy to 45 Gy with concurrent 5-fluorouracil[41] and, in a separate study, also investigated SABR combined with gemcitabine chemotherapy.[42] These studies again demonstrated excellent local control with high rates of metastatic disease. Additional studies have been published on the early experience of SABR for pancreas cancer (**Table 1**).[43–49] Similar to the results seen with SABR of tumors in other organs, local control appears to be excellent, but toxicity remains a concern. In addition, survival has not significantly improved, indicating the need for better systemic therapy.

Future investigations are needed in regard to optimizing the risk/benefit profile and reducing the risk of treatment-related morbidity. However, SABR represents an attractive treatment modality primarily because (1) it can be given in much less time to minimize interruption with systemic chemotherapy delivery, (2) it is much more convenient for patients who spend less time receiving radiation, and (3) it can deliver potentially more intensive and effective radiation to enhance local control.

SUMMARY

Radiation therapy is a rapidly evolving field, and recent technical advances have spurred an increasing number of new treatments as well as marked improvements in previously existing treatments. Despite a growing body of published evidence demonstrating that radiotherapy for the treatment of pancreatic cancer is improving in efficacy and safety, the ultimate effect on patient outcomes remains to be seen. It is an unfortunate fact that the majority of pancreatic cancer patients will ultimately have metastases and succumb to distant disease. Thus, improvements in local tumor control engendered by these recent advances will have little impact on overall survival without the coincident development of better systemic treatment regimens.

REFERENCES

1. Jemal A, Siegel R, Xu J, et al. Cancer statistics. 2010. CA Cancer J Clin 2010;60(5): 277–300.
2. Vincent A, Herman J, Schulick R, et al. Pancreatic cancer. Lancet 2011;378(9791): 607–20.

3. Saif MW. Pancreatic neoplasm in 2011: an update. JOP 2011;12(4):316–21.

4. Wagner M, Redaelli C, Lietz M, et al. Curative resection is the single most important factor determining outcome in patients with pancreatic adenocarcinoma. Br J Surg 2004;91(5):586–94.

5. Abbott DE, Baker MS, Talamonti MS. Neoadjuvant therapy for pancreatic cancer: a current review. J Surg Oncol 2010;101(4):315–20.

6. Kalser MH, Ellenberg SS. Pancreatic cancer. Adjuvant combined radiation and chemotherapy following curative resection. Arch Surg 1985;120(8):899–903.

7. Regine WF, Winter KA, Abrams R, et al. Fluorouracil-based chemoradiation with either gemcitabine or fluorouracil chemotherapy after resection of pancreatic adenocarcinoma: 5-year analysis of the U.S. Intergroup/RTOG 9704 phase III trial. Ann Surg Oncol 2011;18(5):1319–26.

8. Smeenk HG, van Eijck CH, Hop WC, et al. Long-term survival and metastatic pattern of pancreatic and periampullary cancer after adjuvant chemoradiation or observation: long-term results of EORTC trial 40891. Ann Surg 2007;246(5):734–40.

9. Neoptolemos JP, Stocken DD, Dunn JA, et al. Influence of resection margins on survival for patients with pancreatic cancer treated by adjuvant chemoradiation and/or chemotherapy in the ESPAC-1 randomized controlled trial. Ann Surg 2001;234(6):758–68.

10. Oettle H, Post S, Neuhaus P, et al. Adjuvant chemotherapy with gemcitabine vs observation in patients undergoing curative-intent resection of pancreatic cancer: a randomized controlled trial. JAMA 2007;297(3):267–77.

11. Neoptolemos JP, Stocken DD, Bassi C, et al. Adjuvant chemotherapy with fluorouracil plus folinic acid vs gemcitabine following pancreatic cancer resection: a randomized controlled trial. JAMA 2010;304(10):1073–81.

12. Willett CG, Czito BG. Chemoradiotherapy in gastrointestinal malignancies. Clin Oncol (R Coll Radiol) 2009;21(7):543–56.

13. Palta M, Willett C, Czito B. Role of radiation therapy in patients with resectable pancreatic cancer. Oncology (Williston Park) 2011;25(8):715–21,727.

14. Aloia TA, Lee JE, Vauthey JN, et al. Delayed recovery after pancreaticoduodenectomy: a major factor impairing the delivery of adjuvant therapy? J Am Coll Surg 2007;204(3):347–55.

15. Arvold ND, Niemierko A, Mamon HJ, et al. Pancreatic cancer tumor size on CT scan versus pathologic specimen: implications for radiation treatment planning. Int J Radiat Oncol Biol Phys 2011;80(5):1383–90.

16. Ford EC, Herman J, Yorke E, et al. 18F-FDG PET/CT for image-guided and intensity-modulated radiotherapy. J Nucl Med 2009;50(10):1655–65.

17. Murphy JD, Christman-Skieller C, Kim J, et al. A dosimetric model of duodenal toxicity after stereotactic body radiotherapy for pancreatic cancer. Int J Radiat Oncol Biol Phys 2010;78(5):1420–6.

18. Schellenberg D, Quon A, Minn AY, et al. 18Fluorodeoxyglucose PET is prognostic of progression-free and overall survival in locally advanced pancreas cancer treated with stereotactic radiotherapy. Int J Radiat Oncol Biol Phys 2010;77(5):1420–5.

19. Bussels B, Goethals L, Feron M, et al. Respiration-induced movement of the upper abdominal organs: a pitfall for the three-dimensional conformal radiation treatment of pancreatic cancer. Radiother Oncol 2003;68(1):69–74.

20. Chang SD, Main W, Martin DP, et al. An analysis of the accuracy of the CyberKnife: a robotic frameless stereotactic radiosurgical system. Neurosurgery 2003;52(1):140–6 [discussion: 146–7].

21. Park WG, Yan BM, Schellenberg D, et al. EUS-guided gold fiducial insertion for image-guided radiation therapy of pancreatic cancer: 50 successful cases without fluoroscopy. Gastrointest Endosc 2010;71(3):513–8.

22. Kothary N, Dieterich S, Louie JD, et al. Percutaneous implantation of fiducial markers for imaging-guided radiation therapy. AJR Am J Roentgenol 2009;192(4):1090–6.

23. Taremi M, Ringash J, Dawson LA. Upper abdominal malignancies: intensity-modulated radiation therapy. Front Radiat Ther Oncol 2007;40:272–88.

24. Landry JC, Yang GY, Ting JY, et al. Treatment of pancreatic cancer tumors with intensity-modulated radiation therapy (IMRT) using the volume at risk approach (VARA): employing dose-volume histogram (DVH) and normal tissue complication probability (NTCP) to evaluate small bowel toxicity. Med Dosim 2002;27(2):121–9.

25. Milano MT, Chmura SJ, Garofalo MC, et al. Intensity-modulated radiotherapy in treatment of pancreatic and bile duct malignancies: toxicity and clinical outcome. Int J Radiat Oncol Biol Phys 2004;59(2):445–53.

26. Ben-Josef E, Shields AF, Vaishampayan U, et al. Intensity-modulated radiotherapy (IMRT) and concurrent capecitabine for pancreatic cancer. Int J Radiat Oncol Biol Phys 2004;59(2):454–9.

27. Yovino S, Poppe M, Jabbour S, et al. Intensity-modulated radiation therapy significantly improves acute gastrointestinal toxicity in pancreatic and ampullary cancers. Int J Radiat Oncol Biol Phys 2011;79(1):158–62.

28. Bockbrader M, Kim E. Role of intensity-modulated radiation therapy in gastrointestinal cancer. Expert Rev Anticancer Ther 2009;9(5):637–47.

29. Brown MW, Ning H, Arora B, et al. A dosimetric analysis of dose escalation using two intensity-modulated radiation therapy techniques in locally advanced pancreatic carcinoma. Int J Radiat Oncol Biol Phys 2006;65(1):274–83.

30. Yu CX, Tang G. Intensity-modulated arc therapy: principles, technologies and clinical implementation. Physics in medicine and biology 2011;56(5):R31–54.

31. Duthoy W, De Gersem W, Vergote K, et al. Clinical implementation of intensity-modulated arc therapy (IMAT) for rectal cancer. International journal of radiation oncology, biology, physics 2004;60(3):794–806.

32. Yu CX, Li XA, Ma L, et al. Clinical implementation of intensity-modulated arc therapy. International journal of radiation oncology, biology, physics 2002;53(2):453–63.

33. Yu CX, Tang G. Intensity-modulated arc therapy: principles, technologies and clinical implementation. Phys Med Biol 2011;56(5):R31–54.

34. Timmerman R, Paulus R, Galvin J, et al. Stereotactic body radiation therapy for inoperable early stage lung cancer. JAMA 2010;303(11):1070–6.

35. Rusthoven KE, Kavanagh BD, Cardenes H, et al. Multi-institutional phase I/II trial of stereotactic body radiation therapy for liver metastases. J Clin Oncol 2009;27(10):1572–8.

36. Nagata Y, Wulf J, Lax I, et al. Stereotactic radiotherapy of primary lung cancer and other targets: results of consultant meeting of the International Atomic Energy Agency. Int J Radiat Oncol Biol Phys 2011;79(3):660–9.

37. Lax I, Blomgren H, Naslund I, et al. Stereotactic radiotherapy of malignancies in the abdomen: methodological aspects. Acta Oncol 1994;33:677–83.

38. Willett CG, Czito BG, Bendell JC, et al. Locally advanced pancreatic cancer. J Clin Oncol 2005;23(20):4538–44.

39. Koong AC, Le QT, Ho A, et al. Phase I study of stereotactic radiosurgery in patients with locally advanced pancreatic cancer. Int J Radiat Oncol Biol Phys 2004;58(4):1017–21.

40. Hoyer M, Roed H, Sengelov L, et al. Phase-II study on stereotactic radiotherapy of locally advanced pancreatic carcinoma. Radiother Oncol 2005;76(1):48–53.

41. Koong AC, Christofferson E, Le QT, et al. Phase II study to assess the efficacy of conventionally fractionated radiotherapy followed by a stereotactic radiosurgery boost in patients with locally advanced pancreatic cancer. Int J Radiat Oncol Biol Phys 2005;63(2):320–3.
42. Schellenberg D, Goodman KA, Lee F, et al. Gemcitabine chemotherapy and single-fraction stereotactic body radiotherapy for locally advanced pancreatic cancer. Int J Radiat Oncol Biol Phys 2008;72(3):678–86.
43. Didolkar MS, Coleman CW, Brenner MJ, et al. Image-guided stereotactic radiosurgery for locally advanced pancreatic adenocarcinoma results of first 85 patients. J Gastrointest Surg 2010;14(10):1547–59.
44. Mahadevan A, Jain S, Goldstein M, et al. Stereotactic body radiotherapy and gemcitabine for locally advanced pancreatic cancer. Int J Radiat Oncol Biol Phys 2010;78(3):735–42.
45. Mahadevan A, Miksad R, Goldstein M, et al. Induction gemcitabine and stereotactic body radiotherapy for locally advanced nonmetastatic pancreas cancer. Int J Radiat Oncol Biol Phys 2011;81(4):e615–22.
46. Polistina F, Costantin G, Casamassima F, et al. Unresectable locally advanced pancreatic cancer: a multimodal treatment using neoadjuvant chemoradiotherapy (gemcitabine plus stereotactic radiosurgery) and subsequent surgical exploration. Ann Surg Oncol 2010;17(8):2092–101.
47. Rwigema JC, Parikh SD, Heron DE, et al. Stereotactic body radiotherapy in the treatment of advanced adenocarcinoma of the pancreas. Am J Clin Oncol 2011;34(1):63–9.
48. Chang BW, Saif MW. Stereotactic body radiation therapy (SBRT) in pancreatic cancer: is it ready for prime time? JOP 2008;9(6):676–82.
49. Minn AY, Koong AC, Chang DT. Stereotactic body radiation therapy for gastrointestinal malignancies. Front Radiat Ther Oncol 2011;43:412–27.
50. Schellenberg D, Kim J, Christman-Skieller C, et al. Single-fraction stereotactic body radiation therapy and sequential gemcitabine for the treatment of locally advanced pancreatic cancer. Int J Radiat Oncol Biol Phys 2011;81(1):181–8.

Endoscopic Palliation of Pancreatic Cancer

Simon K. Lo, MD[a,b,]*

KEYWORDS

- Pancreatic adenocarcinoma • Palliation
- Biliary decompression • Intestinal stenting
- Celiac plexus neurolysis • Fiducial placement

Pancreatic adenocarcinoma is the fourth leading cause of cancer death in the United States, with a 5-year survival rate of 5.6%.[1] One third of pancreatic cancer patients have local or regional disease at the time the diagnosis is made.[2] The majority of patients are treated with palliation in mind. With the rapid expansion of endoscopic technology, our ability to palliate symptoms of pancreatic cancer has improved significantly over the years.

More than 90% of cancers of the pancreas are ductal adenocarcinomas. Neuroendocrine and intraductal papillary mucinous neoplasm (IPMN) cancers make up the remainder of the malignant diseases of the pancreas.[3] Because of the biological differences between these cancers, their symptoms and presentations may vary significantly. Adenocarcinomas may present early by obstructing the common bile duct, but at the late stages they cause pain and duodenal obstruction. IPMN cancers may cause gastric, duodenal, or biliary fistulae or obstruction of the adjacent organs. Neuroendocrine cancers enlarge slowly as a locally confined disease but may cause jaundice due to extensive liver metastasis or compression of the common hepatic duct with lymph node metastasis. As a result, the modes of palliation differ greatly depending on the nature of these cancers. For instance, the short life spans of patients with adenocarcinoma make endoscopic biliary stenting an appropriate palliative option for obstructive jaundice. On the other hand, a neuroendocrine cancer of the head of the pancreas in a young patient is better palliated by a Whipple resection or surgical biliary bypass. Although a 10-mm-caliber biliary stent is the standard for palliation of adenocarcinoma-related biliary obstruction, it is frequently too small to remain patent or too easy to dislodge within a very large bile duct that is obstructed by the copious, thick mucin of an IPMN cancer. In this case a large-caliber esophageal stent or multiple 10-mm biliary metal stents placed side by side may

---

The author has nothing to disclose.
[a] Cedars-Sinai Medical Center, 8700 Beverly Boulevard, Room 7511, Los Angeles, CA 90048, USA
[b] David Geffen School of Medicine at UCLA, Los Angeles, CA 90095, USA
* Cedars-Sinai Medical Center, 8700 Beverly Boulevard, Room 7511, Los Angeles, CA 90048.
E-mail address: simon.lo@cshs.org

Gastroenterol Clin N Am 41 (2012) 237–253
doi:10.1016/j.gtc.2011.12.005
0889-8553/12/$ – see front matter © 2012 Elsevier Inc. All rights reserved.

Table 1	
Pancreatic malignancy related conditions with possible endoscopic therapies	
Condition	Endoscopic Therapy[a]
Biliary obstruction	
Simple obstruction	ERCP + biliary stenting
Biliary + duodenal obstruction	Biliary + luminal stenting
Obstruction with failed ampullary access	EUS + rendezvous biliary stenting
Gastroduodenal obstruction	Luminal stenting
	Percutaneous gastrostomy drainage
Cancer pain	
Common cancer pain	Celiac nerve block
Pancreatic duct obstruction	Pancreatic stenting
Gastrointestinal bleeding	
Mild to moderate	Endoscopic hemostasis
Severe	Probably none
Postoperative complications	
Afferent limb obstruction	Luminal stenting
Biliary obstruction	Biliary stenting
Pancreaticojejunostomy stricture	Pancreatic ductal dilation and stenting
Pancreatic fistula	Pancreatic stenting ± sphincterotomy
Bleeding: Mild to moderate	Endoscopic hemostasis
Bleeding: Severe	Probably none
Jejunal adhesion-obstruction	Luminal dilation or stenting
Local tumor growth	Fiducial placement

[a] Includes only procedures that are not considered strictly experimental.

provide the best palliation.[4] There are currently many endoscopic options to manage symptoms of pancreatic cancer (**Table 1**).

THE BASIC PRINCIPLE OF PALLIATION

According to the American Cancer Society website, the goal of palliative care is to prevent and relieve suffering and support the best possible quality of life for patients and their families, regardless of the state of the disease. An effective palliation of a cancer is a precisely delivered intervention that brings about prompt symptom relief without incurring serious complications, enormous costs, or redundant treatment. The minimally invasive nature of endoscopy is particularly suited to help pancreatic cancer patients live a good quality life. For obstructive jaundice, stenting with a plastic catheter to relieve biliary obstruction improves liver function, removes the social embarrassment of a yellow appearance, and promotes better appetite and energy. However, metal stenting is preferred if the patient is expected to live longer than 3 months because metal stenting avoids repeated endoscopic retrograde cholangio-pancreatography (ERCP) sessions for stent exchange. The longer duration of stent patency also means less need to visit the doctor's office and undergo blood tests and procedures. In pain management, a mild case of abdominal pain is best treated with the common analgesics on an as-needed basis. However, disabling and constant pain may be better palliated with a slow-release, high-dose narcotic or even celiac neurolysis. As treating physicians, we should constantly assess what is the best way to palliate patients based on proven outcomes, the patient's wish, and our technical ability.

BILIARY OBSTRUCTION

Approximately 70% of pancreatic adenocarcinomas are located in the head region. Some degree of biliary compression may eventually occur in most patients with pancreatic adenocarcinoma; therefore, biliary decompression is the best-known form of pancreatic cancer palliation. At one time, surgical biliary bypass, such as chole-cystojejunostomy or hepaticojejunostomy, was the treatment standard for obstructive jaundice; however, it has largely been replaced by endoscopic stenting because of comparable survivals and effectiveness in relieving jaundice.[5] Procedure-related morbidities are either the same or in favor of endoscopic stenting.[6-8]

Types of Plastic Stents

Most of today's plastic stents are made of a polyethylene material. These stents come in external diameters that range from 5 french to 11.5 french. The most popular stent caliber for distal biliary decompression is 10 french and the most desirable lengths are 7 cm and 10 cm. Both the straight Amsterdam style and double pigtail stents are commercially available for biliary drainage, but virtually all endoscopists choose the straight stents because of their better patency performance relative to the pigtail stents. A single flap near each end of the straight stents provides the anchorage necessary to hold them in place. Unsatisfied with the typical 3-month patency of the polyethylene stents, the Hamburg group introduced a Teflon stent to take advantage of its lower coefficient of friction, compared to common plastic stents, and smaller chance of clogging without any sideholes. This new product was thought to be the ideal plastic stent and the early results showed it to be patent for a median duration of 64 weeks.[9] However, the enthusiasm toward this specially designed stent waned quickly as a randomized prospective study that compared the Tannenbaum Teflon stent to conventional polyethylene stents showed no difference in mean 90-day stent patency.[10]

Plastic Stenting Technique

Plastic stenting begins with guidewire passage through the stricture. A biliary sphincterotomy is not typically required for insertion of a single plastic stent. Likewise, stricture dilation is not usually required for placement of a single plastic stent except when there is an extremely tight blockage; in that case a 4-mm or 6-mm over-the-wire balloon dilator may be used. The length of the stent is selected by estimating the distance between the top of the stricture and the papilla against a known dimension, such as the width of the duodenoscope, based on fluoroscopic assessment. An alternative is to measure the distance of a catheter that has been pulled back from the top of the stricture to the papilla. The plastic stent is then loaded onto the tip of a delivery device. There are three types of stent delivery devices, but they all have an inner guiding catheter and a shorter external pusher catheter. Once the inner catheter has securely passed the stricture, the pusher is advanced forward to push the stent up the bile duct until it reaches the desired location. The guiding catheter and the guidewire are then removed, leaving the stent in place. There are two commercially available modified stenting devices that allow simultaneous removal of the stent and device while leaving the guidewire in place, in case a decision is made to retrieve the stent.

Metallic Stenting

The first commercially available metal biliary stent was introduced in 1989. It was made of individual stainless steel wires that were twined together. One of the first studies reported effectiveness of the 10-mm caliber metal stents without significant problems.[11] A comparison between metallic and plastic stents showed that the median duration of patency (273 days) of the metal stent was significantly longer than that of a polyethylene stent (126 days).[12] However, the overall median survival was 149 days and did not differ significantly between the plastic and metal stent groups. Not only were metallic stents more patent over time than plastic stents, but they were also associated with less cholangitis, shorter duration of hospitalization, and less overall costs than plastic stents.[13] A meta-analysis was performed to analyze seven randomized controlled trials that aimed to compare plastic and metal stents. In total, 724 patients were randomized into one of the treatment arms. The meta-analysis showed that metallic stents were associated with a significantly reduced risk of stent occlusion at 4 months and a lower overall risk of recurrent biliary obstruction.[14] This analysis also showed that the metal stents were more cost effective, as the additional ERCP accounted for substantial cost. But a recent Korean study demonstrated that even in countries where ERCP costs were lower than those of metal stents, metal biliary stents were still the first-line treatment because they offered better palliation without adding a significant cost in palliating the malignant biliary obstruction.[15] Hence, these studies provided strong support for the practice of metal stenting as the first-line palliative modality for malignant biliary obstruction that is typically caused by pancreatic carcinoma. However, these stents were appropriate only when treating definitively unresectable cancers because the strong adherence of these open mesh stents to the biliary tissue made them difficult to remove from the bile duct during dissection and creation of surgical anastomoses.

Early self-expanding metal stents had no covers to prevent tissue penetration through the wire mesh. Indeed, stent failures were noted to be caused by tumor ingrowth across the metal wires.[12] Reactive hyperplastic reactions may also occur at either end of the stent where it is in close contact with the biliary or duodenal tissue.[16] Creating a barrier to tissue ingrowth and, in turn, prolonging stent patency was the driving force that led to the development of partially covered stents.[17] Today, several partially covered metal stents are available. The short, uncovered ends of these stents are designed to provide adherence to the biliary tissue whereas the large, covered portion provides protection from tissue penetration into the stent lumen.

Even though the partially covered stents were designed to prevent tumor ingrowth, occasionally they are still difficult to remove. As neoadjuvant therapy for tumor downstaging and surgical resection becomes an increasingly common practice, the ease of removing these stents is an important consideration in the selection of a metal stent. Fully covered stents became available a few years ago and their removal at the time of a pancreaticoduodenectomy became feasible in virtually all patients.[18]

Multiple studies have compared covered to uncovered metal stents in palliating malignant biliary obstruction. Yoon and colleagues found no significant differences in stent patency at 100, 200, 300, and 400 days between the two groups of metal stents.[19] A randomized trial showed that the median time to recurrent biliary obstruction was 711 days for the uncovered and 357 days for the partially covered self-expanding metal stents.[20] In addition, serious adverse events occurred significantly more frequently with the partially covered stents than with the uncovered stents (62% vs 44%, $P<.05$), mainly due to stent migration (12% vs 0, $P<.01$). Further, a European study that enrolled 400 patients and randomized them to covered or uncovered stents showed no significant differences in stent patency, patient survival, or complication rates between the two groups.[21] The metal stents used in this study were made by a different manufacturer from the metal stents used in the other trials, but the conclusions of these independent studies were identical, disputing any potential advantage of the covered metal stents over their uncovered counterparts. Even though there are the suspicions that the stent cover would contribute to cholecystitis and pancreatitis, there is no evidence that it is the case.[17]

Endoscopic Ultrasound-Guided Bile Duct Stenting

When the bile duct cannot be accessed through the papilla, or when the duodenum is completely obstructed by a large pancreatic tumor, an interventional radiologist or a surgeon is enlisted to perform a drainage or bypass procedure. However, endoscopic ultrasound (EUS) allows gastrointestinal interventionists to puncture the bile duct directly from the duodenal bulb or stomach. This allows the possibility to insert a guidewire pass the stricture and the major papilla to perform biliary stenting and this technique is commonly referred to as the endoscopic or EUS rendezvous procedure.[22,23] Roughly two-thirds of the cases attempted in this manner were reported to be successful in draining the obstructed bile duct, ending with biliary stents crossing the major papillae. EUS-guided choledochoduodenostomy[24–26] and EUS-guided hepatogastrostomy[27,28] have been performed when the duodenum or major papilla cannot be accessed. Plastic or metal stents were inserted directly across the duodenum or stomach into the extrahepatic or intrahepatic bile duct. These highly invasive procedures demand great technical skills and clinical experience and should not be regarded as standard treatment options at the present time.

Drug-Eluting Biliary Stents

Taking biliary stenting one step further, experimental treatment of malignant stricture with drug-eluting metallic stents has been proposed to extend the duration of biliary patency. Paclitaxel, a chemotherapeutic agent, was mixed in a liquid form with polyurethane and tetrahydrofuran to create a stent membrane that slowly released paclitaxel.[29] A low serum level of paclitaxel could be detected in patients stented for longer than 50 days.[29] The mean patency of these covered, paclitaxel-eluting stents was 429 days in 21 patients with unresectable malignant biliary obstruction. This seemingly prolonged patency may serve as supporting evidence to further develop drug-eluting stents in the future.

Metal Stenting Technique

The technique of metal stent placement is similar to that for plastic stenting, although there are some key differences. The first step is to pass a wire across the stricture. As with plastic stenting, dilating a distal bile duct stricture is rarely necessary. Most commercially available metal stents have markings on the proximal and distal ends to guide deployment. Some even have a "point of no return" radio-opaque mark that denotes the position of stent release beyond which the stent cannot be recaptured in case it is necessary to adjust the stenting position. The stainless steel alloy material of some stents is radio-opaque and all wire elements can be seen on fluoroscopy. However, nitinol-based wires are not radio-dense and therefore are marked with radio-opaque spots that are typically placed on both ends of the stents to guide stent release. Virtually all these stents have the tendency to propel forward during deployment; therefore, it is crucial to open up the stent very slowly to avoid inadvertent placement of the entire stent above the stricture. Gradual pullback of the stent is typically needed to compensate for the upward thrust of these stents during deployment. Shortening of the stents is also common as they are allowed to expand. Virtually all metal stents show a temporary waist at the point of maximal obstruction that disappears gradually over the next few days as the stents expand to their full calibers. Although there is no scientific evidence of how the covered metal stents spontaneously migrate, it is logical to assume that the unidirectional expansive force contributes to stent movement. Therefore, if one side of the waist is larger and longer than the other side, there will be the tendency for the stent to shift toward the side that is already more expanded. If a partially or fully covered stent is used, it is best to place the stent such that the waist is located in the center of the stent.

GASTRODUODENAL OBSTRUCTION

Duodenal obstruction eventually occurs in 10% to 20% of patients with pancreatic head cancer.[30] Ampullary cancer and neuroendocrine cancers also tend to involve the duodenum. Because the duodenum is rarely compressed in the initial presentation, most patients with duodenal obstruction are not candidates for curative surgery. As in most malignant obstructions of the gastrointestinal tract, balloon dilation does not produce any lasting improvement of the obstructive symptoms.

Metallic stenting is currently the endoscopic palliation modality of choice. These stents are constructed very similarly to those for the biliary tract, except that they are typically longer (6–12 cm) and of larger calibers (18–23 mm). To prevent spontaneous migration and to avoid compression of the ampullary opening, the stents are uncovered. Duodenal stenting requires some experience and technical skill, but is generally easy to complete. In a four-center study that involved 176 patients with mostly pancreatic cancer obstruction of the gastric outlet and duodenum, stenting was feasible in all patients.[31] Eighty-four percent of these patients were able to resume oral intake for a median of 146 days. The value of duodenal stenting is best demonstrated in a study in which 17 of 25 patients with pancreatic cancer and outlet obstruction were treated with surgical gastrojejunostomy.[32] This group of patients survived for a median duration of 64 days, but their postoperative stay was 15 days. In contrast, six patients received palliation with the Wallstents; they survived 111 days and their postprocedure hospital stay was 4 days. One key advantage of stenting over surgical bypass is avoiding postoperative delayed gastric emptying, which occurred in 59% of the surgical patients. Although other authors did not report such a high rate of delayed gastric emptying, a significant delay in the resumption of oral intake and prolonged hospital stays are still common.[33,34]

It has been suggested that inserting a large-bore gastrostomy tube may be an effective alternative to duodenal stenting when placing a stent is not feasible.[35] Although effective in preventing gastric distention and vomiting, gastrostomy tube decompression is a poor form of palliation of gastric outlet obstruction because of the inability to eat and the required separate feeding jejunostomy or total parenteral nutrition. In the hands of an experienced endoscopist, ineffective duodenal stent decompression may arise only in patients with carcinomatosis, underlying gastric dysmotility, or additional downstream intestinal blockages.

Intestinal Stenting Technique

The technique of intestinal stenting is very similar to biliary stenting, as most of the placement requires endoscopic and fluoroscopic guidance. The procedure must be performed with a large-channeled endoscope, such as a therapeutic upper endoscope or a therapeutic duodenoscope, to allow for passing the stenting device through the instrument channel. On rare occasions, the endoscope can be advanced across the stricture. This allows the inspection of the duodenal wall and placement of a stiff guidewire into the proximal jejunum. More commonly, the endoscope is too large to get through the stricture. In that case, a guidewire in combination with an ERCP catheter allows for injection of contrast to estimate the length of the stricture, while at the same time placing the guidewire. It is preferred that the wire is securely inserted into the proximal jejunum because of the long, stiff leading tip of the stenting device. It is also important to determine if the major papilla is affected by the stent, as postprocedure cholangitis has been noted in 6% of patients.[31] It is always preferred to place the stent clear of the major papilla, but it is not always possible. If the patient also presents with jaundice, a metallic biliary stent placement should be attempted before placement of the duodenal stent. Combined duodenal and biliary stenting has been reported to be successful in 91% of the cases.[36] Very gentle manipulations and excellent ERCP skill are needed in this situation, as it is difficult to approach the major papilla within a tight space. Duodenal perforation is a serious concern because of the possible need to dilate the stricture and then negotiate through it with a side-viewing endoscope. If the stricture is very tight, it may be best to first place the duodenal stent and then perform a transhepatic procedure to insert the biliary stent.

It is also important to avoid resting the ends of the duodenal stent at the corners, such as the duodenal bulb, junction between the second and third portions of the duodenum, and the ligament of Treitz. The duodenal folds in these corners can cover the stent lumen and render the stent ineffective in palliating obstructive symptoms. Mechanical irritation of the intestinal mucosa at these locations may eventually cause bleeding or perforation. Using a stent with smooth or soft ends may also prevent these delayed complications. In deploying the stent, it is important to know the extent of stent shortening during and after its release from the device. Fluoroscopic and endoscopic monitoring is important in achieving optimal stent placement.

POSTOPERATIVE INTESTINAL OBSTRUCTION

Afferent limb obstruction after a Whipple procedure may present as cholangitis, jaundice, pain, or nonspecific discomfort. The median time from pancreaticoduodenectomy to presentation may be as long as 1.2 years.[37] Most of these cases are caused by cancer recurrence, although radiation stricture or kinks caused by adhesions may be the cause as well. Patients with this condition usually have advanced disease and wish to receive a minimal treatment. Endoscopic stenting with a large-caliber (18–22 mm diameter) intestinal stent is a simple way to palliate this condition.[38] However, a variety of treatment modalities have been used, including balloon dilation and plastic or metallic biliary stent placement, alone or in combination. The results of such palliation are quite variable, ranging from immediate relief to persistent symptoms until death.[37]

DISABLING ABDOMINAL AND BACK PAIN

Pain is typically a late symptom of pancreatic cancer but can be a very difficult problem to manage. Even the most intensive narcotic analgesics may fail to control the discomfort. When conventional analgesic therapy becomes ineffective, or when a patient cannot tolerate the side effects of heavy doses of narcotics, an alternative treatment modality is typically desperately needed. As pancreatic stenting became technically feasible, endoscopists began to report that pancreatic ductal stenting might improve pancreatic cancer pain due to ductal obstruction.[39] It has been suggested that pancreatic duct stenting plays a role in 15% of pancreatic cancer pain.[40] Carr-Locke and colleagues proposed that pain brought on by oral intake might be best treated in this manner.[41] The plastic stents used for ductal decompression for pain control ranged from 7 french to 10 french in caliber.[40] Some authors even proposed using metallic stents for pain control.[41,42] The risk of acute and chronic pancreatitis is a genuine concern in treating patients who are already suffering a great deal from their incurable cancer. Limited available data show that about 60% of carefully chosen patients with successful pancreatic stent placement will experience significant resolution of pain and that another 20% to 25% of patients will be able to decrease their use of narcotics.[40] But the series that reported success of stenting are few and small, and the limited evidence cannot be used to support its widespread use.

A more proven and less invasive procedure to control pancreatic cancer pain when narcotic analgesics fail is neurolytic celiac nerve blocks. Patients with cancer in the head of pancreas may experience significantly more benefit in pain control than those with cancer in the body or tail of the pancreas. In one study using fluoroscopy or computed tomography (CT)-guided percutaneous neurolysis, 92% of 36 patients with cancer in the head of pancreas achieved improvement of pain, with a mean duration of relief of 119 days.[43] In contrast, only 29% of 14 patients with body and tail lesions experienced relief for a duration of 65 days. As expected, patients with a large tumor load do not have satisfactory pain control.

There are at least three routes of delivering celiac block or neurolysis: percutaneous, operative, and endoscopic. When performed endoscopically, ultrasound guidance is used. For cancer pain control, the objective is permanent damage of the nerve ganglia; therefore, alcohol is used to achieve neurolysis. By far, the most common route of treatment today is the percutaneous method. There are few studies that address the superiority of one method over the other. Gress and colleagues published a small randomized, prospective series on the treatment of chronic pancreatitis pain with celiac nerve block using bupivacaine and triamcinolone comparing the effectiveness of pain control between the CT and EUS-guided blocks.[44] While pain control of chronic pancreatitis cannot be regarded as the same as that for cancer pain, this study showed that the EUS-guided method provided significantly more persistent pain relief than the CT technique. A meta-analysis evaluated the results of percutaneous celiac neurolysis for pancreatic cancer based on five randomized controlled trials.[45] A total of 302 patients were evaluated. Compared with control patients who were treated with nonsteroidal anti-inflammatory drugs (NSAIDs) and narcotics, patients treated with neurolysis had lower pain scores and opioid usage at 2, 4, and 8 weeks. The patients in the neurolysis arm also reported a reduction in constipation. While most studies reported improvement of pain control with neurolysis, some actually dispute the efficacy of either celiac block or splanchnicectomy.[46] It appears that celiac neurolysis may bring about only mild to moderate pain relief in patients with pancreatic pain. As noted elsewhere, this form of pain therapy should be considered an adjunct to opioid use and an adjuvant therapy in patients with pancreatic cancer pain.[47]

Most recent publications on celiac neurolysis for pancreatic cancer have evolved around EUS-guided neurolysis, which may be a reflection of the development of technology, enthusiasm of endoscopists, or advantage of EUS over the conventional percutanueous modality. A meta-analysis showed that EUS neurolysis had provided pain relief in 80.1% of patients with pancreatic cancer pain.[48] The review further showed that the technique of bilateral injections provided superior pain relief relative to the unilateral injection technique (85% vs 46%). A more recent randomized, single-blind study showed no significant difference in pain relief (81% for two injections vs 69% for one injection), median onset of pain relief (1 day for both groups), median duration of pain relief (14 weeks for two injections vs 11 weeks for one injection) or patients with complete pain relief (8% both groups).[49] Until more definitive studies become available, the single and double injection methods should be considered interchangeable.

EUS Neurolysis Technique

The basic technique of EUS neurolysis has been described elsewhere.[50] Preprocedure intravenous hydration and antibiotic are usually given. The procedure itself begins with passage of a curved linear-array echoendoscope into the proximal stomach. Once the celiac artery is identified, neurolysis is performed with the single midline or bilateral approach. The midline method targets a location slightly anterior and cephalad to the origin of the celiac artery. The bilateral approach uses equal, split doses to inject both sides of the origin of the celiac artery. Because the individual nerve ganglia can be visualized on EUS, some endoscopists have advocated direct ganglion injection. The evidence for this approach is reported in a retrospective review of 64 patients with pancreatic cancer pain. Of eight potential predictors of symptom improvement, visualization of the ganglia for direct injection was the best predictor of response, as those patients with visible ganglia were 15 times more likely to respond.[51] Fine-needle aspiration (FNA) needles of 19-, 20-, 22-, and 25-gauge have been used for this purpose, although there is significant resistance to overcome in using the 22-gauge and 25-gauge needles. A spray needle that can produce an even and wide distribution of the liquid agents has recently been made available.

The needle is usually prefilled with saline without a stylet in place. When the desired location is punctured, aspiration is performed to confirm that the needle is not inside the vasculature. To reduce alcohol-induced pain, 5 mL of a long-acting local anesthetic, such as 0.25%.bupivicaine, is then delivered. Finally, 20 mL of absolute ethanol is infused in the midline method to achieve neurolysis. Split doses of ethanol are used if the bilateral technique is applied. As the alcohol exits the needle tip, an echogenic cloud is produced at the affected tissue. Sakamoto and colleagues introduced a new technique of neurolysis that aimed at the tissue adjacent to the superior mesenteric artery (broad plexus neurolysis) rather than nearby the celiac artery and reported that the new method provided superior pain relief.[52] Although promising, this broad plexus neurolysis procedure should not be considered a standard treatment modality until more data become available.[53] A few precautions must be taken when attempting a neurolysis block. The patient must be well sedated to avoid accidental needle injury of the nearby vascular structures. This is best achieved with monitored anesthesia care. Vital sign monitoring is crucial at baseline, throughout, and after the procedure because of the deep sedation and the tendency for significant drops in blood pressure.

GASTROINTESTINAL HEMORRHAGE

Gastrointestinal bleeding may occur de novo or after surgical treatment. Early cancer presentation as gastrointestinal hemorrhage is rare and is usually caused by direct involvement of the duodenum or stomach. The cause of bleeding after a pancreatic surgery for cancer may be due to the exposure of skeletonized vessels to erosive enzymes, inflammatory or traumatic pseudoaneurysms, and pancreatic pseudocysts.[54] Anastomosis ulcer bleeding may occur as well. The common endoscopic hemostasis techniques should be attempted for mild bleeding cases.[55] However, most massive bleeding or recurrent tumor bleeding is best managed surgically or with interventional radiology.

POSTOPERATIVE PANCREATIC FISTULA

Fistula occurs most often after resection of the tail of the pancreas. Although surgical mortality in the experienced surgeon's hands is quite low,[56] 5% to 60% of distal pancreatectomy may be complicated by pancreatic fistula.[57] Pancreatic stenting with or without sphincterotomy is highly effective, with the median duration to closing of fistula of 4 days.[58]

LOCAL CANCER GROWTH

There is no proven endoscopic role in controlling local tumor growth of any pancreatic malignancies. However, a number of intriguing endoscopic procedures have been proposed. Iodine-125 seeds of 4.5 mm by 0.8 mm may be inserted in pancreatic tissue using an EUS-guided 18-gauge or 19-gauge needle.[59] Small-scale pilot studies have been performed on humans with minimal but encouraging results.[60–62] Similarly, direct intratumor injection of a replication-defective adenovirus vector carrying the human tumor necrosis factor (TNF)-alpha gene is thought to have the potential for control of tumor growth. A case of a large cancer with metastasis was treated with percutaneous TNFerade injection and regression was noted and the patient was able to undergo cancer resection subsequently.[63] Even though there is no proven therapeutic efficacy today, this type of direct tumor treatment by EUS is appealing and worth further exploration.

Another brachytherapy approach is to take advantage of ERCP access to the pancreatic duct. Nine patients were treated with pancreatic duct brachytherapy with reasonably good tolerance.[64] Clinical efficacy was difficult to determine in this small early study. Recently, a polyurethane plastic stent loaded with iodine-125 seeds has been manufactured to deliver brachytherapy in an experimental model.[65] Its application on humans has yet to be tested.

Finally, on the horizon of endoscopic palliation of pancreatic cancer improved targeting for stereotactic radiosurgery with real-time guidance using small reference fiducials. To our knowledge, the first report of the use of EUS-guided needle delivery of fiducials aiming at the pancreas was reported by Pishvaian and colleagues in 2006.[66] Fiducials of 3 mm or 5 mm were delivered with 19-gauge needles, with three or four fiducials placed in each of these pancreatic cancer lesions. A thinner set of fiducials (10 mm × 0.35 mm) that can be loaded onto a 22-gauge FNA needle has also become commercially available.[67,68] Only one or two fiducials are needed to highlight the tumor for stereotactic radiotherapy. The ability to use a relatively flexible 22-gauge needle undoubtedly makes fiducial placement a much easier procedure than with a stiff, 19-gauge needle. There has been no report on the influence of EUS fiducials on the outcome of radiotherapy.

COMPLICATIONS OF ENDOSCOPIC THERAPY

As endoscopists seek to expand their ability to palliate pancreatic cancer, they need to be reminded that their procedures must be minimally invasive, effective, and reasonably safe. Nonetheless, complications inherently accompany interventional procedures. Before performing these procedures, the endoscopist must fully inform the patient of the risks and their likelihood. All alternative treatment modalities must also be considered. Procedure experience, knowledge of potential complications, and early recognition and the ability to manage adversities are necessary to avoid adding misery to these terminally ill patients.

1. **Endoscope passage.** Although it is not a therapeutic intervention, the mere passage of an endoscope can be risky. This is particularly true when passing a duodenoscope through a narrow duodenum. Side-viewing scope passage through a Billroth II intestine is particularly prone to induce perforation, with reported incidents as high as 18%.[69,70] Special attention must be paid when advancing a scope through a freshly dilated duodenal or jejunal stricture. Many endoscopists are inexperienced in negotiating the post-Whipple or Roux-en-Y anatomy and they should be careful not to cause injury to the anastomosis or intestinal wall.

2. **ERCP and biliary stenting.** Most complications of biliary stenting occur as a result of the ERCP. In 21 selected prospective studies that included 16,855 patients, ERCP complications occurred in 6.9% of cases, with 1.7% being severe in nature.[71] The most common complication was pancreatitis (3.5%), followed by infections (1.4%), bleeding (1.3%), and perforations (0.6%). Data collected in prospective studies indicated that procedure-related morbidity related to stenting may range from 4% to 12% and mortality from 0 to 3.9%, with biliary sepsis, pancreatitis, and sphincterotomy bleeding as the main causes.[72,73] Duodenal perforation due to pressure necrosis is known to occur with plastic stents that protrude excessively from the papilla. Cholecystitis has been reported as a complication as well. Stent migration is a unique problem of partially or fully covered metal stents, reported to occur in 6% of cases.[74] Intestinal or colonic perforation, vascular fistula, and intestinal obstruction are rare complications of migrated biliary metal stents.[75–77] The one late complications of biliary stenting that is inevitable is clogging if the stent is left in place indefinitely. Stent caliber, material, length, and design all may influence the time it takes to become clogged. The same factors may also influence the likelihood of stent migration.

3. **EUS-guided biliary decompression procedures.** In spite of the seemingly simple concept, the decompression is actually rather technically challenging. The potential issues encountered during the multistep procedure include bleeding, perforation, and false puncture during the initial step to access the obstructed bile duct with a needle. The needle-guidewire exchange may cause sheering of the coating of the standard guidewire by the sharp beveled needle tip. A deformed guidewire may make it impossible to pass other therapeutic instruments over it. If a broken wire is removed, bile leak will probably occur.

   The next step of inserting a dilating catheter or balloon may be the most challenging step, as it can be very difficult to force these instruments through the thick gastric wall. Finally, bile fluid or gastrointestinal fluid may leak around a well-placed stent and lead to peritonitis. While the internal rendezvous procedure seems relatively safe, the complication rate of the transgastric hepatogastrostomy has been reported as 14%. Complications include ileus, bilioma, cholangitis, and stent migration.[78] A similar rate of complications due to bile peritonitis and pneumoperitoneum has been reported.

4. **Gastrointestinal luminal stenting.** Stricture dilation is an integral part of management of intestinal obstruction. Perforation or transient septicemia should always be considered. Stenting of a firm stricture may cause pain, as does excessive rubbing of duodenal tissue by an end of the intestinal stent. Some stents do not result in resolution of symptoms because of poor positioning and need to be replaced or removed. Late complications include clogging, migration, and perforation. Baron and colleagues examined a 19-case series that included reporting of complications, which occurred in roughly 20% of the cases.[79]

5. **Celiac plexus neurolysis.** Abscess formation as a result of celiac neurolysis has been reported.[80] A meta-analysis of the literature on celiac neurolysis before

EUS-neurolysis became available showed that transient adverse events were very common,[81] including back pain (96%), diarrhea (44%), and hypotension (38%). Serious complications occur in 2% of injections and they include neurologic complications such as lower extremity weakness and paresthesia (l%) and nonneurologic events such as pneumothorax, hiccoughing, and hematuria (1%). No mortality was reported. On the other hand, transient hypotension occurred in 20% and diarrhea was noted in 10 of 58 patients who underwent neurolysis with the aid of EUS.[82] It appears that EUS-guided neurolysis may be associated with fewer adverse events than the percutaneous method, although more data are needed to confirm this observation.

6. **Pancreatic stenting**. Some pancreatic ductal cannulations are exceedingly difficult and pancreatitis can occur simply from instrument probing. Excessive contrast injection and guidewire puncture of pancreatic tissue through a ductal radical may result in diffuse or focal pancreatitis. A poor choice of stent, awkward stent positioning, or prolonged stenting may result in pancreatic irritation or stricture formation. Inward stent migration is technically very difficult to remove, with a success rate of less than 80% in a major interventional endoscopy center.[83] Finally, stenting may convert a sterile pancreatic fistula into tissue infection or abscess formation.

7. **Fiducial insertion.** This is a new procedure with limited clinical experience. Thus far, it is reported to be very safe. In one series of 30 subjects, one (3%) patient developed transient fever and elevation of liver enzymes.[68] An infected porta hepatis mass was noted within the first 30 days after the fiducial placement in one patient (8%).[66] In another report of 51 patients who underwent the procedure using the 19-gauge needles for fiducial delivery, one (2%) patient experienced mild pancreatitis.[84] Three of 57 (5%) cases in another report encountered minor intraprocedure complications including malfunctioning of the instrument and bleeding.[85] Finally, fiducial migration may occur soon after placement, thus potentially misdirecting tumor therapy. Until more experience is accumulated, a reasonable protocol is to give prophylactic antibiotic and place more than one fiducial to compensate for the potential of subsequent marker migration.

SUMMARY

There is no doubt that our long-range goal is to cure pancreatic cancer. Realistically, most of what we can do currently is treat the disabling symptoms of this dreadful disease. Biliary decompression, intestinal stenting, celiac plexus neurolysis, and fiducial placement are some of the endoscopic procedures that aim to provide better quality of life to patients suffering from this disease. A thorough understanding of these options will help patients make good decisions in choosing the proper treatment. Endoscopists who perform these procedures must possess great skills, but importantly, they must also be compassionate and act with good judgment.

REFERENCES

1. National Cancer Institute. SEER Cancer Statistics Review 1975–2006. Bethesda (MD): National Cancer Institute. Available at: http://seer.cancer.gov/csr/1975_2006. Accessed January 9, 2012.
2. Merrill RM, Hunter BD. Conditional survival among cancer patients in the United States. Oncologist 2010;15:873–82.
3. Saif MW. Pancreatic neoplasm in 2011: an update. JOP 2011;12(4):316–21.

4. Seynaeve L, Van Steenbergen W. Treatment, by insertion of multiple uncovered metallic stents, of intraductal papillary mucinous neoplasm of the pancreas with biliary obstruction by mucus impaction. Pancreatology 2007;7:540–3.
5. Cipolletta L, Rotondano G, Marmo R, et al. Endoscopic palliation of malignant obstructive jaundice: an evidence-based review. Dig Liver Dis 2007;39:375–88.
6. Shepherd HA, Royle G, Ross AP, et al. Endoscopic biliary endoprosthesis in the palliation of malignant obstruction of the distal common bile duct: a randomized trial. Br J Surg 1988;75:1166–8.
7. Andersen JR, Sorensen SM, Kruse A, et al. Randomised trial of endoscopic endo-prosthesis versus operative bypass in malignant obstructive jaundice. Gut 1989;30:1132–5.
8. Smith AC, Dowsett JF, Russell RC, et al. Randomised trial of endoscopic stenting versus surgical bypass in malignant low bile duct obstruction. Lancet 1994;344:1655–60.
9. Binmoeller KF, Seitz U, Seifert H, et al. The Tannenbaum stent: a new plastic biliary stent without side holes. Am J Gastroenterol 1995;90:1764–8.
10. Catalano MF, Geenen JE, Lehman GA, et al. "Tannenbaum" Teflon stents versus traditional polyethylene stents for treatment of malignant biliary stricture. Gastrointest Endosc 2002;55:354–8.
11. Huibregtse K, Cheng J, Coene PP, et al. Endoscopic placement of expandable metal stents for biliary strictures—a preliminary report on experience with 33 patients. Endoscopy 1989;21:280–2.
12. Davids PH, Groen AK, Rauws EA, et al. Randomised trial of self-expanding metal stents versus polyethylene stents for distal malignant biliary obstruction. Lancet 1992;340:1488–92.
13. Knyrim K, Wagner HJ, Pausch J, et al. A prospective, randomized, controlled trial of metal stents for malignant obstruction of the common bile duct. Endoscopy 1993;25:207–12.
14. Moss AC, Morris E, Leyden J, et al. Do the benefits of metal stents justify the costs? A systematic review and meta-analysis of trials comparing endoscopic stents for malignant biliary obstruction. Eur J Gastroenterol Hepatol 2007;19(12):1119–24.
15. Yoon WJ, Ryu JK, Yang KY, et al. A comparison of metal and plastic stents for the relief of jaundice in unresectable malignant biliary obstruction in Korea: an emphasis on cost-effectiveness in a country with a low ERCP cost. Gastrointest Endosc 2009;70:284–9.
16. Han YM, Jin GY, Lee SO, et al. Flared polyurethane-covered self-expandable nitinol stent for malignant biliary obstruction. J Vasc Interv Radiol 2003;14:1291–301.
17. Willingham FF. All wrapped up: metal biliary stents and the effects of stent coverings. Gastrointest Endosc 2010;72:924–6.
18. Siddiqui AA, Mehendiratta V, Loren D, et al. Fully covered self-expandable metal stents are effective and safe to treat distal malignant biliary strictures, irrespective of surgical resectability status. J Clin Gastroenterol 2011;45:824–7.
19. Yoon JW, Lee JK, Lee KH, et al. A comparison of covered and uncovered Wallstents for the management of distal malignant biliary obstruction. Gastrointest Endosc 2006;63:996–1000.
20. Telford JJ, Carr-Locke DL, Baron TH, et al. A randomized trial comparing uncovered and partially covered self-expandable metal stents in the palliation of distal malignant biliary obstruction. Gastrointest Endosc 2010;72:907–14.
21. Kullman E, Frozanpor F, Söderlund C, et al. Covered versus uncovered self-expandable nitinol stents in the palliative treatment of malignant distal biliary obstruction: results from a randomized multicenter study. Gastrointest Endosc 2010;72:915–23.

22. Kim YS, Gupta K, Mallery S, et al. Endoscopic ultrasound rendezvous for bile duct access using a transduodenal approach: cumulative experience at a single center. A case series. Endoscopy 2010;42:496–502.

23. Maranki J, Hernandez AJ, Arslan B, et al. Interventional endoscopic ultrasound-guided cholangiography: long-term experience of an emerging alternative to percutaneous transhepatic cholangiography. Endoscopy 2009;41:532–8.

24. Hara K, Yamao K, Mizuno N, et al. Endoscopic ultrasound-guided choledochoduodenostomy. Dig Endosc 2010;22:147–50.

25. Yamao K, Bhatia V, Mizuno N, et al. EUS-guided choledochoduodenostomy for palliative biliary drainage in patients with malignant biliary obstruction: results of long-term follow-up. Endoscopy 2008;40:340–2.

26. Kahaleh M, Hernandez AJ, Tokar J, et al. Interventional EUS-guided cholangiography: evaluation of a technique in evolution. Gastrointest Endosc 2006;64:52–9.

27. Bories E, Pesenti C, Caillol F, et al. Transgastric endoscopic ultrasonography-guided biliary drainage: results of a pilot study. Endoscopy 2007;39:287–91.

28. Park do H, Koo JE, Oh J, et al. EUS-guided biliary drainage with one-step placement of a fully covered metal stent for malignant biliary obstruction: a prospective feasibility study. Am J Gastroenterol 2009;104:2168–74.

29. Suk KT, Kim JW, Kim HS, et al. Human application of a metallic stent covered with a paclitaxel-incorporated membrane for malignant biliary obstruction: multicenter pilot study. Gastrointest Endosc 2007;66:798–803.

30. Lillemoe KD, Cameron JL, Hardacre JM, et al. Is prophylactic gastrojejunostomy indicated for unresectable periampullary cancer? A prospective randomized trial. Ann Surg 1999;230:322–8.

31. Telford JJ, Carr-Locke DL, Baron TH, et al. Palliation of patients with malignant gastric outlet obstruction with the enteral Wallstent: outcomes from a multicenter study. Gastrointest Endosc 2004;60:916–20.

32. Wong YT, Brams DM, Munson L, et al. Gastric outlet obstruction secondary to pancreatic cancer: surgical vs endoscopic palliation. Surg Endosc 2002;16(2):310–2.

33. Maetani I, Tada T, Ukita T, et al. Comparison of duodenal stent placement with surgical gastrojejunostomy for palliation in patients with duodenal obstructions caused by pancreaticobiliary malignancies. Endoscopy 2004;36:73–8.

34. Mehta S, Hindmarsh A, Cheong E, et al. Prospective randomized trial of laparoscopic gastrojejunostomy versus duodenal stenting for malignant gastric outflow obstruction. Surg Endosc 2006;20:239–42.

35. Kruse EJ. Palliation in pancreatic cancer. Surg Clin North Am 2010;90:355–64.

36. Maire F, Hammel P, Ponsot P, et al. Long-term outcome of biliary and duodenal stents in palliative treatment of patients with unresectable denocarcinoma of the head of pancreas. Am J Gastroenterol 2006;101:735–42.

37. Pannala R, Brandabur JJ, Gan SI. Afferent limb syndrome and delayed GI problems after pancreaticoduodenectomy for pancreatic cancer: single-center, 14-year experience. Gastrointest Endosc 2011;74:295–302.

38. Akaraviputh T, Trakarnsanga A, Tolan K. Endoscopic treatment of acute ascending cholangitis in a patient with Roux-en-Y limb obstruction after a Whipple operation. Endoscopy 2010;42(Suppl 2):E335–6.

39. Harrison MA, Hamilton SW. Palliation of pancreatic cancer pain by endoscopic stent placement. Gastrointest Endosc 1989;35:443–5.

40. Costamagna G, Mutignani M. Pancreatic stenting for malignant ductal obstruction. Dig Liver Dis 2004;36:635–8.

41. Tham TC, Lichtenstein DR, Vandervoort J, et al. Pancreatic duct stents for "obstructive type" pain in pancreatic malignancy. Am J Gastroenterol 2000;95:956–60.

42. Keeley SP, Freeman ML. Placement of self-expanding metallic stents in the pancreatic duct for treatment of obstructive complications of pancreatic cancer. Gastrointest Endosc 2003;57:756–9.
43. Rykowski JJ, Hilgier M. Efficacy of neurolytic celiac plexus block in varying locations of pancreatic cancer: influence on pain relief. Anesthesiology 2000;92(2):347–54.
44. Gress F, Schmitt C, Sherman S, et al. A prospective randomized comparison of endoscopic ultrasound- and computed tomography-guided celiac plexus block for managing chronic pancreatitis pain. Am J Gastroenterol 1999;94:900–5.
45. Yan BM, Myers RP. Neurolytic celiac plexus block for pain control in unresectable pancreatic cancer. Am J Gastroenterol 2007;102:430–8.
46. Johnson CD, Berry DP, Harris S, et al. An open randomized comparison of clinical effectiveness of protocol-driven opioid analgesia, celiac plexus block or thoracoscopic splanchnicectomy for pain management in patients with pancreatic and other abdominal malignancies. Pancreatology 2009;9:755–6.
47. Chak A. What is the evidence for EUS-guided celiac plexus block/neurolysis? Gastrointest Endosc 2009;69:S172–3.
48. Puli SR, Reddy JB, Bechtold ML, et al. EUS-guided celiac plexus neurolysis for pain due to chronic pancreatitis or pancreatic cancer pain: a meta-analysis and systematic review. Dig Dis Sci 2009;54:2330–7.
49. Leblanc JK, Al-Haddad M, McHenry L, et al. A prospective, randomized study of EUS-guided celiac plexus neurolysis for pancreatic cancer: one injection or two? Gastrointest Endosc 2011;74(6):1300–7.
50. Penman ID. Basic technique for celiac plexus block/neurolysis Gastrointest Endosc 2009;69:S163–5.
51. Ascunce G, Ribeiro A, Reis I, et al. EUS visualization and direct celiac ganglia neurolysis predicts better pain relief in patients with pancreatic malignancy (with video). Gastrointest Endosc 2011;73:267–74.
52. Sakamoto H, Kitano M, Kamata K, et al. EUS-guided broad plexus neurolysis over the superior mesenteric artery using a 25-gauge needle. Am J Gastroenterol 2010;105:2599–606.
53. Virtue MA, Levy MJ. Editorial: Neurolysis for pancreatic cancer pain: same song, different verse? Am J Gastroenterol 2010;105:2607–9.
54. Tsirlis T, Vasiliades G, Koliopanos A, et al. Pancreatic leak related hemorrhage following pancreaticoduodenectomy. A case series. JOP 2009;10:492–5.
55. Standop J, Schäfer N, Overhaus M, et al. Endoscopic management of anastomotic hemorrhage from pancreatogastrostomy. Surg Endosc 2009;23:2005–10.
56. Lillemoe KD, Kaushal S, Cameron JL, et al. Distal pancreatectomy: indication and outcome in 235 patients. Ann Surg 1999;229:693–700.
57. Rieder B, Krampulz D, Adolf J, et al. Endoscopic pancreatic sphincterotomy and stenting for preoperative prophylaxis of pancreatic fistula after distal pancreatectomy. Gastrointest Endosc 2010;72:536–42.
58. Goasguen N, Bourrier A, Ponsot P, et al. Endoscopic management of pancreatic fistula after distal pancreatectomy and enucleation. Am J Surg 2009;197(6):715–20.
59. Sun S, Qingjie L, Qiyong G, et al. EUS-guided interstitial brachytherapy of the pancreas: a feasibility study. Gastrointest Endosc 2005;62:775–9.
60. Sun S, Xu H, Xin J, et al. Endoscopic ultrasound-guided interstitial brachytherapy of unresectable pancreatic cancer: results of a pilot trial. Endoscopy 2006;38:399–403.
61. Jin Z, Du Y, Li Z, et al. EUS-guided interstitial implantation of iodine 125 seeds combined with chemotherapy in the treatment of unresectable pancreatic carcinoma: a prospective pilot study. Endoscopy 2008;40:314–20.

62. Du YQ, Li ZS, Jin ZD. Endoscope-assisted brachytherapy for pancreatic cancer: from tumor killing to pain relief and drainage. J Interv Gastroenterol 2011;1:23–7.

63. Chadha MK, Litwin A, Levea C, et al. Surgical resection after TNFerade therapy for locally advanced pancreatic cancer. JOP 2009;10(5):535–8.

64. Mutignani M, Shah SK, Morganti AG, et al. Treatment of unresectable pancreatic carcinoma by intraluminal brachytherapy in the duct of Wirsung. Endoscopy 2002; 34:555–9.

65. Liu Y, Liu JL, Cai ZZ, et al. A novel approach for treatment of unresectable extrahepatic bile duct carcinoma: design of radioactive stents and an experimental trial in healthy pigs. Gastrointest Endosc 2009;69:517–24.

66. Pishvaian AC, Collins B, Gagnon G, et al. EUS-guided fiducial placement for CyberKnife radiotherapy of mediastinal and abdominal malignancies. Gastrointest Endosc 2006;64(3):412–7.

67. Ammar T, Coté GA, Creach KM, et al. Fiducial placement for stereotactic radiation by using EUS: feasibility when using a marker compatible with a standard 22-gauge needle. Gastrointest Endosc 2010;71:630–3.

68. DiMaio CJ, Nagula S, Goodman KA, et al. EUS-guided fiducial placement for image-guided radiation therapy in GI malignancies by using a 22–gauge needle (with videos). Gastrointest Endosc 2010;71:1204–10.

69. Faylona JM, Qadir A, Chan AC, et al. Small-bowel perforations related to endoscopic retrograde cholangiopancreatography (ERCP) in patients with Billroth II gastrectomy. Endoscopy 1999;31:546–9.

70. Kim MH, Lee SK, Lee MH, et al. Endoscopic retrograde cholangiopancreatography and needle knife sphincterotomy in patients with Billroth II gastrectomy: a comparative study of the forward-viewing endoscope and the side-viewing duodenoscope. Endoscopy 1997;29:82–5.

71. Andriulli A, Loperfido S, Napolitano G, et al. Incidence rates of post-ERCP complications: a systematic survey of prospective studies. Am J Gastroenterol 2007;102: 1781–8.

72. Kaassis M, Boyer J, Dumas R, et al. Plastic or metal stents for malignant stricture of the common bile duct? Results of a randomized prospective study. Gastrointest Endosc 2003;57:178–82.

73. Prat F, Chapat O, Ducot B, et al. A randomized trial of endoscopic drainage methods for inoperable malignant strictures of the common bile duct. Gastrointest Endosc 1998;47:1–7.

74. Kahaleh M, Tokar J, Conaway MR, et al. Efficacy and complications of covered Wallstents in malignant distal biliary obstruction. Gastrointest Endosc 2005;61: 528–33.

75. Garcia Figueiras R, Otero Echart M, Garcia Gonzalez R, et al. Colocutaneous fistula relating to the migration of a biliary stent. Eur J Gastroenterol Hepatol 2001;13: 1251–3.

76. Lee TH, Park DH, Park JY, et al. Aortoduodenal fistula and aortic aneurysm secondary to biliary stent-induced retroperitoneal perforation. World J Gastroenterol 2008;14: 3095–7.

77. Ikeda T, Nagata S, Ohgaki K. Intestinal obstruction because of a migrated metallic biliary stent. Gastrointest Endosc 2004;60:988–9.

78. Hara K, Yamao K, Mizuno N, et al. Interventional endoscopic ultrasonography for pancreatic cancer. World J Clin Oncol 2011;2(2):108–14.

79. Baron TH, Harewood GC. Enteral self-expandable stents. Gastrointest Endosc 2003; 58:421–33.

80. Muscatiello N, Panella C, Pietrini L, et al. Complication of endoscopic ultrasound-guided celiac plexus neurolysis. Endoscopy 2006;38(8):858.
81. Eisenberg E, Carr DB, Chalmers TC. Neurolytic celiac plexus block for treatment of cancer pain: A meta-analysis. Anesth Analg 1995;80:290–5.
82. Gunaratnam NT, Sarma AV, Norton ID, et al. A prospective study of EUS guided celiac plexus neurolysis for pancreatic cancer pain. Gastrointest Endosc 2001;54:316–24.
83. Price LH. Good stents gone bad: endoscopic treatment of proximally migrated pancreatic duct stents. Gastrointest Endosc 2009;70(1):174–9.
84. Sanders MK, Moser AJ, Khddalid A, et al. EUS-guided fiducial placement for stereotactic body radiotherapy in locally advanced and recurrent pancreatic cancer. Gastrointest Endosc 2010;71:1178–84.
85. Park WG, Yan BM, Schellenberg D, et al. EUS-guided gold fiducial insertion for image-guided radiation therapy of pancreatic cancer: 50 successful cases without fluoroscopy. Gastrointest Endosc 2010;71:513–8.

Index

Note: Page numbers of article titles are in **bold face** type.

A

Adjuvant chemotherapy, for pancreatic cancer, 190–193
Adrenocorticotropic hormone, tumors secreting, 122
Alcohol cessation
  for acute pancreatitis, 5
  for chronic pancreatitis, 64
Allopurinol, for chronic pancreatitis, 66
American Joint Committee on Cancer, neuroendocrine tumor staging system of, 123
Analgesics, for chronic pancreatitis, 64–65
Anomalous pancreaticobiliary union, ERCP for, 30
Antibodies, in autoimmune pancreatitis, 14–15
Antidepressants, for chronic pancreatitis, 65
Antioxidants, for chronic pancreatitis, 66
APACHE II score, for pancreatitis, 1–2
Arc therapy, for pancreatic cancer, 228–229
Arterial resection and reconstruction, for pancreatic cancer, 217–218
Atherosclerosis, pancreas transplantation impact on, 137
Atrophy, pancreatic, in autoimmune pancreatitis, 12
Autoimmune pancreatitis, **9–22**
  as multisystem disease, 15–16
  clinical features of, 11–12
  diagnosis of, 16–17
  differential diagnosis of, 11–12
  histology of, 11
  imaging for, 12–14
  incidence of, 11–12
  pathophysiology of, 10–11
  serology of, 14–15
  subtypes of, 9–10
  terminology of, 9
  treatment of, 17–18
Autonomic neuropathy, pancreas transplantation impact on, 138
Axitinib, for pancreatic cancer, 200
Azathioprine, for autoimmune pancreatitis, 18

B

Bacteremia, in acute pancreatitis, 5
Balloon dilation, for pseudocysts, 50–51, 54
BAY 12-9566, for pancreatic cancer, 200
Bedside Index of Severity in Acute Pancreatitis (BISAP), 1–2
Beger procedure, for chronic pancreatitis, 86–87

Gastroenterol Clin N Am 41 (2012) 255–270
doi:10.1016/S0889-8553(12)00026-X
0889-8553/12/$ – see front matter © 2012 Elsevier Inc. All rights reserved.

gastro.theclinics.com

Moving?

Make sure your subscription moves with you!

To notify us of your new address, find your **Clinics Account Number** (located on your mailing label above your name), and contact customer service at:

Email: journalscustomerservice-usa@elsevier.com

800-654-2452 (subscribers in the U.S. & Canada)
314-447-8871 (subscribers outside of the U.S. & Canada)

Fax number: 314-447-8029

Elsevier Health Sciences Division
Subscription Customer Service
3251 Riverport Lane
Maryland Heights, MO 63043

*To ensure uninterrupted delivery of your subscription, please notify us at least 4 weeks in advance of move.

Printed and bound by CPI Group (UK) Ltd, Croydon, CR0 4YY

03/10/2024

01040459-0009